Human T Cell Clones

Experimental Biology and Medicine

HUMAN T CELL CLONES

A New Approach to Immune Regulation

Edited by

Marc Feldmann,
Jonathan R. Lamb,
and James N. Woody

Humana Press · **Clifton, New Jersey**

Library of Congress Cataloging in Publication Data

Main entry under title:

Human T cell clones.

(Experimental biology and medicine)
"Proceedings of a conference held at Trinity College,
Oxford, on September 22-26, 1984"—Introd.
Includes index.
1. T cells—Congresses.   2. Clone cells—Congresses.
3. Cell receptors—Congresses.   4. Antigens—Congresses.
5. HLA histocompatibility antigens—Congresses.
6. Immunopathology—Congresses.   I. Feldmann, Marc.
II. Lamb, Jonathan R.   III. Woody, James N.   IV. Series:
Experimental biology and mediciine (Clifton, N.J.)
[DNLM: 1. Autoimmune Diseases—congresses.   2. Clone Cells
—congresses.   3. HLA Antigens—congresses.   4. Immunity,
Cellular—congresses.   5. Receptors, Antigen, T-Cell—
congresses.   6. T Lymphocytes—congresses.
QW 568 H918 1984]
QR185.8.L9H849 1985   616.07'9   85-8079
ISBN 0-89603-084-9

©1985 The Humana Press Inc.
Crescent Manor
PO Box 2148
Clifton, NJ 07015

Printed in the United States of America

PREFACE

Most complex biological systems, such as enzyme pathways, are effectively controlled near the beginning of the process. There is increasing evidence that the same is true for the immune system, with the initial interactions between antigen, antigen-presenting cells, and T cells having a paramount influence on the ensuing events. Thus, analysis of the early stages of the immune responses has been a preoccupation of many immunologists. This has been considerably aided by the capacity to expand these early events, and 'immortalize' them as clones of T cells, for detailed analysis.

The discovery by Morgan, Ruscetti, and Gallo (*Science* **193,** 1007, 1976) of T-cell growth factor (now termed interleukin-2 or IL-2) has had a major impact in immunology that is far from over. The greater ease of handling murine tissues experimentally, with the availability of more precisely defined reagents such as inbred strains. has meant that, to date, most of the work on long-term T-cell cultures has been performed in the mouse, as summarized by Fathman and Fitch (eds., *Isolation, Characterization and Utilization of T Lymphocyte Clones*, Academic Press, NY, 1982). However, the limitations of working with human tissues are counterbalanced by the great long-term importance of understanding disorders of human immune regulation, especially since it is becoming evident that these are far from rare.

Immune deficiencies such as agammaglobulinemia and T-cell deficiencies are not common, but immune hyperresponsiveness occurring in allergy and allergic diseases (e.g., asthma, eczema), and in autoimmunity (e.g., rheumatoid arthritis, thyroid autoimmunity, and juvenile diabetes), is common. The immunological hyporesponsiveness found in cancer patients still needs to be understood. A number of laboratories have embarked on studies of human immune regulation that apply to various diseases, using T-cell cloning as the major tool, and a sample of these are represented in this book. It is evident that practical applications of new information are still distant, but a clear understanding of pathogenesis and mechanisms of immune dysregulation could revolutionize our approaches to the management of immune dysfunction in a fairly short period of time.

T-cell cloning has been achieved in a variety of ways apart form the use of IL-2. In murine systems, much information has been obtained from T-cell hybridomas and some from virus-induced leukemias, but in human systems these other techniques of cloning have not as yet been useful. These techniques will doubtless improve and will be valuable in future research.

From the table of contents it is clear that the major role and use of T-cell clones at the moment is still that of a major research technique, providing homogeneous material for increasing our understanding of immunology, of T-cell receptors, of the interaction of T cells with antigen-presenting cells, with HLA antigens, of the role of non-receptor cell surface molecules in T-cell function, and in the study of the T-cell products released by T cells. This is desirable, since a deeper understanding of normal immune mechanisms will make the task of those wishing to unravel the pathogenesis of diseases all the easier.

This book encompasses the proceedings of a conference held at Trinity College, Oxford on September 22–26, 1984, organized scientifically by a committee comprised of ourselves, aided by Dr. P. C. L. Beverley, Dr. M. Crumpton, Dr. A. McMichael, and Dr. A. Williamson, and locally organized by Dr. A. McMichael. In order to make sessions easier to penetrate by nonspecialists in this field, we have made a brief summary of some of the key points of each session. This meeting was made possible by generous contributions from the Office of Naval Research, US Navy, Imperial Cancer Research Fund, Sandoz, I.C.I., Hoffman La Roche, Wellcome Foundation, Glaxo, and Johnson and Johnson. We are grateful to our friends within these organizations for their considerable help, and to our numerous colleagues for their great assistance with the multiple tasks involved in organizing and running such a conference.

Marc Feldmann
Jonathan R. Lamb
James N. Woody

PARTICIPANTS

ORESTE ACUTO · Dana Farber Cancer Institute, Department of Medicine, Harvard Medical School, Boston, Massachusetts

ISTVAN ANDO · Imperial Cancer Research Fund, HumanTumour Immunology Group, University of College Hospital, London, UK

PHIL ASKENASE · Department of Internal Medicine, School of Medicine, Yale University, New Haven, Connecticut

ITA ASKONAS · MRC, NIMR, London, UK

P. BEVERLEY · Imperial Cancer Research Fund, Human Tumour Immunology Group, University College Hospital, London, UK

BILL BIDDISON · NINCDS, NIH, Bethesda, Maryland

BARRY BLOOM · Department of Microbiology and Immunology, Albert Einstein College of Medicine, Bronx, New York

W. BODMER · Imperial Cancer Research Fund, London, UK

J. BODMER · Imperial Cancer Research Fund, London, UK

R. BOLHUIS · Rotterdam Radio Therapeutisch Inst. afd. Immunologie, Rotterdam, Netherlands

FRANCO BOTTAZZO · Department of Immunolgy, Middlesex Hospital Medical School, London, UK

STEVEN J. BURAKOFF · Department of Pediatrics, Harvard Medical School, Dana Farber Cancer Institute, Boston, Massachusetts

VIRGINIA CALDER · Institute of of Neurology, London, UK

IRUN COHEN · Department of Cell Biology, Weizmann Institute of Science, Rehovot, Israel

MARY K. L. COLLINS · Imperial Cancer Research Fund, Tumour Immunology Unit, Department of Zoology, University College London, London, UK

M. CRUMPTON · Imperial Cancer Research Fund, London, UK

ERIC CULBERT · Corporate Bioscience Group, Central Toxicology Laboratory, Cheshire, UK

DAVE ECKELS · Immunogenetics Research Section, The Blood Center of Southeastern Wisconsin, Milwaukee, Wisconsin

ED ENGLEMAN · Department of Pathology and Medicine, Stanford, University School of Medicine, Stanford, California

G. ESSERY-RICE · Imperial Cancer Research Fund, Tumour Immunology Unit, Department of Zoology, University College London, London, UK

M. FELDMANN · Imperial Cancer Research Fund, Tumour Immunology Unit, Department of Zoology, University College London, London, UK

ALAIN FISCHER · Groupe de Recherche d'Immunologie et Rheumatologie Pediatriques, Hôpital des Enfants Malades, Paris, France

R. C. GALLO · Laboratory of Tumour Cell Biology, National Cancer Institute, National Institutes of Health, Bethesda, Maryland

R. GEHA · Division of Allergy, Children's Hospital Medical Center, Boston, Massachusetts

GILLIAN HARCOURT · Department of Neurological Science, Royal Free Hospital, School of Medicine, London, UK

K. HASKINS · Department of Medicine, National Jewish Hospital and Research Center, National Asthman Center, Denver, Colorado

G. HILDICK-SMITH · Corporate Office of Science and Technology, Johnson and Johnson, New Brunswick, New Jersey

DOUG KILBURN · Department of Microbiology, University of British Columbia, Vancouver, British Columbia, Canada

TADAMITSU KISHIMOTO · Department of Medicine, Osaka University School of Medicine, Osaka, Japan

SIRKKA KONTIAINEN · Municipal Bacteriological Laboratory, Aurora Hosptial, Helsinki, Finland

PHIL LAKE · Immuno-Oncology Division, Lombardi Cancer Center, Georgetown University School of Medicine, Washington, D.C.

J. LAMB · MRC Tuberculosis and Related Infections, Hammersmith Hosptial, London, UK

MARCO LONDEI · Imperial Cancer Research Fund, Tumour Immunology Unit, Department of Zoology, Unviersity College London, London, UK

P. LYDYARD · Middlesex Hospital Medical School, London, UK

R. N. MAINI · Clinical Immunology Division, Kennedy Institute of Rheumatology, Hammersmith, London, UK

J. MAJDE · Cellular Biosystems Program, Department of the Navy, Office of Naval Research, Arlington, Virginia

CLAUDE MAWAS · Centre d'Immunologie INSERM-CNRS, de Marseille-Luminy, Marseille, France

A. J. McMICHAEL · Nuffield Department of Surgery, John Radcliffe Hospital, Oxford, UK

STEFAN C. MEUER · Klinikum der Johannes Gutenberg Universitat, Mainz, Federal Republic of Germany

A. MORETTA · Ludwig Institute of Cancer Research, Epalinges, Switzerland

P. MORRIS · Nuffield Department of Surgery, John Radcliffe Hospital, Oxford, UK

ERIK QVIGSTAD · Tissue Typing Lab, Rikshospitalet, The National Hospital, Oslo, Norway

A REES · MRC Unit of Laboratory Studies of Tuberculosis, RPMS, London, UK

M. ROBERTSON · *Nature,* MacMillan Journals, London, UK

I. M. ROITT · Department of Immunology, Arthur Stanley House, Middlesex Hospital Medical School, London, UK

T. ROZZELL · Cellular Biosystems Program, Department of the Navy, Office of Naval Research, Arlington, Virginia

TAKEHIKO SASAZUKI · Department of Human Genetics, Medical Research Institute, Tokyo Medical and Dental University, Tokyo, Japan

MAX SCHREIER · Preclinical Research, Sandoz, Basel, Switzerland

CLAIRE SHARROCK · Royal Postgraduate Medical School, Hammersmith Hospital, London, UK

KENDALL A. SMITH · Department of Medicine, Dartmouth Medical School, Hanover, New Hampshire

BRUNO SPIRE · Institut Pasteur, Paris, France

HERGEN SPITS · Division of Immunology, Netherlands Cancer Institute, Amsterdam, Netherlands

T. SPRINGER · Department of Membrane Immunochemistry, Dana-Farber Cancer Institute, Boston, Massachusetts

ERIK THORSBY · Tissue Typing Lab, Rikshospitalet, The National Hospital, Oslo, Norway

ALAN TOWNSEND · Department of Medicine, John Radcliffe Hosptial, Oxford, UK

J. TROWSDALE · Imperial Cancer Research Fund, London, UK

D. VOLKMANN · Clinical Physiology Section, Lab of Clinical Investigation, NIAID, NIH, Bethesda, Maryland

BRENT VOSE · Corporate Bioscience Group, Central Toxicology Group, ICI, Cheshire, UK

ANNA VYAKARNAM · Ludwig Institute for Cancer Research, Cambridge, UK

H. WAGNER · Institute of Medical Microbiology, University of Mainz, Mainz, Federal Republic of Germany

TOM WALDMANN · National Cancer Institute, National Institute of Health, Bethesda, Maryland

L. WALLACE · Cancer Research Campaign Labs, Department of Cancer Studies, The Medical School, University of Birmingham, Birmingham, UK

A. WILLIAMS · MRC Cellular Immunology Unit, Sir William Dunn School of Pathology, Oxford University, Oxford, UK

A. WILLIAMSON · Glaxo Group Research Ltd, Greenford, Middlesex, UK

J. WOODY · Tissue Bank, Naval Medical Research Institute, Bethesda, Maryland

E. ZANDERS · Department of Immunobiology, Glaxo Group Research, Greenford, Middlesex, UK

CONTENTS

SESSION IV: ROLE OF CELL SURFACE MOLECULES IN T CELL FUNCTION
M. J. Crumpton and A. J. McMichael

SECTION V: T CELL CLONES AND THE ANALYSIS OF DISEASE
I. Roitt and R. N. Maini

SESSION VI: IMMUNEREGULATION
K. Smith and H. Wagner

SESSION VIII: T CELL CLONES AND ANTI-TUMOR IMMUNITY
P. W. Askenase and M. Feldmann

SESSION I
T Cell Receptor

Chairmen: A. Williamson and A. Williams

The most striking difference between lymphocyte physiology and that of other cell types rests in the diversity of clones of lymphocytes, due to their possession of different receptors for antigen. Thus understanding T cell receptor function is crucial and due to the recent progress in the past 2 years in this area, it was felt essential to start discussions of T cell clones with a firm grounding on the current status of T cell receptors, both at the protein and genetic level.

Concerning the protein chemistry of the T cell receptor, as revealed by 'clonotypic' monoclonal antibodies, reacting with only a single T cell clone, both groups which first described such antibodies, in man and mouse were represented. In the first presentation Dr Acuto began with a summary of the effect of anti clonotypic and anti T3 antibodies on T cell function and demonstrated that the antigen specific receptor on cytotoxic inducer and suppressor T cells is the Ti/T3 complex. The analysis of receptor structure by protein chemistry and molecular genetics suggested that the Tiβ subunit is similar to the murine Tβ chain comprising of a variable and constant extracellular domain each with a disulphide loop, a hydrophobic transmembrane region and a cytoplasmic tail. Partial NH_2 terminal amino acid sequencing revealed that the Tiα and Tiβ subunit lacked homology but have overall a domain structure similar to immunoglobulin V region. Dr Haskins described both idiotypic and allotypic antireceptor antibodies to murine T cells. Distribution of the allotypic determinant was investigated on thymocytes and peripheral T cell being found on both Class I (20%) and Class II (34%) specific T cells.

The molecular approach to the murine T cell receptor was reviewed by Dr Gascoigne representing Mark Davis' group, which had been the first to isolate T cell β chains using subtraction libraries. At the meeting he concentrated on the mechanisms for generating diversity using V D J genes, which could be spliced in different ways, e.g. VDJ or VJ, or even possibly 2 D's together due to different spacing of signal sequences in T cell receptor genes than in B receptors genes.

1

Sequence analysis of a number of T_β V regions indicated that there are more than the 3 hypervariable "complementary determining" sites present in immunogloblin V regions, possibly enabling a single T cell V_β region to bind to a far larger portion of antigen than Ig, possibly encompassing both antigen and MHC. But that leaves little role for the $T\alpha$ chain, not described at the time of the conference but reported independently soon after by both Davis' group and Tonegawa's, the $T\alpha$ chain being very similar in overall plan to the T_β chain.

The human T_β chain was discussed by Dr Collins and its chromosomal assignment, on the long arm of chromosome 7 indicates that the linkage of mouse T_β on chromosome 6, the same chromosome as the K immunoglobulin light chain locus is probably not important, as it is not conserved between species.

MOLECULAR AND FUNCTIONAL ANALYSIS OF THE HUMAN T CELL ANTIGEN/MHC RECEPTOR

Oreste Acuto,[*] Marina Fabbi & Ellis L. Reinherz

Dana-Farber Cancer Institute and Harvard Medical School
44 Binney Street, Boston, MA   02115

INTRODUCTION

T lymphocytes, unlike B lymphocytes, predominantly recognize antigen when it is associated with membrane-bound products of the major histocompatibility complex (MHC)(1-4). This "dual" recognition is important for activation of both cytotoxic effector T cells and immunoregulatory T cells. T cells act as inducers or suppressors for interactions between T cells, B cells, macrophages and other cells (8-13).

The specificity of T cells is determined by their cell surface receptors, and therefore, knowledge of these receptors is particularly useful in understanding the cellular interactions that underlie the different activities of T cells. Because T lymphocytes recognize antigen in a precise fashion, certain receptors on their surface were thought to be specific to single T cell clones (i.e. clonotypic). The ability to propagate human T lymphocyte clones in vitro (14-18) has made it possible to identify these clonotypic recognition determinants. Using T cell clones as immunogens, murine monoclonal antibodies specific to single clones have been generated and used to define a novel class of clonotypic molecules found on the surface of all T cells (19,20).

3

FUNCTIONAL EFFECTS OF ANTI-Ti MONOCLONAL ANTIBODIES

Earlier studies indicated that the human T3 molecule
present on all peripheral T cells and mature thymocytes
played an important role in immune recognition (21-26).
Specifically, anti-T3 monoclonal antibodies were able to
inhibit T cell function at the effector and induction phase
and in the presence of macrophages to provide a mitogenic
stimulus for resting T cells. Biochemical analysis of the
T3 molecule showed that it was comprised of at least three
subunits (27-29)(25-28KD, 21-23KD and 19KD, respectively)
without detectable "variability" in subunits of T3 molecules derived from different T cell lines. Since the latter
is an essential prerequisite for an antigen/MHC receptor
molecule, it was concluded that T3, although intimately
linked to the antigen recognition process, did not itself
contain the Ag/MHC binding site.

To identify "clonotypic" molecules in the initial studies, we produced monoclonal antibodies against two distinct
human T cell cytotoxic clones (CT8$_{III}$ and CT4$_{II}$) derived
from the same individual and developed a screening strategy
that selects for anticlonotypic antibodies. In this way, a
series of non-crossreactive monoclonal antibodies that reacted only with the respective immunizing clone but not with
a large number of additional T cell clones or peripheral T
cells from the same donor were generated (19,20). These
were termed anti-Ti.

Since the unique reactivities of anti-Ti monoclonals
suggested that the surface structures defined were involved
in the individual clonal specificity, it was determined
whether these antibodies in soluble form could block recognition of antigen. To this end, effector cells were incubated with one or another monoclonal antibody for varying
periods prior to assay of the clones' cytolytic and proliferative capacities. It was shown that cytolytic activity
and the proliferative response of such clones were affected
only by their respective anticlonotypic antibodies (19).
That these effects were not simply due to an inactivation
of the clones as a result of antibody treatment was clear
from the fact that the same anti-Ti treatment augmented
proliferation to IL-2 (20).

If anti-Ti monoclonal antibodies defined variable regions of the T cell receptor, then we reasoned that under

the appropriate conditions, anti-Ti antibodies might induce
clonal T cell activation in a fashion analogous to that of
antigen itself. Because the alloantigens that serve as
receptor ligands are membrane bound and likely interact via
multi-point surface attachment, and because anticlonotypic
monoclonal antibodies, by themselves, were not mitogenic,
the functional effects of purified monoclonal antibodies
bound to a solid surface support (Sepharose beads) was investigated (30). A number of important points emerged from
these experiments: a) Sepharose linked anti-Ti and Sepharose linked anti-T3 caused very similar functional effects,
initiating clonal proliferation and secretion of lymphokines including IL-2; b) triggering of a single clonally
unique epitope appears to be sufficient to induce antigen
specific functions and to substitute for antigen plus MHC
determinant; c) multimeric interactions between ligand and
antigen receptor was an essential requirement for the initiation of clonal T cell responses; and d) these clones produced and responded to IL-2.   In addition, immunofluorescence studies showed that T3 modulation was accompanied by
loss of anti-Ti reactivity (20). These data imply that both
T3 and Ti have a role in antigen recognition and suggest a
relation between the cell surface structures defined by
these two antibodies.

Ti: A 90,000 DALTON DISULFIDE LINKED HETERODIMER

Because all studies described above demonstrated a
close functional and phenotypic relation between T3 glycoproteins and the Ti clonotype, it was important to biochemically define the surface molecules detected by clonotypic
antibodies. Therefore we selected two effector clones,
$CT4_{II}$ and $CT8_{III}$, for which we had specific monoclonal
anti-Ti antibodies (anti-Ti_{1B} and anti-Ti_{2A}, respectively)
and surface labelled cells from these clones with ^{125}I Na.
Cell membranes were solubilized, immunoprecipitated with
the appropriate anticlonotypic antibody and electropheresed
to enable protein bands to be visualized (Fig. 1)(19).

The two anticlonotypic antibodies were noncrossreac-
tive by immunofluorescent studies and specifically precipitated material only from the clone to which they were directed (Fig. 1). Furthermore, neither antibody reacted
with peripheral T cells ,or with a total of 80 other clones
derived from the same donor. Immunoprecipitated $CT8_{III}$ mem-

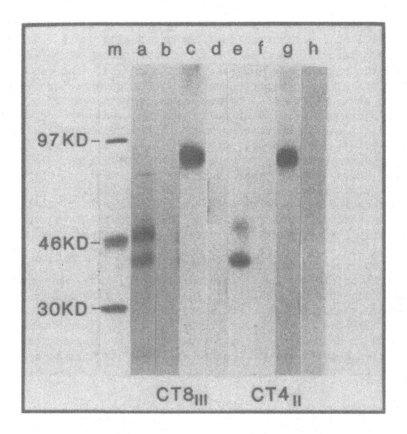

FIG. 1. SDS-PAGE analysis of anti-Ti immune precipitates from ^{125}I surface labelled CT8$_{III}$ and CT4$_{II}$. Lanes a to d depict immunoprecipitated proteins from CT8$_{III}$ membranes with anti-Ti1$_B$ antibody (a and c) and anti-Ti2$_A$ antibody (b and d) under reducing (a and b) and nonreducing conditions (c and d). Lanes e to h depict proteins immunoprecipitated from CT4$_{II}$ with anti-Ti1$_B$ antibody (e and g) and anti-Ti2$_A$ antibody (f and h) under reducing (e and f) and nonreducing conditions (g and h).

branes yielded two specific bands when electropheresed under reducing conditions (conditions that break disulfide bonds)(Fig. 1): a 49KD α chain and a 43KD β chain (lane a). Under nonreducing conditions (lane c) this structure appears as a single band at approximately 90KD. Anti-Ti2$_A$ antibody precipitates a similar molecule from ^{125}I labelled CT4$_{II}$ with subunits of 51KD and 49KD under reducing conditions,

and 90KD under nonreducing conditions. Thus, although the
Ti_1 and Ti_2 antigens can be defined by non-crossreactive
monoclonal antibodies, they both appear to be disulfide
linked heterodimers with distinct structural similarities.

The receptor for antigen on inducer and suppressor
clones is also a T3 associated disulfide linked heterodimer. Moreover, when anti-T3 antibody was used to precipi-
tate surface antigens from these effector or regulatory
clones, electropheresis (reducing) produced four bands: a
major protein band at 20KD, a band at 25KD and two higher
molecular weight (41-43KD and 49-52KD) bands identical to
those precipitated by anti-Ti antibody. Under nonreducing
conditions, the latter two bands migrated as a single band
at 90KD and the smaller molecular weight bands were unchanged. These results suggested that anti-T3 antibody
precipitated a T3-Ti complex, whereas clonotypic antibodies
disassociated the T3 subunits from the Ti structure. Together, these data show that each functional T cell population (cytotoxic, suppressor or inducer) expresses a T3-Ti
complex.

PEPTIDE VARIABILITY IN Ti MOLECULES

Ti_1 molecules immunoprecipitated from $CT4_{II}$ and sub-
jected to two dimensional gel electropheresis migrated at
pI 4.4 (α subunit) and pI 6.0 (β subunit). In contrast, Ti_2
α and β subunits from $CT8_{III}$ migrated at pI 4.7 and 6.2,
respectively (32). However, in both clones each subunit
migrated as a tight cluster of spots. To determine if the
microheterogeneity we observed within an individual clone
represented actual peptide differences, we pretreated the
Ti molecules with neuraminidase. After such treatment,
subunits from both Ti molecules resolved into single distinct spots, implying that the slight intraclonal microheterogeneity represented different degrees of sialyation,
whereas the intraclonal differences in isoelectric point
resulted from actual peptide differences(unpublished observation).
These data suggested to us that like the immunoglobulin molecule, Ti molecules might be composed of constant
and variable domains. To test this hypothesis, we compared
peptide maps obtained from isolated ^{125}I labelled subunits
after digesting them with proteolytic enzymes (32). The
tryptic peptide maps of the α chains from clones $CT4_{II}$ and

and CT8$_{III}$ were similar yet distinct and at least one minor and one major peptide were clearly identical in both clones. Of the remaining peptides, a group of six migrated minimally in both directions and although distinct, appeared to be related. All other peptides were clearly different.

The β subunits were not well digested with trypsin and therefore proteolysis with pepsin was required. Out of 11 to 13 peptides, two were identical and the rest migrated as a single large cluster. These data may indicate that variability in the β subunit is confined to a single region. Note that when peptides from both subunits were compared, no similarities were found (33 and unpublished data), indicating that they are products of different genes without apparent homology. These peptide map studies show unequivocally that Ti structures are analogs, and support the notion that both α and β subunits of Ti have constant and variable domains.

PARTIAL N-TERMINAL AMINO ACID SEQUENCING OF THE Ti β SUBUNIT

To obtain amino acid sequence data of the β subunit of Ti protein, we isolated microgram amounts of this structure from the REX thymic tumor cell line using immune affinity chromatography and polyacrylamide gel electrophoresis (34). Using a gas-liquid-solid phase protein sequenator, we obtained unambiguous amino acid sequence of 17 out of 20 residues in the N-terminal sequence of this subunit. A peptide with a sequence identical to that postulated for residues 2-11 was synthetized and used to produce a rabbit antiserum. This antiserum immunoprecipitated the isolated denatured β subunit of REX Ti, confirming that the postulated protein sequence was indeed that of the Ti β subunit.

To determine if homologies existed between this N-terminal sequence (residues 2-11 and 2-20) and known proteins, we did a computer search using the Dayhoff protein data bank. As shown with the representative amino acid sequence in Table 1, homologies with the first framework of the variable region of the immunoglobulin λ and k light chains were found. Lambda homology was evident with the shorter 2-11 peptide, and k homology was obvious with residues 2-20. In total, 44 of 60 matches were made with human and mouse light chain framework.

GENES ENCODING THE T CELL RECEPTOR

By using a novel techniqiue of cDNA cloning known as subtractive hybridization, two groups recently isolated cDNA clones encoding putative membrane proteins that are expressed uniquely in human and murinei T cell clones (35,36).

Restriction enzyme ·analysisi showed that those genes are
rearranged in T cells but not in B cells (36). The N-
terminus of the gene product predicted by the complementary
human DNA clones was completely consistent with the 17 amino
acids we had identified unambiguously in the N-terminal
sequence of the human Ti β subunit. This predicted N-
terminal sequence began at residue 22, identifying the first
21 residues as the leader signal peptide. In addition, the
cDNA deduced amino acid sequence shows remarkable homology to
the human immunoglobulin chain in both N-terminal (variable)
and C-terminal (constant) regions, particularly in the location of cysteine residues. These results are consistent with
our peptide map and N-terminal amino acid sequence data of
the Ti β subunit.

The correspondence of sequence data obtained by two different approaches and the additional fact that the molecular
weight of the polypeptide predicted for thé protein encoded
by the cDNA clone (35KD) corresponded closely with that of
the membrane form of Ti (43KD) strongly suggest that this DNA
clone is the gene for the β subunit of the human Ti molecule.
Differences in the molecular weight of the predicted and
observed protein can be explained by glycosylation; Ti is
known to be a glycoprotein and at least two potential
glycosylation sites for complex oligosaccharides are
predicted from the complete amino acid sequence deduced from
the cDNA clone (35).

Based on NH_2-terminal amino acid determinations and the
predicted protein sequence, the 291 amino acid human Ti β
subunit appears to contain four domains. Two extracellular
domains, one variable and one constant, each of which is
comprised within a disulfide loop, a carboxyterminal hydrophobic transmembrane region and a cytoplasmic tail. The high
degree of homology between the 3´ regions in the human and
mouse cDNA clones (80% between residues 134-306), and the
apparent lack of homology between the α and β subunits as
inferred from peptide map analysis indicates that the protein
encoded is the mouse equivalent of the Ti β subunit.

PARTIAL AMINO ACID SEQUENCE OF A CnBr FRAGMENT OF THE Ti α
SUBUNIT

To acquire data on the primary structure of the Ti α
chain, we purified the latter to a degree of purity suitable
for amino acid sequencing (37). Attempts to obtain NH_2-
terminus amino acid sequence gave negative results, indicating that the amino-terminal was blocked. To circumvent this
problem, CnBr cleared fragments were generated and sequenced

(37). Of three fragments obtained, only one of 25KD yielded sequence information. As shown in Fig. 2, unambiguous amino acid residue assignment could be made for 16 of 19 residues. Note that a methionine has been placed in the first portion as CnBr cleavage occurs at methionyl peptide bands.

To determine whether there were any homologies between known proteins and the REX Ti α sequence, we searched the Dayhoff protein data base. Of the 23 best matches, 15 were with variable regions of immunoglobulin heavy and light chains, including rabbit immunoglobulin k variable (V) region, mouse immunoglobulin heavy chain V (V_H) region and human, rabbit and murine immunoglobulin λ V region. Fig. 2 shows several representative examples. Note that the REX α chain sequence shows 42-47% similarity to a stretch of amino acids in framework 3 of the immunoglobulin V regions. Specifically, the homology involves the amino acids around and including the cysteine at about position 100, which corresponds to the second residue forming the intrachain disulfide bond within the variable region. This location is just NH_2-terminal of the third hypervariable region of immunoglobulin and is the most highly conserved sequence of immunoglobulin variable regions' (38). Moreover, Fig. 2 shows that the REX Ti α sequence is 36% homologous with the Ti β chain sequence obtained from the same tumor deduced from a cDNA clone (39). Again, this involves residues around the cysteine at position 90 which forms a putative intrachain disulfide bond to the cysteine at position 21 within the Ti β V region.

As noted previously peptide mapping analysis provided evidence of variability at the protein level in Ti α subunits derived from clones of differing specificities. The homology between the REX Ti α sequence and the sequences of immunoglobulin heavy, k and λ chains and the Ti β V region around the central cysteine (residues 80-100) reported here suggests that a structurally similar V region domain is contained within the Ti α subunit. Our data also support the notion that the Ti α subunit may be part of the gene superfamily encoding immunoglobulin, class I and II MHC products, Thy1, polyvalent Ig receptor and Ti β subunit. The presence of an immunoglobulin-like V region in the Ti α and β subunits suggests that both chains are required for antigen and/or MHC recognition, as is the case for immunoglobulin heavy and light chains. In this respect it is interesting to speculate that the fundamental structural basis of T and B cell recognition may be similar.

ACKNOWLEDGEMENTS

This work was supported by NIH grants AI 19807, AIGM 21226, and AI 12069-11.

REFERENCES

(1) Benacerraf, B. & McDevitt, H. Science 175, 273 (1979).

(2) Schlossman, S.F. Transplant. Rev. 10, 97 (1972).

(3) Zinkernagel, R.M. & Doherty, J.M.   J. Exp. Med. 141, 1427 (1975).

(4) Corradin, G. & Chiller, J.M.   J. Exp. Med. 149, 436 (1979).

(5) Hunig, T. & Bevan, M. Nature 294, 460 (1981).

(6) Cerottini, J.C. Prog. Immunol. 4, 622 (1980).

(7) Doherty, P.C. Prog. Immunol. 4, 563 (1980).

(8) Quinnan, G.V. et al. N. Engl. J. Med. 307, 7 (1982).

(9) Wallace, L.E., Rickinson, A.B., Rose, M. & Epstein, M.A. Nature 297, 413 (1982).

(10) Meuer, S.C. et al. J. Immunol. 131, 186 (1983).

(11) Gershon, R.K. Contemp. Top. Immunol. 3, 1 (1974).

(12) Cantor, H. & Boyse, E.A.   Cold Spring Harbor Symp. Quant. Biol. 41, 23 (1977).

(13) Cohen, S., Pick, E. & Oppenheim, J.J. In: Biology of the Lymphokines (Oppenheim, J.J. ed), Academic Press, New York, pp. 179-195.

(14) Morgan, D.A., Ruscetti, R.W. & Gallo, R.C. Science 1983, 1007 (1976).

(15) Kurnick, J.T. et al. J. Immunol. 122, 255 (1979).

(16) Bonnard, G.D., Yasaka, K. & Maca, R.D.   Cell. Immunol. 51, 390 (1980).

(17) Sredni, B., Tse, H.Y. & Schwartz, R.H. Nature 283, 581 (1980).

(18) Meuer, S.C., Schlossman, S.F. & Reinherz, E.L.   Proc. Natl. Acad. Sci. USA 79, 4395 (1982).

(19) Meuer, S.C. et al. Nature 303, 808 (1983).

(20) Meuer, S.C. et al. J. Exp. Med. 157, 705 (1983).

(21) Reinherz, E.L., Hussey, R.E. & Schlossman, S.F. Eur. J. Immunol. 10, 758 (1980).

(22) van Wauwe, F.P., DeMay, J.R. & Goossener, J.G. J. Immunol. 124, 2708 (1980).

(23) Chang, T.W., Kung, P.C., Gingras, S.P. & Goldstein, G. Proc. Natl. Acad. Sci. USA 78, 1805 (1981).

(24) Burns, G.F., Boyd, A.E. & Beverley, P.C.L. J. Immunol. 124, 1451 (1982).

(25) Reinherz, E.L. et al. Cell 30, 735 (1982).

(26) Umiel, T. et al. J. Immunol. 129, 1054 (1982).

(27) Borst, J., Prendiville, M.A. & Terhorst, C. J. Immunol. 128, 1560 (1982).

(28) Borst, J., Alexander, S., Elder, J. & Terhorst, C. J. Biol. Chem. 258, 5135 (1982).

(29) Kannelloplos, J.M., Wigglesworth, N.M., Owen, M.J. & Crumpton, M.J. Embo. J. 2, 1807 (1983).

(30) Meuer, S.C. et al. J. Exp. Med. 158, 988 (1983).

(31) Meuer, S.C. et al. Science 218, 471 (1982).

(32) Acuto, O. et al. J. Exp. Med. 158, 1368 (1983).

(33) Acuto, O. et al. Cell 34, 717 (1983).

(34) Acuto, O. et al. Proc. Natl. Acad. Sci. USA 81, 3851 (1984).

(35) Yanagi, Y. et al. Nature 308, 145 (1984).

(36) Hedrick, S.M., Cohen, D.I., Nielsen, E.A. & David, M.M. Nature 308, 153 (1984).

(37) Fabbi, M., Acuto, O., Smart, J. & Reinherz, E.L. Nature 312, 269 (1984).

(38) Kabat, E.A. et al. Sequences of Proteins of Immunological Interest (U.S. Dept. of Health and Human Services)(1983).

(39) Royer, H.D. et al. Cell, in press.

TABLE 1. Ti β AND IMMUNOGLOBULIN LIGHT CHAINS ARE HOMOLOGOUS IN PORTIONS OF THEIR N–TERMINAL AMINO ACID SEQUENCES

Protein	1				5					10					15				
Ti	X	V*	I	Q	S	P	R	H	E	V	T	E	X	G	X	E	V	L	R
Bvr: VλII		V	S	G	S	P	G	H	S	V	T								
Tro: VλII		V	S	G	S	P	G	Q	S	V	T								
Nig48:λV VI		V*	S	E	S	P	G	K	T	V	T								
Ag: VκI		M	T	Q	S	P	S	S	L	S	A	S	V	G	D	R	V	T	I	T
Ni: VκI		M	T	Q	S	P	S	S	L	S	A	T	V	G	D	R	V	T	L	L
Pom: VκIV		M	T	Q	S	P	V	T	L	S	V	P	G	E	S	R	A	T	L	S
MOPC21: Vκ		M	T	Q	S	P	K	S	M	S	V	G	E	R	V	T	L	T

(Ti: V* annotated *10; Nig48: V* annotated *4)

Note that all protein homologies shown are with human immunoglobulin except for MOPC21 (mouse). Single amino acid nomenclature is utilized with bound areas showing homology.
*Denotes amino acid positions corresponding to start of sequence homology in the immunoglobulin proteins.

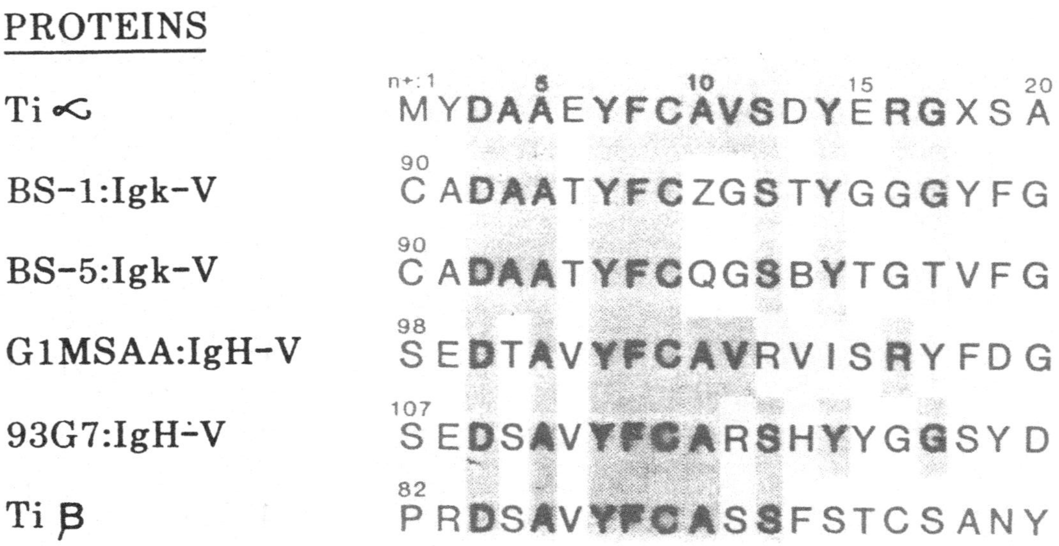

PROTEINS

Ti α	n+1	MYDAAEYFCAVSDYERGXSA	(positions 5, 10, 15, 20)
BS-1:Igk-V	90	CADAATYFCZGSTYGGGYFG	
BS-5:Igk-V	90	CADAATYFCQGSBYTGTVFG	
G1MSAA:IgH-V	98	SEDTAVYFCAVRVISRYFDG	
93G7:IgH-V	107	SEDSAVYFCARSHYYGGSYD	
Ti β	82	PRDSAVYFCASSFSTCSANY	

Fig. 2. Amino acid sequence determination of REX Ti α CnBr fragments. The amino acid sequences are given in the single letter code. The Ti α and β subunits are derived from the REX tumor; BS-1 is a rabbit immunoglobulin κ V region, as is BS-5; G1MSAA is a mouse immunoglobulin heavy chain V region; 93G7 is a mouse immunoglobulin heavy chain V region. Numbers on the left indicate the position of the residue in the molecule. Numbers above the top line indicate the positions of the assigned residues in the REX Ti α fragments. Shading indicates homology.

THE MURINE T CELL RECEPTOR

Kathryn Haskins, Neal Roehm, Charles Hannum,
Janice White, Ralph Kubo, Philippa Marrack
and John Kappler

National Jewish Hospital & Research Center/National
Asthma Center, Department of Medicine
3800 E. Colfax Avenue
Denver, CO 80206

IDENTIFICATION OF THE T CELL RECEPTOR
BY CLONE-SPECIFIC ANTIBODIES

In the past two years, the major histocompatibility complex (MHC)-restricted receptor for antigen on T cells has been identified by several laboratories through the use of clone-specific antibodies which recognize idiotypic determinants on T cell antigen receptors. Studies with these antibodies, summarized in a recent review (1) have established that the antigen/MHC recognition structures on T cells (a) are idiotypic molecules as indicated by the highly specific nature of their binding to the anti-receptor antibodies; (b) can be functionally inhibited or stimulated through interaction with clone-specific antibodies, suggesting that the specific recognition of antigen and MHC involves a single binding site; (c) are 85-90,000 dalton glycoproteins consisting of two hetero-dimeric disulfide-linked subunits; and (d) contain variable and constant peptide regions in both the alpha and the beta chains. The biochemical characterization of the receptor with the clone-specific antibodies has since been confirmed and extended by recent reports on the genomic organization of the receptor β chain (2-6).

15

The clone-specific anti-receptor antibodies produced in our laboratory are listed with the murine T cell hybridomas to which they were made in Table I. KJ1-26 was the first antibody we isolated and is specific for the antigen-specific MHC-restricted T cell hybridoma DO-11.10 (7). This hybrid responds to chicken ovalbumin (cOVA) in the context of I-A^d by making interleukin 2 (IL-2); the antibody KJ1-26 specifically blocks the IL-2 response of DO-11.10. The antibody reacts in identical fashion with a second T cell hybridoma, 7DO-286, which has antigen/MHC specificities identical to those of DO-11.10 but which was independently selected (8). 3DT-52.5 is a Class I-restricted T cell hybridoma which produces IL-2 in response to D^d (9) and is inhibited by the clone-specific antibody KJ12-98 (10).

TABLE 1

Anti-Receptor Antibodies to Murine T Cells

Monoclonal Antibody	Type	T Cell Specificity
KJ1-26	Idiotypic	DO-11.10 (cOVA, I-A^d)
		7DO-286 (cOVA, I-A^d)
KJ12-98	Idiotypic	3DT-52.5 (D^d)
KJ16-133	Allotypic	20% of T cells

REACTIVITY OF AN ANTI-RECEPTOR ANTIBODY
DIRECTED TOWARD AN ALLOTYPIC DETERMINANT

In addition to these clone-specific antibodies which have been very useful in studying the receptor on single clones of T cells, we have recently described another anti-receptor antibody which is directed toward an allotypic determinant present on about 20% of murine T cells (11). This antibody, KJ16-133, was produced by immunizing a rat with receptor material isolated from the T cell hybridoma DO-11.10 with the clone-specific antibody KJ1-26. The antibody-receptor complex was precipitated with Staphylococcus aureus and the resulting preparation was used as the immunogen. The presence of anti-receptor antibodies in the rat antiserum was detected by immuno-precipitation studies in which it was shown that the 85,000 MW band characteristic of the receptor could be precipitated not only from lysates of DO-11.10 but also from lysates of normal BALB/c T cells. Spleen and lymph node cells of this animal were fused to the mouse myeloma, P3-X63Ag8.653/3, and resulting hybrids were tested for receptor binding activity by ELISA. One hybrid, KJ16-133, was found that precipitated from both DO-11.10 and normal BALB/c T cells an 85,000 MW band which migrated to ~43,000 MW upon reduction. Sequential immunoprecipitation studies showed that the KJ16-133 antibody recognized the same molecule on DO-11.10 as did the clone-specific antibody KJ1-26.

In further characterizing the reactivity of the new antibody, immunoprecipitation studies and cytofluoro-graphic analysis showed that KJ16-133 bound T cells from most strains of mice. Exceptions included the SJL, SJA/20, SWR, C57L and C57BR strains. Reactivity with a wide range of T cell hybridomas and tumors was also investigated and KJ16-133 was found to bind about 20 percent of hybrids tested. Over twenty hybrids with different specificities and origins were examined for reactivity with the antibody, and in some cases where the antibody tested positive for binding, it also was found to affect functional activity of the hybrid by either blocking or stimulating the antigen/MHC response. No correlation, however, could be made between antigen/MHC specificity of the reactive hybrid and reactivity with the antibody, as illustrated by some examples listed in Table 2 (11).

TABLE 2

Reactivities of T Cell Hybridomas
and Tumors with KJ16-133

Cell Line	Specificity	Reactivity with KJ16-133
DO-11.10	cOVA/I-A^d, I-A^b cOVA/I-A^b	+
3DO-18.3	cOVA/I-A^d	−
3DO-20.10	cOVA/I-A^d	−
3DT-18.11	TGAL/I-A^d	−
3DT-52.5	D^d	+
MDK 16	I-A^k	+
S18.4	I-A^d	+
SKK 2.3	KLH/I-A^k	−
SKK 45.10	KLH/I-A^k, I-A^b	+
AODH-3.4	cOVA/I-A^k, I-A^b	−
BW5147	−	−

DISTRIBUTION OF THE ALLOTYPIC DETERMINANT ON PERIPHERAL T CELLS AND ON THYMOCYTES

In the cytofluorometric analysis of peripheral T cells from BALB/c mice, it was found that the KJ16-133 antibody bound in a uniform manner a discrete population of cells amounting to about 20 percent of the total. SJL peripheral T cells, which are not bound by the KJ16-133 antibody, were used as negative controls. As T cells are thought to acquire specificity in the thymus, we were very interested in determining the pattern of KJ16-133 reactivity with thymocytes. To carry out these experiments, thymocytes from BALB/c mice were separated into mature and immature thymocyte populations by peanut agglutinin (PNA) or lobster agglutinin 1 (LAg 1) fractionation and these were compared to thymocytes from mice pretreated with cortisone. Immunoprecipitation experiments showed that the receptor molecule was precipitated from lysates of all of the populations tested, although bands precipitated from whole and immature thymocyte populations were much lighter than those observed in mature populations, suggesting that fewer receptors were present on immature cells (12).

To examine more quantitatively the amount of KJ16-133 determinant expressed on thymocytes, flow cytometric analysis was carried out on both fractionated and total thymocyte populations. Staining of total thymocytes showed that the distribution of the KJ16-133 determinant was very heterogeneous in the thymus overall, and that thymocytes bound the antibody at considerably lower levels (~10%) than those observed with peripheral T cells (~20%). Analysis of the different thymocyte populations showed that the distribution of the allotypic determinant recognized by KJ16-133 on mature thymocytes was quite similar to that of peripheral T cells, with about 20 percent of the mature cells showing strong reactivity with the antibody. On the other hand, in the immature, PNA$^+$, population the pattern of KJ16-133 staining indicated that only about 9 percent of these cells reacted with the antibody and showed varying levels of staining intensity, reflecting the pattern of reactivity observed with total thymocyte populations. It appeared from these studies then that the T cell receptor is expressed on some immature thymocytes, but in varying amounts and at about half the frequency observed in mature thymocytes or peripheral T cells. Flow cytometric analysis of fetal thymocytes showed that the appearance of the KJ16-133 determinant was detectable in 17 day embryos and increased gradually to almost adult thymocyte levels in newborn mice. These results suggested that thymocytes do not bear antigen/MHC receptors initially but only acquire these molecules during maturation. Moreover, the number of receptors per cell of fetal and newborn thymocytes is considerably lower than that observed with mature thymocytes or peripheral T cells (12).

Lastly it was of interest to look at the distribution of the KJ16-133 determinant on Class I versus Class II restricted T cells. BALB/c peripheral T cells were analyzed for reactivity to the KJ16-133 antibody in the presence of either fluoresceinated anti-L3T4 (Class II-specific T cells) or anti-Lyt2 (Class I-specific T cells). KJ16-133 receptors were found on both classes of T cells and at even higher levels (34%) on $Lyt2^+$ cells than on $L3T4^+$ cells (20%), a result contrary to our expectations that the antibody might show preferential reactivity with Class II-restricted T cells since it was raised to the Class II-specific T cell hybridoma, DO-11.10 (12). A summary of the distribution of the KJ16-133 determinant is presented in Table 3.

TABLE 3

Distribution of the KJ16-133 Determinant on
Peripheral T cells and Thymocytes

T cell population	Percent of cells reactive with KJ16-133
Peripheral T cells	15-20%
Whole thymocyte population	10%
Mature thymocytes (PNA^-)	20%
Mature thymocytes (CRT)	19%
Immature thymocytes (PNA^+)	9%
$L3T4^+$ Peripheral T cells	20%
$Lyt2^+$ Peripheral T cells	34%

NATURE OF THE KJ16-133 DETERMINANT

Although the KJ16-133 antibody precipitates the same 85,000 MW molecule from DO-11.10 as the clone-specific antibody KJ1-26, the determinant recognized by KJ16-133 is different (11). This was first suggested by the observation that binding of the KJ16-133 antibody to the receptor was temperature sensitive, but binding of KJ1-26 was not. That KJ16-133 was reacting with a site distinct from the receptor idiotype bound by KJ1-26 was also apparent from experiments in which affinity-purified receptor was reduced and alkylated and then tested for precipitation with both antibodies. The KJ16-133 antibody still precipitated both chains of the receptor but the clone-specific antibody showed very low reactivity with the reduced receptor chains, indicating that the site recognized by this antibody is sensitive to reduction and alkylation procedures, unlike the KJ16-133 determinant. Further indication that the two antibodies recognize different sites on the receptor was provided by antibody blocking experiments in which it was found that binding of one antibody to the receptor is inhibited only partially or not at all by the other antibody.

EXPRESSION OF THE ALLOTYPIC DETERMINANT

Recent mapping studies suggest that the KJ16.133 determinant on the T cell receptor is allelically excluded and that the locus which controls the presence of this allele is on chromosome 6 in the mouse (13).

Cytofluorographic analysis was carried out on T cells from CBA/J, SJL, or (CBA/J x SJL)F_1 mice. SJL T cells are negative for expression of the KJ16-133 determinant but are positive for the codominantly-expressed Lyt 2 allele, Lyt 2.2. Conversely, CBA/J T cells are reactive with the KJ16-133 antibody but not with anti-Lyt 2.2 antibodies. When T cells from the (CBA/J x SJL)F_1 mice were analyzed for binding to either KJ16-133 or anti-Lyt 2.2, it was found that the anti-Lyt 2.2 antibody bound the same percentage of T cells as in the parent but at half the intensity, as might be expected with a codominantly-expressed determinant. A different binding profile was observed with KJ16-133; the antibody bound to F_1 T cells as well as it bound to the parent T cells, but the frequency with which the antibody bound F_1 T cells was a little over half that observed in the parent. One interpretation of this result is that the gene which codes for the KJ16-133 determinant is controlled by allelic exclusion.

To gain further information about the gene that codes for the KJ16-133 determinant, we looked in (CBA x SJL)F_2 mice for linkage of the KJ16 allele to Ly-2 which has been shown to be in close proximity to the receptor beta chain on chromosome 6 (14). Our results showed that the two loci were linked, thus suggesting that the KJ16-133 antibody is reacting with a site on the beta chain of the T cell receptor. Other studies on the expression of the KJ16-133 determinant in recombinant inbred mice have yielded preliminary information which indicates that there may also be genetic influence on the frequency of KJ16-133 expression. Most notably, the frequency of expression of the KJ16-133 determinant seems to be correlated with Igh on chromosome 12, β_2m on chromosome 2 and Mls on chromosome 1. Further examination of these loci is in progress and should reveal more about their influence on how frequently the KJ16 allotypic determinant is expressed.

REFERENCES

1. Haskins, K., Kappler, J. & Marrack, P. Ann. Rev. Immunol. 2, 51-66 (1984).

2. Yanagi, Y., Yoshikai, Y., Leggett, K., Clark, S.P., Aleksander, I. & Mak, T.W. Nature 308, 145-149 (1984).

3. Hedrick, S.M., Cohen, D.I., Nielsen, E.A. & Davis, M.M. Nature 308, 149-153 (1984).

4. Hedrick, S.M., Nielsen, E.A., Kavaler, J., Cohen, D.I. & Davis, M.M. Nature 308, 153-158 (1984).

5. Chien, Y., Gascoigne, N., Kavaler, J., Lee, N. & Davis, M. Nature 309, 322-326 (1984).

6. Gascoigne, N., Chien, Y., Decker, D.M., Kavaler, J. & Davis, M.M. Nature 310, 387-391 (1984).

7. Haskins, K., Kubo, R., White, J., Pigeon, M., Kappler, J. & Marrack, P. J. Exp. Med. 157, 1149-1169 (1983).

8. Marrack, P., Shimonkevitz, R., Hannum, C., Haskins, K. & Kappler, J. J. Exp. Med. 158, 1635-1646 (1983).

9. Endres, R.O., Marrack, P. & Kappler, J.W. J. Immunol. 131, 1656-1662 (1983).

10. Kappler, J., Kubo, R., Haskins, K., White, J. & Marrack, P. Cell 34, 727-737 (1983).

11. Haskins, K., Hannum, C., White, J., Roehm, N., Kubo, R., Kappler, J. & Marrack, P. J. Exp. Med. 160, 452-471 (1984).

12. Roehm, N., Herron, L., Cambier, J., DiGiusto, D., Haskins, K., Kappler, J. & Marrack, P. Cell 38, 577-584 (1984).

13. Roehm, N., Carbone, A., Kushnir, E., Taylor, B.A., Riblet, R., Marrack, P. & Kappler, J. Manuscript submitted for publication (1984).

14. Caccia, N., Kronenberg, M., Saxe, D., Haars, R., Bruns, G.A.P., Goverman, J., Malissen, M., Willard, H., Yoshikai, Y., Sunon, M., Hood, L. & Mak, T.W. Cell 37, 1091-1099 (1984).

THE GENES OF THE MURINE T CELL RECEPTOR

Nicholas R.J. Gascoigne, Yueh-hsiu Chien, Phillip Patten,
Daniel M. Becker, Tullia Lindsten, Joshua Kavaler,
Nadine E. Lee and Mark M. Davis

Department of Medical Microbiology, Fairchild Building,
Stanford University School of Medicine
Stanford, CA 94305, USA.

INTRODUCTION

T cells recognize antigen in a way fundamentally different from B cells. It has been known now for a decade (1-
3) that the T cell receptor sees the antigen, not alone, but
in association the major histocompatibility complex (MHC,
H-2 in the mouse). As a general rule cytotoxic T (Tc) cells
recognize antigen in association with Class I MHC molecules
and helper T (Th) cells do so with Class II structures
(4,5).

The nature of the T cell antigen receptor has only been
investigated with any success in the last two years, since
the development of monoclonal antibodies to idiotypic
(clonotypic) structures on the T cell surface (6-9). The
receptor is an heterodimer of two 40-45 kd chains linked by
a disulphide bridge. Both chains have variable and constant
portions as judged by tryptic peptide analysis (10,11). Although Tc and Th cells are known to have different restriction specificities, no clear difference between their
receptor molecules has emerged from these protein studies
(6-12).

The work described below follows the isolation of a
cDNA clone for one chain of the T cell receptor (13-15). We
now know this to encode the β-chain of the heterodimer since
N-terminal amino acid sequence of the human β-chain (16)
corresponds with the variable region of the human cDNA clone

25

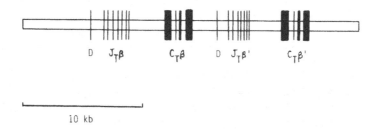

D $J_T\beta$ $C_T\beta$ D $J_T\beta'$ $C_T\beta'$

|———————————————|

10 kb

<u>Figure 1. Genomic organization of the β-chain gene on</u>
<u>chromosome six</u>

(15) which is ~80% homologous to mouse. This gene was originally shown to have variable (V), joining (J) and constant
(C) regions as judged by homology to the respective immunoglobulin genes (14, 15). The α-chain of the receptor is now
known to have similar properties (17) and has been confirmed
as the α-chain by protein sequence (N.Jones, J.Strominger
personal communication).

RESULTS AND DISCUSSION

Genomic Organization and Rearrangement of the β-chain

The sequence organization of the β-chain is summarised
in Fig. 1. There is a tandem arrangement: DJC/DJC, covering
a region of about 15kb (18-22) of chromosome 6 (23,24). The
V region elements are positioned an indeterminate distance
upstream of the region shown. Only one D region in each
position has so-far been identified but the total number may
be above ten (25). Each is about 0.6kb upstream of the respective J region cluster (21,22), which consists of seven
distinct elements (18-20). The D region immediately 5' to
the more 5' J region cluster bears strong homology to the
D_{Q52} region of immunoglobulin (26).

J regions. One J region in each cluster is clearly a
pseudogene-J_T7 has no suitable RNA splice site (19) and J_T6'
a stop codon in the coding sequence (18,20). Figure 2 shows
the coding sequences of the twelve possibly functional J
regions and indicates the nine that have so-far been found
expressed in cDNA clones (27). The regions of homology are
boxed and show that the carboxy end of the J regions are far

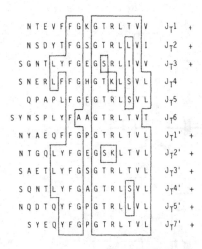

Figure 2. J region homo-
logies. Those known to
be expressed in cDNAs are
indicated with a "+" sign

more homologous than the amino ends. Immediately 5' to each
J region element is a conserved heptamer (NNNTGTG), a spacer
of 10-14 nucleotides and a relatively conserved nonamer
(characterized by several T residues) (18-20). These may
(by analogy to immunoglobulin) constitute the signal sequences for the DNA rearrangements that occur to generate
functional variable regions. No clear T cell specificity is
found in these signal sequences. J_T1' for instance has the
same heptamer as ~90% of immunoglobulin J regions (CACTGTG).

     Rearrangement.   In immunoglobulin heavy chain genes,
the functional gene is formed by somatic rearrangements that
juxtapose the V region to a D region to a J region. Diversity in the antibody binding site is therefore generated not
just by the sequence of the different V, D and J regions,
but also by the indeterminate position of the joints.
Immunoglobulin light chain genes behave in a similar fashion
except that they have no D regions and bind directly from V
to J (28) (fig.3). We have shown for the murine system
(18), as others have in the human system (29), that rearrangement in the β-chain occurs as the immunoglobulin
heavy chains: V-D-J

     The rearrangements are believed to be controlled by the
heptamer and nonamer sequences that are (as mentioned above)
found immediately 5' to the J regions. Complementary sequences are present 3' to the D regions and similarly on the
5' end of D and 3' end of V. The length of the spacer sequ-

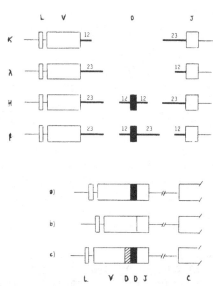

Figure 3. "12/23" nucleotide spacer arrangements and the three possible outcomes (a,b,c) of β-chain rearrangement

ences appears very important, since, in immunoglobulin genes an element with a 12 (∓1) nucleotide spacer may only join to one with a 23 (∓1) spacer. This ensures that in light chains a V region joins to a J, and in heavy chains that a D is inserted between V and J (Fig. 3). In the β-chain however, the "12/23 rule" allows two other possibilities than exist for heavy chains; either direct V-J joining (fig.3b) or the sequential joining of D regions (fig.3c). Evidence for the former from a cDNA has now been reported (30) and a possible example of the latter also (25). It is also worth noting that the only case in which the 12/23 rule would prohibit rearrangement of a V_β to an immunoglobulin J is with κ. Since, in mouse, κ is on the same chromosome as β, this may represent an insurance against accidental rearrangement between these two loci.

A further nuance in the pattern of rearrangement is that there is a very high frequency of an alternate transcript. This occurs when a D is joined to a J region without any involvement of a V region (22). The region immediately upstream of the D region, including the heptamer and nonamer sequences is transcribed, providing a strongly hydrophobic leader-like sequence in the approximately 50 amino acids of open reading frame. A similar phenomenon has also been

found in immunoglobulin and in this case a protein appears
to be translated (31). On northern blots this "DJ" message
is seen as a 1.0kb band distinct from the complete "VDJ"
message at 1.3kb (22,32). It is found in thymus and spleen
cell RNA, but only in some functional T cell clones (32,
NRJG unpublished observations). Its significance is unknown, though its presence in B cells makes it unlikely that
it is involved in thymic learning or any other T cell specific phenomenon.

The Constant Regions

There are two C region loci for the β-chain (fig. 1),
but a comparison of their sequences (19) shows them to have
only minor differences. Each locus consists of four exons,
with most of the variation between them occurring at the
more 3' end of the gene. The first exon (C_T1) encodes the
globular domain, most of the external part of the C
region. C_T2 is a short (18 nucleotides, 6 amino acids) exon
that encodes the cysteine of the interchain disulphide bond,
C_T3 the transmembrane region and C_T4 the intracytoplasmic
tail and 3' untranslated region. There are a total of four
amino acid changes between the two loci, three in C_T3 and
one in C_T4. Of these, only one (glutamine:histidine at position 249) is likely to be outside the membrane (19) and
therefore available as an isotypic determinant. Only one
possible allotypic determinant has so-far been described;
lysine 164 (19) (within C_T1 of $C_Tβ'$ from the B10.A mouse) is
changed to an arginine in BALB/c (33).

The transmembrane regions of all the three T cell specific, rearranged genes isolated to date (14,17, 33) have
significant homology to each other (fig.4a). In particular
they all have a lysine within the region which is rather unusual. Since T3 has a negative charge in the transmembrane
region (C.Terhorst, personal communication), this suggests
that it is of some importance, perhaps forming a salt bridge
to the mouse T3 molecule (14,19). These transmembrane regions have no homology to those of immunoglobulin, which are,
in turn, highly homologous to each other (34).

A T cell receptor hinge region? The hinge region of
immunoglobulins has two known functions: to provide the cys-
teine(s) for the inter heavy chain bond(s) and to provide
flexibility. There is some homology between the C_T2 exon of

a)

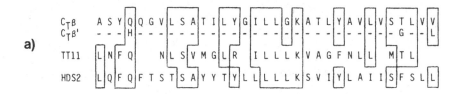

b)

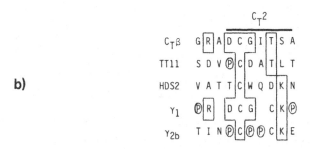

Figure 4. Homologies in (a) the transmembrane region and (b) the hinge region. (a) The two $C_T\beta$ alleles are compared with the comparable region of the α-chain (TT11, ref.17) and another T cell specific, rearranged gene (HDS2, ref.33). (b) Comparisons of these genes with immunoglobulin hinge regions. The region encoded by C_T2 in C_T is indicated. Homologies are boxed and prolines circled.

the β-chain with the γ1 hinge region (fig.4b), though not to other hinges. The γ1 hinge has been shown to be the least flexible of the immunoglobulin hinges (35) and thus the homology of C_T2 and its lack of prolines (thought very important for flexibility) probably indicates that this region of the β-chain does not confer flexibility on the molecule. The region around this cysteine in the other two T cell specific, rearranged genes is also shown. The gene of Saito et al. (HDS2) (33), which is probably not the α-chain (17, 36,37) has no notable homology to immunoglobulin hinges and no prolines, however, that of Chien et al. (TT11) (17), a likely candidate for the α-chain, does have a proline next to the cysteine. Again there is no particular homology to the immunoglobulin hinges, but the presence of a proline in this region may indicate a relationship. Thus if C_T2 does represent a β-chain hinge region, there may also be one present in the α-chain.

Variable Regions and the Generation of Diversity

Patten et al. (38) have recently analyzed a set of β-chain V regions and compared them to an array of heavy and light chain V regions. There were several striking findings: the β-chain V regions were far more diverse than the immunoglobulins (18-51% amino acid homology as opposed to 45->90% for immunoglobulins). Although the three regions of V_β sequence which correspond to the classical V_κ hypervariable (HV) regions were observed to be hypervariable, four new HVs were identified.

Though the β-chain primary structure was very different from immunoglobulin (25-35% homologous to immunoglobulin V regions), the Chou and Fasman algorhythm predicted strong secondary structure conservation relative to immunoglobulin. Since β-chain V regions are most homologous to κ V regions, these V regions were modelled on the α-carbon skeleton of a κ Fab fragment. This revealed that the new putative HVs were arranged, not around the immunoglobulin binding site, but on another surface of the protein. The altered regions of immunoglobulin framework correspond to: two external loops between antiparallel β-sheets (this is a similar structure to that of classical immunoglobulin HVs), one β-turn and sheet which in V_κ interacts with solvent and another turn/sheet which would make hydrogen bonds and hydrophobic interactions with the heavy chain. This last region is highly conserved in V_κ. These differences in V_β lead to the prediction (38) that there may be separated binding regions on the β-chain molecule. Two models consistent with this interpretation of the placing of these new HVs are sketched in figure 5b/c. The classical binding site in the T cell receptor should be larger than in immunoglobulin (fig.5a) and the other putative binding site might make contact with MHC molecules. In these models conformational changes caused by interactions with MHC molecules could alter the internal binding site and thus responses against the same antigen but restricted by different MHC alleles would be likely to use different V regions. This is the case for the response of B10.A and B10.S(9R) mice to pigeon cytochrome c (S.M. Hedrick, personal communication). These models also suggest that there may be some affinity for self MHC and antigen individually. While there is very little data to support such an idea, there has recently been a report of direct antigen binding to the receptor (39).

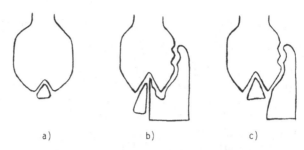

Figure 5. (a) The classical interaction of antibody with antigen. (b,c) Two models for T cell receptor interaction with antigen.

Generation of Diversity. Another finding of Patten et al. (38) was that 4 out of 5 murine V_βs hybridize to single bands on genomic southern blots at moderate stringency and thus are probably single copy genes. The 5th V region repr- esents a small (~2-3) family. This is in contrast to imm- unoglobulin Vs where large families are common. They also found that four of these V regions were able to account for about 40% of all V region-bearing β-chain clones in a cDNA library derived from thymus. Thus perhaps less than 10 V regions predominate in thymus.

However, one of the V regions tested, that of 2B4, a functional, anti-cytochrome c hybridoma, was not detected amongst 250,000 clones screened. This may indicate that although there is a set of very common V regions present in thymus, there is also a less common set present at much lower frequencies. This is in agreement with the work of Eichmann's group (40,41) who have found three frequencies of antigen reactive T cells: a frequent set at 1/40-90, an int- ermediate set at 1/600-3000 and a rare set at 1/20,000- 100,000. Although these authors interpreted their results as due to suppressor cells active in vivo they may rather indicate that there are groups of T cell receptor V genes that occur at very different frequencies.

Thus the contribution of the V region elements to the generation of T cell diversity is still unresolved. In immunoglobulin there are a large number of V regions (38, 42), several D regions and a few J regions (~4 each for H, κ and λ). There are three HV regions in immunoglobulin, the third being at the VDJ or VJ boundary. The D region in heavy chains is therefore very important for diversity. The

5' end of the J region also encodes part of HV 3. In the β-chain the D and J regions are therefore also likely to be responsible for a large measure of the diversity. It is important to note that they have substantially more capacity for generation of diversity than do the homologous immuno-globulin regions. There is a larger number of β-chain J regions (nine functional at the very least) and they are significantly more varied than their immunoglobulin counter-parts (19). There is considerable variability in the length of the J regions, both from their sequence and from the var-iable positions of rearrangement (19). In addition there are three possible ways of recombining V to J: with a D region (fig.3a), with more than one D region (fig.3c) and without a D region (fig.3b). These options do not exist for immunoglobulins. The existence of "N" regions (somatically generated nucleotides added between the join of the VD or DJ regions, probably by the enzyme teminal deoxynucleotidyl transferase (43)) may also provide for variation (18,21), though the extent of its activity is unclear. Should it turn out that there are in fact comparatively few V regions for the β-chain, this would not preclude that T cells have a large repertoire, but it would reside more around the HV 3 of immunoglobulin and rely more on combinatorial events than does the diversity of B cells. At present it is not poss-ible to comment on the generation of diversity in the α-chain and its contribution to the binding site. This must await further studies which are now in progress.

NRJG is supported by the Cancer Research Institute, New York and TL by a Damon Runyon/Walter Winchell fellowship.

REFERENCES

1. Zinkernagel, R.M., Doherty, P.C. (1974) Nature **248**: 701
2. Gordon, R.D., Simpson, E., Samelson, L.E. (1975) J. Exp. Med. **142**: 1108
3. Bevan, M.J. (1975) J. Exp. Med. **142**: 1349
4. Zinkernagel, R.M., Doherty, P.C. (1979) Adv. Immun. **27**: 52
5. Sprent, J., et al. (1980) Springer Semin. Immunopath. **3**: 213
6. Allison, J.P., MacIntyre, B.W., Block, D. (1982) J. Immun. **129**: 2293
7. Meuer, S. et al. (1983) J. Exp. Med. **157**: 705
8. Haskins, K. et al. (1983) J. Exp. Med. **157**: 1149
9. Samelson, L.E., Germain, R.N., Schwartz, R.H. (1983)

Proc. Natl. Acad. Sci. USA **80**: 6972
10. MacIntyre, B.W., Allison, J.P. (1983) Cell **34**: 739
11. Kappler, J.W. et al. (1983) Cell **35**: 295
12. Kappler, J.W. et al. (1983) Cell **34**: 727
13. Hedrick, S.M. et al. (1984) Nature **308**: 149
14. Hedrick, S.M. et al. (1984) Nature **308**: 153
15. Yanagi, Y. et al. (1984) Nature **308**: 145
16. Acuto, O. et al. (1984) Proc. Natl. Acad. Sci. USA **81**: 3851
17. Chien, Y., Becker, D.M., Lindsten, T., Okamura, M., Cohen, D.I., Davis, M.M. (1984) Nature **311**: in press
18. Chien, Y., Gascoigne, N.R.J., Kavaler, J., Lee, N.E., Davis, M.M. (1984) Nature **309**: 322
19. Gascoigne, N.R.J., Chien, Y., Becker, D.M., Kavaler, J., Davis, M.M. (1984) Nature **310**: 387
20. Malissen, M. et al. (1984) Cell **37**: 1101
21. Kavaler, J., Davis, M.M., Chien, Y. (1984) Nature **310**: 421
22. Siu, G. et al. (1984) Nature **311**: 344
23. Caccia, N. et al. (1984) Cell **37**: 1091
24. Lee., N.E. et al. (1984) Nature **160**: 905
25. Chien, Y., Kavaler, J., Davis, M.M. (1984) Proc. Natl. Acad. Sci. USA in press
26. Sakano, H. et al. (1980) Nature **286**: 676
27. Davis, M.M. (1985) Ann. Rev. Immun. **3**: in press
28. Honjo, T. (1983) Ann. Rev. Immun. **1**: 499
29. Siu, G. et al. (1984) Cell **37**: 393
30. Yoshikai, Y. et al. (1984) Nature in press
31. Reth, M., Alt, F.W. (1984) Nature in press
32. Hedrick, S.M. et al. (1984) Proc. Natl. Acad. Sci. USA in press
33. Saito, H. et al. (1984) Nature **309**: 757
34. Komaromy, M. et al. (1983) Nucleic Acids Res. **11**: 6775
35. Oi, V.T. et al. (1984) Nature **307**: 136
36. McIntyre, B.W., Allison, J.P. (1984) Cell **38**: 459
37. Robertson, M. (1984) Nature **311**: 305
38. Patten, P., et al. (1984) Nature **311**: in press
39. Rao, A. et al. (1984) Cell **36**: 879
40. Melchers, I., Fey, K., Eichmann, K. (1982) J. Exp. Med. **156**: 1587
41. Hamann, U., Eichmann, K., Krammer, P. (1983) J. Immun. **130**: 7
42. Brodeur, P.H., Riblet, R. (1984) Eur. J. Immun. **14**: in press
43. Alt F.W., Baltimore, D. (1982) Proc. Natl. Acad. Sci. USA **79**: 4118

MOLECULAR STUDIES OF THE HUMAN T-CELL ANTIGEN RECEPTOR

Mary K.L. Collins, A. Maija Kissonerghis, M. Jenny Dunne
and Michael J. Owen

Imperial Cancer Research Fund
Tumour Immunology Unit, Department of Zoology
University College London
Gower Street, London WC1E 6BT.

The T cell receptor for antigen has been identified in both mouse and man as a 90-kd disulphide-linked heterodimer comprised of one α chain ($\sim$ 50,000 mol.wt.) and one β chain ($\sim$ 40,000 mol.wt.) (1-3). Recently, cDNA clones encoding one of the chains of the T-cell antigen receptor have been isolated from mouse (4) and human (5) T-cell libraries. Sequence analysis of these cDNA clones demonstrates that they contain variable, joining and constant regions similar to those encoding immunoglobulins (5,6). Furthermore, the cDNA clones hybridise to gene sequences capable of undergoing somatic rearrangements in T-cells (4). The mouse and human cDNA probes most probably detect the β chain family of the T-cell antigen receptor since partial protein sequence analysis of a human T-cell β chain agrees with the translated nucleotide sequence of the human cDNA clone (7).

We have used the mouse cDNA clone, 86T1 (6) to determine the chromosomal location of the human T-cell receptor β chain genes. A Southern blot of an EcoRI digest of human and mouse DNA revealed different size restriction fragments hybridising with the 86T1 probe (Figure 1). Two bands (2.7 kb and 11.7 kb) were observed with EcoRI-digested mouse L cell DNA (Figure 1, track A). With DNA prepared from a mouse T-cell line (BW5147) a 2.3-kb band was observed in addition to the 2.7-kb and 11.7-kb bands, reflecting the somatic rearrangement of the gene, from which the 86T1 probe is derived, in T-cell lymphomas

35

FIGURE 1

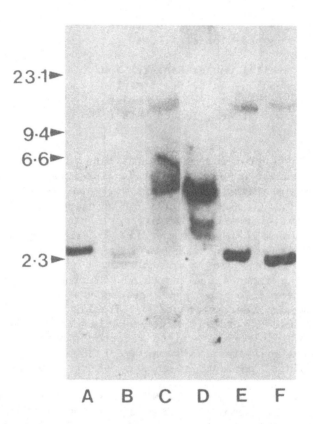

Southern hybridisation analysis of human, mouse and somatic cell hybrid DNA.

(Figure 1, track B). A Southern blot of human cell DNA, when probed at low stringency (2 x SSC) with the 86T1 insert showed two bands, at 11.7-kb and 4.7-kb (Figure 1, track C) with EcoRI. These bands correspond to a human T-cell antigen receptor β chain gene since they showed somatic rearrangement when DNA from a human T-cell lymphoma was used (Figure 1, track D).

The restriction fragment size differences between human and mouse EcoRI-cut DNA enabled us to determine which human chromosome contained the gene encoding the β chain, using the mouse probe and Southern blot analysis of DNA prepared from human-mouse somatic cell hybrids. The use of a panel of such hybrids is shown in Table I. Using an initial panel of hybrids the β chain gene was shown to segregate with chromosome 7. This was confirmed using DNA from the hybrid clone 21, which contains chromosome 7 as its only human material (Figure 1E).

These results demonstrate that a human β chain is localised on chromosome 7 in agreement with another report (8). This localisation excludes a linkage in the human system with the immunoglobulin heavy chain, kappa or lambda gene clusters (located on chromosomes 14, 2 and 22 respectively) (9-11), despite the striking similarities of the β chain genes with immunoglobulin heavy chain genes. This contrasts with a mouse T-cell antigen receptor β chain which has been localised to chromosome 6 (8), which also carries the mouse kappa chain gene cluster (12). The results presented here, however, would appear to rule out any functional importance for such a linkage since it has not been maintained in the human system. More precise chromosomal localisation was obtained using DNA from a hybrid, FIR5, containing a translocation chromosome t(x;7)(q13;q22). This hybrid retains the 7pter7q22 segment of human chromosome 7. Southern blot analysis failed to reveal a human specific band with FIR5 (Figure 1F). The human β gene is, therefore, localised to the q22-qter region of the long arm of chromosome 7. This localisation disagrees with that obtained by in situ hybridisation (8) which locates this gene to chromosome 7 bands p13-21. The reason for this discrepancy is unclear, but a precise localisation is of importance as chromosomal translocations involving the T-cell receptor gene loci may occur in T-cell tumourigenisis by analogy to those seen in Burkitt's lymphoma involving the Ig gene clusters (13).

We have confirmed the mapping results obtained with the mouse clone 86T1 using pB400, a human cDNA clone,

TABLE 1

Hybrid	Human chromosomal contribution[a]	Presence of human-specific[b] bands
CTP41.P2[c]	2, 3, 6, <u>7</u>, 14, 16, 17, 20, X	+
HORP27R C14[d]	4, <u>7</u>, 10, 11, 12, 14, 15, 21	+
3W4 C15[e]	<u>7</u>, 10, 11, 12, 14, 15, 17, 21, X	+
2W1R70[e]	<u>7</u>, 13	+
Clone 21E[f]	<u>7</u>	+
DUR4.3[g]	3, 5, 10, 11, 12, 13, 14, 15, 17, 18, 20, 21, 22. X	−
DT1.2[h]	3, 8, 10, 11, 13, 15, 17, 18, 20, 21, 22, X	−
SIR74ii[i]	1, 2, 3, 12, 14, 18, 21. 22, X	−
FIR5[j]	7pter-1q22, 14, 18, Xqter-Xq13	−
Controls		
IR[e]	Mouse L cell	−
BW5147[k]	Mouse thymoma	−
PCC4[l]	Mouse embryonal carcinoma	−
Maja[m]	Human B-lymphoblastoid line	+
JY[m]	Human B-lymphoblastoid line	+
MOLT 4[n]	Human T-cell line	+
HSB2[o]	Human T-cell line	+

Segregation of a human β-chain gene in somatic cell hybrids

isolated from a library constructed in the vector λ GT10 from the human T-cell Jurkat. The sequence of pB400 and a further overlapping cDNA clone p3L5, identical to pB400 in the region of overlap, is shown in Figure 2. Comparison of the predicted amino acid sequence with that of the β-chain clone isolated from MOLT 3 (5) shows that this transcript encodes a joining (J) region and a β-chain constant region. In addition 15 bases 5' to the joining region are present. Analysis of genomic clones hybridising with a constant region probe has localised the mouse β-chain genes into two clusters of joining regions and two constant regions (14). There are multiple base changes and several amino acid changes between the two constant region genes (14,15). The sequence shown here clearly corresponds to the previously published β sequence from Molt 3, now ascribed to $C\beta_1$ (15). However comparison of these constant region sequences reveals two silent base changes, indicated by arrows in Figure 2. This demonstrates that there is variation in $C\beta_1$ transcripts, analysis of further $C\beta_1$ sequences will determine whether this is the result of somatic mutation or allelic polymorphism.

In contrast to the near identity of the constant region, the 45 nucleotides of the J region exhibit multiple changes when compared to the corresponding sequence from MOLT 3 and the previously described Jurkat β-chain cDNA clone (5,16). The 3' end of the J region presented here is highly homologous to the other human joining regions (16) and the mouse joining regions (14) previously reported, with the exception of the Trp in place of an almost invariant Arg at amino acid 11. There are further conserved features, including the sequence Phe-Gly-X-Gly at amino acids 6-9. At the 5' end of the joining region a stop codon has been introduced at the exact point of predicted D-J joining which therefore makes this transcript unable to code for a protein.

Recognition sequences for V-D and D-J recombination follow rules first established for immunoglobulin (17). The sequences in the T-cell receptor β-chain locus include a highly conserved heptamer with the bases TGTG situated immediately 5' to every J region in both human (16) and mouse (14). Inspection of the sequence shown in Figure 2 reveals that no such sequence exists immediately 5' to the boundary of the J region. We conclude therefore that this transcript results from a non-functional (generating a stop codon) D-J joining.

FIGURE 2

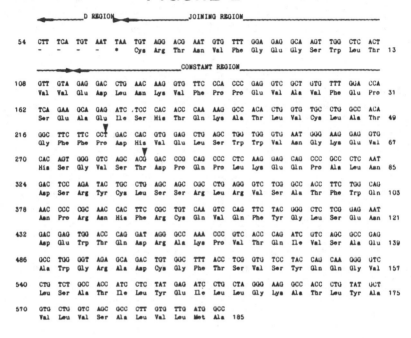

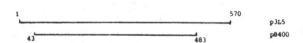

DNA sequence of Jurkat cDNA clones p3L5 and PB400. Arrows indicate the position of nucleotide differences when the constant region sequence is compared with that previously published for MOLT 3 (5).

Northern blot analysis of various mRNA populations hybridised with pB400 is shown in Figure 3. Tracks A and C show the human T-cells Jurkat and MOLT 4 respectively. Track B contains mRNA from the B-cell BR1-8. This experiment revealed the presence of two sizes of β-chain transcript in Jurkat, in agreement with a previous report (18). The 1.3 kb transcript has been ascribed to a functional V-D-J re-arrangement, since it is present in every mature T-cell (4,5), and hybridises with a V-region specific probe (19). The 1.1 kb transcript has been observed at varying levels in other human T-cells (5, Figure 3 and data not shown). We have observed no correlation between the maturity in phenotype of human T-cells and the presence of this RNA species (manuscript in preparation). Clark et al (19) have demonstrated that such shorter transcripts, in RNA from human thymus and a human tumour line, lack a V region, and that some proportion of them include a D region. It therefore appears that the transcript which we have sequenced, which is clearly not the functional T-cell receptor mRNA from Jurkat (16) comprises at least part of the 1.1 kb RNA. Similar transcripts lacking a variable region have been isolated from a mouse thymocyte cDNA library (4, 20). Further data in support of this hypothesis comes from a primer extension experiment, using a synthetic oligonucleotide comprising bases 135-155 of the sequence of Figure 2. This demonstrated two predominant sites of initiation of transcription in Jurkat mRNA. One approximately 583 bases 5' to the primer presumably represents the functional V-D-J transcript. The other 138 bases 5' to the primer corresponds almost exactly to the 5' end of the insert in the cDNA clone p3L5.

A summary of potential human β-chain transcripts is shown in Figure 4. On the left hand side the complete V-D-J rearrangement in T-cell DNA produces a transcript encoding the functional T-cell receptor β chain. On the left unrearranged T-cell DNA, or partial D-J rearrangements could theoretically allow a variety of truncated transcripts. However as transcripts from un-rearranged joining regions have not been observed it appears that partial D-J rearrangements must in some way stimulate transcription from a promoter located 5' to the D region. Our analysis of β-chain gene restriction enzyme fragments in Jurkat has found only one change compared to the germ-line configuration. Figure 5 shows an EcoRI digest of Jurkat DNA (track B) compared to germ line DNA (track A)

FIGURE 3

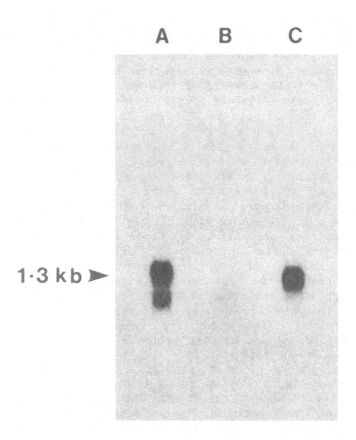

Northern hybridisation analysis of T-cell receptor β-chain mRNA.

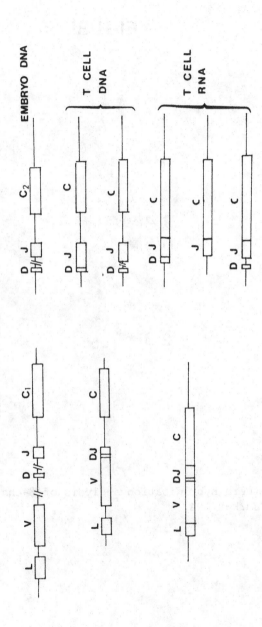

FIGURE 4

HUMAN β CHAIN TRANSCRIPTS

FIGURE 5

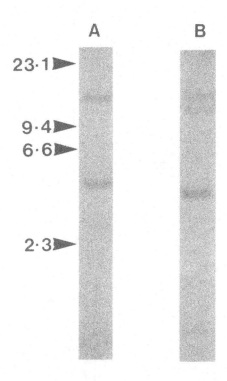

Southern hybridisation analysis of β-chain re-arrangements in Jurkat DNA.

hybridised with pB400. It is clear that in Jurkat the 11Kb EcoRI fragment is partially re-arranged, as previously described (21). As V-D joining involves a much larger distance than D-J (14) we assume that this difference that we can detect is the allele of $c\beta_1$ that has undergone V-D-J joining, and that the 11Kb EcoRI fragment therefore corresponds to the $C\beta_1$ gene. It is likely that we have not managed to detect D-J joining with the restriction enzymes that we have used. It is therefore a possibility that as well as a D-J rearrangement at the second $C\beta_1$ allele which has given rise to the transcript described here, further D-J rearrangements at either or both of the $C\beta_2$ alleles may have occured in Jurkat. Such partial re-arrangements have been detected in murine T-cells (22).

The function of such β-chain transcripts, resulting from D-J joining and lacking a variable region, as we have described here, remains unclear. It is significant that the RNA which we have isolated from Jurkat contains a stop codon immediately 5' to the J region and clearly therefore cannot encode a protein. Not all 11Kb transcripts are necessarily similarly non-coding and some could give rise to the proposed truncated polypeptides (22). However any potential regulatory role in T-cell function of the transcript that we have characterized must involve the RNA molecule itself.

REFERENCES

1.   Allison, J.P., McIntyre, R.W. and Black, D.   J. Immunol. **129**, 2293 (1982).
2.   Haskins, K., Kubo, R., White, J., Pigeon, M., Kappler, J. and Marrack, P.   J. Exp. Med. **157**, 1149 (1983).
3.   Meuer, S.C., Fitzgerald, K.A., Hussey, R.E., Hodgdon, J.C., Schlossman, S.F. and Reinherz, E.L.   J. Exp. Med. **155**, 705 (1983).
4.   Hedrick, S.M., Cohen, D.I., Nielson, E.A. and Davis, M.M.   Nature **308**, 149 (1984).
5.   Yanagi, Y., Yoshikai, Y., Leggett, K., Clark, S.P., Aleksander, I. and Mak, T.   Nature **308**, 145 (1984).
6.   Hedrick, S.M., Nielsen, E.A., Kavaler, J., Cohen, D.I. and Davis, M.M.   Nature **308**, 153 (1984).
7.   Acuto, O., Fabbi, M., Smart, J., Poole, C., Protentis, J., Roger, H., Schlossman, S. and Reinherz, E.   Proc. Natl. Acad. Sci. USA. **86**, 3851.

8. Caccia, N., Kronenberg, M., Saxe, D., Haars, R., Bruns, G.A.P., Goverman, J., Malissen, M., Willard, H., Yoshikai, Y., Simon, M., Hood, L. and Mak, T.W. Cell, **37,** 1091 (1984).

9. Croce, C.M., Shander, M., Martinis, J., Cicurel, L., D'Ancona, G.G., Dolby, T.W. and Koprowski, H. Proc. Natl. Acad. Sci. USA. **76,** 3416 (1979).

10. Malcolm, S., Barton, P., Murphy, C., Ferguson-Smith, M.A., Bentley, D.K. and Rabbits, T.H. Proc. Natl. Acad. Sci. USA **79,** 4957 (1982).

11. McBride, O.W., Heiter, P.A., Hollis, G.F., Swan, D., Otey, M.C. and Leder, P. J. Exp. Med. **157,** 705 (1982).

12. Hengartner, H., Mes, T. and Muller, E. Proc. Natl. Acad. Sci. USA **75,** 4494 (1977).

13. Perry, R.P. Cell **33,** 647 (1983).

14. Gascoigne, N.R.J., Chien, Y., Becker, D.M., Kavaler, J. and Davis, M.M. Nature **310,** 387 (1984).

15. Yoshikai, Y., Antoniou, D., Clark, S.P., Yanagi, Y., Sangster, R., Nelson, D., Terhorst, C. and Mak, T.W. Nature (in press) (1984).

16. Siu, G., Clark, S.P., Yoshikai, Y., Malissen, M., Yanagi, Y., Strauss, E., Mak, T.W. and Hood, L. Cell **37,** 393 (1984).

17. Early, P., Huang, M., Davis, M., Calame, K. and Hood, L. Cell **19,** 981 (1980).

18. Yoshikai, Y., Yanagi, Y., Suciu-Foca, N. and Mak, T.W. Nature **310,** 506 (1984).

19. Clark, S.P., Yoshikai, Y., Taylor, S., Siu, G., Hood, L. and Mak, T.W. Nature **311,** 387 (1984).

20. Kavaler, J., Davis, M.M. and Chien, Y-L. Nature **310,** 421 (1984).

21. Toyonaga, B., Yanagi, Y., Suciu-Foca, N., Minchen, M. and Mak, T.W. Nature **311,** 385 (1984).

22. Siu, G., Kronenberg, M., Strauss, E., Maars, R., Mak, T.W. and Hood, L. Nature **311,** 344 (1984).

SESSION II
HLA Antigens and Their Recognition

Chairpersons: W. Bodmer and P. Morris

Human T cells recognize HLA antigens, with or without associated extrinsic antigens. Thus this session began with a review by Dr J. Trowsdale of the genetic structure of the HLA region, especially of the HLA-D gene cluster. This has undergone a recent change in nomenclature, with HLA-DR remaining as is, but HLA-DQ replacing HLA-DC, and HLA-DP replacing HLA-SB. Some surprises were revealed, especially that some gene products in a highly polymorphic region are conserved, e.g. HLA-DR$_\alpha$ chain, but can associate with any of 3 ß chains. The importance of structural analysis lies in its underpinning of functional analyses: initial experiments of this type were described, transfecting cosmid clones containing human DP$_\alpha$ and DP$_\beta$ genes into mouse L cells which were then capable of presenting antigen to T cell clones. This supports observations on the capacity of transfected mouse L cells to activate a variety of murine T cell clones specific for allo- or soluble antigen.

Dr Biddison analysed the interaction between DP restricted cytolytic clones and their targets, using antibodies against cell surface antigens such as T4, MHC Class II and LFA-1. Considerable heterogeneity was revealed, correlating with avidity: highly avid clones being difficult to inhibit.

Dr Eckels discussed his extensive analysis of HLA-D restricted clones demonstrating that each of the 3 HLA-D regions acted as a restricting element for T helper clones, suggesting that all 3 regions may be functionally homologous, and that none is related to the I-J region of the mouse.

The remaining papers by Dr Thorsby and Dr Wallace focussed in the use of T cells to probe deeper into the functional complexity of sites on MHC molecules which are capable of being recognized in conjunction with antigen act as 'restriction elements'. For this purpose, clonal analysis permits far greater resolution than the previous use of heterogeneous T cells, but may not be definitive until single gene products can be studied, using either transfection or deletion mutants. However as a complete understanding of what T cells recognize will not be realized until the target antigen and MHC structures are defined, this work is of importance.

47

CLONED HLA-D GENES: CHARACTERISATION AND APPROACHES

TO EXPRESSION AND ANALYSIS OF FUNCTION

John Trowsdale, Penelope Austin, Susan Carson, Adrian Kelly,
Jonathan Lamb* and John Young

Imperial Cancer Research Fund, Lincoln's Inn Fields, London
and, * Tumour Immunology Unit, Department of Zoology,
University College, London.

The HLA-D region (Class II) genes determine cell
surface glycoproteins which are heterodimers of an α and β
chain, and which function in the immune response.   This
brief paper contains a summary of some of the current
studies in this laboratory on the organisation of human
Class II genes.   Details on the characterisation of six
different Class IIα chain genes are presented, including a
new gene, DZα, which does not fit into any of the three
most clearly established sets of loci: DP,DQ and DR(1).
The genes for which we have most sequence information, and
the most detailed map, are in the DP region(2).   We have
succeeded in transferring some of these cloned HLA-DP genes
into mouse L cells and can detect expression of DP antigens
on the cell surface.   The transfectants are apparently
capable of inducing a human T lymphocyte clone to
proliferate specifically in response to presentation of the
neuraminidase glycoprotein of influenza A virus along with
DPw2 ClassII determinants(3).

Six HLA-D region chain genes

      Analysis of cosmid clones containing sequences which
hybridised to an HLA-DRα chain cDNA probe indicated that
there are at least six different HLA-ClassII genes (1).
All of these genes are known to map onto human chromosome
6, by analysis of somatic cell hybrids, and are thus
presumably all in the HLA region (1) (4).   Southern blot
analysis of DNA from a variety of HLA-homozygous cell
lines, using probes made from fragments of the six α chain
genes, confirmed that the genes were non-allelic, and
revealed some associated polymorphisms with the genes.
These data are summarised on Table 1.   Most of them have
been discussed before (1).

TABLE 1 Summary of characterisation and polymorphism of
HLA-D region α chain genes*

Gene	Characteristic·band sizes in kb			Polymorphism
	EcoRI	PstI		
DRα	3.2,4.5	2.0,5.8	–	no fuctional polymorphism found
DQα	variable (15.5)	variable (12.5)	++	extensive polymorphism in coding region
DXα	5.0	variable (6.6)	+	some polymorphism e.g. with PstI and TaqI-domain not known
DPαI	11.0	1.9,2.3.	+	polymorphic in coding region from sequencing
DPα2	5.5	3.2	–	non-polymorphic from limited study so far
DZα	10.0	2.0	–	non-polymorphic from limited study so far

*These data are taken from recent work from this laboratory,
 except for the column on the right – sequences from
 several laboratories have been used to assess the
 polymorphism of the DRα and DQα chains (see Text).   We
 have also sequenced the DZα chain gene but there are no
 data yet on comparison of different alleles.

The DZα gene was discovered comparatively recently in
this laboratory(1).   It appears to be homologous to a
gene reported by another group(5).   The sequence of the DZ
gene, which we have almost completed, shows that it is as
different from the genes at the DR,DQ and DP loci as they
are from each other.   At the nucleotide level, for example,
the DZα2 domain is about 70% homologous to sequences from
these other loci.   The only exception is in the α1 domain
where there is more resemblance (67%) to some of the DQα
alleles than to those at other loci (about 60% homology at
the nucleotide level; Trowsdale, J. and Kelly, A., in
preparation).

Most of the polymorphism of Class II glycoproteins
was thought by biochemical studies to reside on the β chain
(6) (7).   The DNA cloning studies showed that the DQα
chain was extensively polymorphic, particularly in the α1
domain (1) (2) (3).   The combination of a polymorphic α
and β chain obviously provides for increased diversity of
Class II molecules in the population.   It is puzzling
however, that some of the loci are not polymorphic.   In DRα,
for example, only one allelic difference has been found from
analysis of several cDNA sequences published so far - a
conservative amino acid change(a LEU to VAL at position
217; See, for example, refs. 9 and 10).   From
recent work in our laboratory, the DPαI gene is also
polymorphic. (Young, J. & Trowsdale J. in preparation;
Table 1).   From the two alleles sequenced so far there is
about 5% variation in amino acids in the domain, compared
with about 20% for an equivalent region in some DQα alleles
but, as mentioned above, none in DRα.

To explain these differences in degree of variation
between different Class IIα chain loci one could propose
that it is of evolutionary advantage to have some polymorphic loci whilst at the same time maintaining some of
them constant.   One constant product could guarantee a
Class II molecule of a more usual shape and charge.   The
other products (DQ,DP) can then be of more experimental
design without compromising the immune system if the
particular combination of α and β chains is not satisfactory.
This is only speculation and there are other plausible
explanations.   For example,   different Class II molecules
may be expressed sequentially in ontogeny (11), and they may
each have evolved individually to fit a precise role.

Alternatively, the degree of variation permitted by each
chain may be restricted by the structure of its partner.
There is probably little, if any, interlocus combination
of α and β chains, which must be due to structural
differences, since trans-combination is permissible
between α and β chains from alleles at the same locus
(12).

Organisation of the DP genes

Our current map of the DP genetic region is shown in
Figure 1.   An interesting feature of this organisation is
the inverted configuration of the genes, also found in the
mouse I-A and I-E genes, suggesting an α-β duplication unit
(14).   The Class I genes of both species are, in contrast,
aligned in the same direction (8).   From sequencing,
DPα1 and DPβ1 matched protein sequence data for the major
expressed (previously SB) product (16), and it is not known
if the other two genes, DPα2 and DPβ2 are functional.

We have done DNA sequencing on one of the cosmids
indicated on Figure 1, LC11, which includes the
whole of the DPβ1 gene as well as the junction between this
gene and the adjacent DPα1 gene.   These studies will be
published elsewhere.   The distance between the 5' ends
of the two genes is about 2 kb. Upstream of the initiator
methionine codons of both genes, and incidentally the DZα
gene, are blocks of sequences similar to those in the
promoter region of the I-Eα, I-Eβ, and DPα genes described
by Saito et al (17).   This sequence from the DPβ1 gene
does not match the others so closely.

The DPβ1 gene contains two candidate signal sequences
although the sequence nearest to the β1 domain has not been
found on a cDNA clone so far, and it is not preceded by the
aforementioned promoter sequences (See Ref.2).

Functional expression of HLA-DP genes

One of the major objectives of the gene cloning
studies is to express protein products from these genes so
that their functions can be studied after manipulation of
either the gene sequences or the cells in which they are
contained.   We have started these studies by introducing
the cosmid clones into a mouse fibroblast cell line.

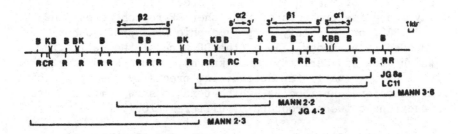

Figure 1. Restriction map of the DP (formerly SB) region.
Overlapping cosmids covering almost 90kb of DNA were isolated
from three different libraries.   Boxes indicate the approximate
extents of each gene.   The orientations of the genes were
determined using 3' and 5' end probes (from cDNA clones for α
genes and from genomic and M13 clones for β genes).   The libraries
used were: JG (placental library) and LC (lung carcinoma library)
from Frank Grosveld, MRC, Mill Hill, London (4), and MANN, made
from homozygous lymphoblastoid cell line (A29, B12, CW4, DR7, SB2)
SC, this laboratory.   Restriction enzymes were as follows:
                                    B, Bam HI; K, KpnI; R, EcoRI,
C, ClaI.

Cosmid JG8a, containing the DPα1 and DPβ1 genes, was
introduced into mouse L cells by co-precipitation with
calcium phosphate, followed by selection with thymidine
kinase (Figure 1).   Northern blot analysis of mRNA from
the TK+ transfectants showed that transcription was
occurring from all three genes.   A monoclonal antibody,
DA6.231 (anti-DR,DQ and DP) was used to select for transfectants with comparatively high levels of cell surface DP
antigen expression. (see Refs.18-21 for a summary of the
antibodies used).
     The ELISA binding assays on one clone of transfected
cells are shown in Figure 2.   The patterns of binding with
the antibodies shown are consistent with the locus assign-
ments previously determined.   Indeed, positive binding of
antibody B7/21 supports the view that this antibody detects

DP-region molecules, previously termed FA(18).   The lack
of binding of MHM4 questions its specificity for DP.   It
may recognise products of the other DP region genes DPα2
and DPβ2, or, possibly, a polymorphic DPβ1 product not
encoded by the cosmid JG8a (the DP type of the cells from
which JG8a was derived is not known).   This kind of study
will be invaluable for determining precisely the specificity
of monoclonal antibodies, which tend to show complex cross-
reactions between products of different loci.

Confirmation of the presence of the DP antigen in
iodine-labelled cell transfected mouse cell lysates came
from immunoprecipitation using the antibodies SG171 and
B7/21 and analysis by 2D NEPHGE/SDS-PAGE electrophoresis.

The main purpose of the study was to see if the Class
II antigen on the JG8a transfectants could function in
vitro.   This was assessed using a human T cell clone,
TLC 71, which has been shown to proliferate in response to
DPw2 Class II determinants and the neuraminidase glycoprotein of influenza A virus. (for details of T cell clones
used, see refs. 22-25).   In the presence of intact
influenza virus, or neuraminidase, the L cell transfectant
was able to induce clone TLC71 to proliferate, as shown on
Figure 3.   Further experiments showed that this T cell
activation by the DP transfectants is both HLA dependent
and antigen specific (Figure 3) and may be inhibited by
Class II HLA antibodies (data not shown).

The capacity of the DP-expressing mouse fibroblasts to
activate human T cells in the presence of the appropriate
antigen indicates that antigen presentation is a property
that is not necessarily restricted to the macrophage/
monocyte or B cell lineages, and provides a simplified
system in which the role of secondary signals such as Il-1
can be investigated.   These experiments are the beginning
of a study of the function of the HLA antigens, which should
now progress rapidly from studies of the sequence and organisation of the genes to the structure and function of the
proteins.   These studies will complement studies of the T
cell receptor molecule when it is possible to study the
interaction of both expressed receptor and Class II molecule
in in vitro systems.

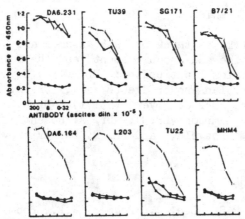

Figure 2. ELISA assay for binding of HLA Class II monoclonal
antibodies to transfectants. A standard binding assay was
performed using cells fixed with glutaraldehyde and assayed
using mouse monoclonal antibodies as shown, plus goat anti-mouse
Ig and peroxidase-antiperoxidase immune complexes, followed by
substrate as described (3). o———o control EBV transformed B cell
line; ●———● control mouse L cell line; ▲———▲ L cell clone
transfected with cosmid JG8a.

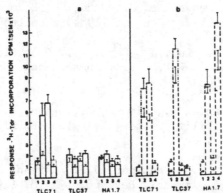

Figure 3.
        Antigen presentation assay. The T cell clones and the
functional assays have been decribed in detail elsewhere.(4,22–25).
Briefly, TLC71 is DPw2 restricted, neuraminidase specific. Clone
HA1.7 is DQ restricted and specific for peptide 20; and, TLC37
is DR restricted and specific for matrix protein. To determine
antigen-specific proliferation cloned T cells and antigen were
cultured together in the absence of antigen (column 1) or with
intact virus (column 2), neuraminidase (column 3) or peptide 20
(column 4). The following were used as presenting cells: Panel a:
DP L cell transfectant (———); DQ L cell transfectant (non-
expressing due to truncated gene, ...); Panel b: autologous PBLs
(—.—.—.); EBV transformed autologous B cells (— — —).
Proliferation was measured by 3H TdR incorporation.

ACKNOWLEDGEMENTS

We would like to thank Dr. W.F. Bodmer and Dr. M. Feldman for advice and encouragement, and the following people for monoclonal antibodies: Dr. V.Van Heyningen (DA 6.164); Dr. Ian Trowbridge (B7/21); Dr. A. Zeigler (TU39 and TU22); Dr. S. Goyert (SG171); Dr.A. McMichael (MHM4); Dr. L. Lampson (L203); Dr. A. Rosenthal, Dr. R. Webster, Dr. F. Grosveld, and Dr. R. Lerner provided other essential regants.

REFERENCES

1.   Spielman, R.S., Lee, J., Bodmer, W.F., Bodmer, J.G. & Trowsdale, J.   Proc. natn. Acad. Sci. U.S.A. 81, 3461-3465 (1984).

2.   Trowsdale, J., Kelly, A., Lee, J., Carson, S., Austin, P. & Travers, P.   Cell 38, 241-249 (1984).

3.   Austin, P., Trowsdale, J., Rudd, C., Bodmer, W.F., Feldmann, M & Lamb, J.   Nature (1984) submitted.

4.   Trowsdale, J., Lee, J., Carey, J., Grosveld, F., Bodmer, J. & Bodmer, W.F.   Proc. natn. Acad. Sci. U.S.A. 80, 1972-1976 (1983).

5.   Inoko, H., Ando, A., Kimura, M., Ogata, S. & Tsuji, K. In: Histocompatibility Testing 1984 (ed. E. Albert) Springer Verlag (in Press).

6.   Shackelford, D.A., Kaufman, J.F., Korman, A.J. & Strominger, J.L.   Immunol. Rev. 66, 133-187 (1982).

7.   De. Kretser, T.A., Crumpton, M.J., Bodmer, J.G. & Bodmer, W.F.   Eur. J. Immunol. 12, 600-606 (1982).

8.   Auffray, C., Lillie, J.W., Arnot, D., Grosberger, D., Kappes, D., Strominger, J.L.   Nature 308, 327-333 (1984).

9.   Lee, J.S., Trowsdale, J., & Bodmer, W.F.   Proc. natn. Acad. Sci U.S.A. 79, 545-549 (1982).

10. Larhammar, D., Gustafsson, K., Claesson, L., Bill, P., Wiman, K., Schenning, L., Sundelin, J., Widmark, E.,

Peterson, P.A. & Rask, L.   Cell, 30, 153-161 (1982).

11. Guy, K. & Van Heyningen, N., Immunol. Today 4, 186-189 (1983).

12. Travers, P., Blundell, T.L., Sternberg, M.J.E. & Bodmer, W.F.   Nature 235, 235-238 (1984).

13. Charron, D.J., Lotteau, V. & Turmel, P.   In Histocompatibility Testing 1984 (ed. E. Albert) Springer Verlag (in Press).

14. Steinmetz, M. & Hood, L.   Science 222, 727-733 (1983).

15. Malissen, M., Damotte, M., Bimbaum, D., Trucy, J. & Jordan, B.R.   Gene 20, 485-489 (1982).

16. Hurley, C.K., Shaw, S., Nadler, L., Schlossman, S. & Capra, J.D.   J.Exp. Med. 156,1557-1562 (1982).

17. Saito, H., Maki, R.A., Clayton, L.K. & Tonegawa, S. Proc. natn. Acad. Sci U.S.A. 80, 5520-5524.

18. Watson, A.J. DeMars, R., Trowbridge, I.S. & Bach, F.C. Nature 304, 358-361 (1983).

19. Shaw, S., Ziegler, A. & DeMars, R.   Human Immunology (submitted).

20. Bodmer, J.G. & Bodmer W.F.   Brit. Med. Bull, in press.

21. Crumpton, M.J., Bodmer, J.G. Bodmer, W.F., Heyes, J.M. Lindsay, J. & Rudd, C.E.   In: Histocompatibility Testing 1984. (ed. E. Albert, W. Mayr) Springer Verlag, in press.

22. Eckels, D.D., Lake, P., Lamb, J.R. et al. Nature 301, 716-718 (1983).

23. Lamb, J.R., Eckels, D.D., Phelan, M. & Woody, J.N. J. Immunol. 128,1428-1432 (1982).

24. Lamb, J.R. & Feldmann, M.   Nature 308,72-74 (1984).

25. Lamb, J.R., Eckels, D.D., Lake, P., Woody, J.N. & Green, N.   Nature 300, 66-69 (1982).

SB-Specific CTL Clones Exhibit Functional Heterogeneity in their Susceptibility to Blocking by Anti-T3
and Anti-T4 Antibodies.

William E. Biddison and Stephen Shaw

From: The Neuroimmunology Branch, National Institute
of Neurological, Communicative Disorders and Stroke,
and the Immunology Branch, National Cancer Institute,
National Institutes of Health, Bethesda, MD   20205

INTRODUCTION

Human T cells which recognize class II major
histocompatibility complex (MHC) antigens are almost
exclusively contained within a subpopulation of T
cells that bear the T4 (Leu 3) cell surface marker
[1-3]. Antibodies that bind the T4 molecule have been
shown to block the proliferative and cytotoxic
responses of T4[+] cells to class II MHC antigens
[2,4,5]. Studies that have partitioned the cytolytic
process into binding and post-binding phases have
demonstrated that anti-T4 antibodies block cytolysis
by interfering with formation of functional conjugates
[6,7]. These and other findings have led to the
hypothesis that the function of the T4 molecule is to
bind to a non-polymorphic epitope on class II
molecules and to thereby act as an ancillary structure that can facilitate T cell-target cell interactions [2,6,8].

The T3 molecular complex has been found on all mature
functional peripheral T cells [9]. The T3 complex
consists of two 20 KD chains and one 16 KD chain that
are noncovalently associated with the α and β chains
of the antigen-specific receptor [9,10]. Antibodies
specific for the T3 complex can either inhibit or
induce T cell functions, depending on their concentration and whether they are present in solution

or immobilized on beads [11-13]. Anti-T3 antibodies
in conjunction with phorbol esters can induce an
influx of calcium into T cells [14]. Taken together
these observations suggest that the function of the T3
molecular complex is to act as a signal transducer for
the antigen-specific receptor.

Recent studies have demonstrated that there are
differences between clones in their susceptibility to
inhibition by anti-T3 and anti-T4 antibodies, and have
raised the possibility that there are differences
between clones in their requirements for these
molecules [6,15]. We have recently shown that the
overall avidity of individual T cell clones for target
cells, as assessed in a conjugate dissociation assay,
correlates with their susceptibility to blocking by
anti-T3 and anti-T4 antibodies: the highest avidity
clones are the least susceptible to blocking, while
the opposite is true for the lowest avidity clones
[6]. These results imply that there may not
necessarily be fundamental differences between clones
in their requirements for the functions of the T3 and
T4 molecules, but that there are avidity-dependent
factors that determine the ability to block T cell
functions with antibodies to these molecules. We have
used two additional approaches that involve
antibody-mediated inhibition of T cell-target
interaction and its susceptability to inhibition by
anti-T3 and anti-T4 antibodies. Those studies are
detailed elsewhere [16] and summarized in this report.

MATERIALS AND METHODS

Immunochemical reagents. The monoclonal antibodies
used in the present experiments have been described
previously [6]. The OKT series of antibodies was
kindly provided by Dr. G. Goldstein (Ortho
Pharmaceuticals, Raritan, NJ). The anti-LFA-1
antibody TS1/22 [17] was kindly supplied by Dr. T.
Springer (Dana Farber Cancer Institute, Boston, MA)
and the broadly reactive anti-Ia antibody SG171 [18]
was kindly provided by Dr. J. Silver (Hospital for
Joint Diseases, NY).
SB-specific cytotoxic T lymphocyte (CTL) clones. The
generation and maintenance of the SB-specific CTL
clones have been described in detail elsewhere [6].

Cytolytic activity was measured 4-6 days following
specific antigen stimulation.

Cytotoxic assays. A standard 51Cr release assay was
performed using Epstein-Barr virus transformed
lymphoblastoid B cell lines as target cells [6]. In
antibody blocking experiments effector cells were
preincubated with antibodies at 37°C for 15-20 min
before addition of target cells; in the experiments
with limiting doses of anti-Ia antibodies, the target
cells were preincubated with anti-effector antibodies.

Conjugate dissociation assay. This assay was
performed as adapted by us [6] from the procedure
originally described by Balk and Mescher [19]. The
procedure essentially involves formation of
effector-target conjugates by centrifugation for 5 min
in media with 5mM EGTA, followed by gentle
resuspension with varying numbers of unlabelled
competitor cells. The cells are maintained in
suspension at 23°C for 3 hrs in media with EGTA.
The cell suspension is then transferred to media
containing Ca++ without EGTA (to permit lysis of bound
targets) and a viscous solution of dextran (to
prohibit formation of new conjugates), incubated for 4
hrs at 37°C, and the amount of 51Cr released into
the medium is measured.

RESULTS

Heterogeneity of SB2-specific CTL clones. A panel of
nine T3+, T4+, T8- SB2-specific CTL clones has
been generated and characterized as previously
described [6]. Figure 1 summarizes the results of
antibody blocking studies using the OKT3 and OKT4A
monoclonal antibodies to inhibit cytotoxic effector
function. There is a wide disparity in the
susceptibility of the different clones to inhibition
by both OKT3 and OKT4A, and there is a good
correlation between susceptibility to blocking by OKT3
and OKT4A. Some clones, such as 8.4 and 8.9, are
almost totally resistant to blocking by OKT3 and OKT4A
at an antibody concentration which completely inhibits
other clones (e.g. 8.6 and 8.8).

Correlation of susceptibility to blocking with clonal
avidity. To test the hypothesis that variations in
susceptibility to antibody blocking would correlate

with differences in clonal avidity for target cells,
the same panel of SB2-specific CTL clones was assayed
for relative avidity by a conjugate dissociation
assay. This assay quantitates the number of
unlabelled target cells that are required to induce
dissociation of preformed conjugates between CTL
clones and 51Cr-labelled target cells. High avidity
clones, as opposed to low avidity clones, will require
more unlabelled targets to induce conjugate
dissociation (as measured by a loss of 51Cr release
from labelled target cells initially bound during
conjugate formation). Figure 2 presents the results
of comparing the amount of OKT4A antibody required to
inhibit 50% of CTL activity with the number of
unlabelled target cells required to induce 50%
conjugate dissociation. The results indicate that
there is a wide variation between clones in the number
of unlabelled target cells required to induce
conjugate dissociation. There is a good correlation
between clonal susceptibility to blocking with OKT4A
and differences in the amount of target cells required
to induce conjugate dissociation: those clones that
are least susceptible to antibody blocking require the
most unlabelled target cells to induce conjugate
dissociation. This type of comparison was also made
with susceptibility to blocking by OKT3, and similar
results were obtained [16]. A good correlation was
seen between susceptibility to blocking by OKT3 and
induction of conjugate dissociation. These results
indicated that high avidity clones were least
susceptible to blocking by both OKT3 and OKT4A, and
low avidity clones were the most susceptible to
blocking by both antibodies.

An alternate approach for the assessment of whether
the failure to block certain clones with anti-T3 and
anti-T4 antibodies was due to the high avidity with
which those clones interacted with antigen is to test
a single clone on two different targets that are
recognized with different avidities. Such an approach
was possible with clone 8.4, which exhibited a low
level cross-reaction on three SB2-negative cells [16].
A comparison of the susceptibility to blocking of
clone 8.4 was examined on either an SB2-positive
target (M16B) or one of the three SB2-negative targets
(K7B) (Figure 3). The cytolytic activity of 8.4 on

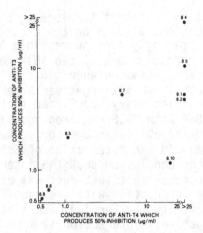

Figure 1. Correlation of susceptibility to blocking of CTL effector function by OKT3 and OKT4A. Each clone (8.1,8.2, etc.) was assayed on the SB2+ target M16B.

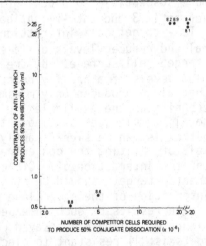

Figure 2. Correlation of susceptibility to blocking of SB-specific CTL clones by OKT4A and the number of unlabel-led competitor cells required to produce 50% conjugate dissociation. Conjugate dissociation assays were performed as described in reference 6.

M16B was completely resistant to blocking by OKT3 or
OKT4A. The same clone assayed on the cross-reactive
target K7B was strikingly more susceptible to blocking
by OKT4A, and moderately more susceptible to OKT3.
Similar results were obtained when clone 8.4 was
assayed on the other two SB2-negative targets [16].
Conjugate dissociation assays confirmed that the
interaction of 8.4 with M16B required approximately
5-fold more cold targets to induce conjugate
dissociation than did the interaction of 8.4 with K7B
[16], confirming the conclusion that the interaction
of 8.4 with the cross-reactive target was of lower
avidity than the interaction with the specific
target. These results further indicate that a lower
avidity CTL-target cell interaction is more
susceptible to blocking by anti-T3 and anti-T4
antibodies than is a higher avidity interaction.

One additional approach to test whether lower avidity
interactions are more susceptible to blocking is to
assess the amount of anti-T3 and anti-T4 antibodies
required to block CTL - target cell interactions under
conditions of normal and reduced levels of Ia antigen
expression on the target cell surface. By treating
target cells with low levels of a broadly reactive
anti-Ia antibody that alone produces only minimal
blocking of CTL recognition, the available
concentration of total Ia molecules available to T
cells on such target cells can be significantly
reduced. As a result of limiting the concentration of
target cell antigen, the interaction of a CTL clone
with antibody-pretreated targets should be of lower
avidity than the interaction of the same clone with
untreated targets. The results of such an experiment
are presented in Figure 4. Clone 8.4 assayed on
untreated M16B targets is: 1) resistant to blocking by
OKT3 and OKT4A antibodies; 2) very slightly blocked by
the chosen concentration of anti-Ia antibody (SG171);
and 3) partially blocked by an anti-LFA-1 antibody.
The same clone assayed on M16B targets that were
pretreated with anti-Ia are markedly more susceptible
to blocking by OKT3 and OKT4A. In contrast, blocking
with anti-LFA-1 is not stronger on anti-Ia treated
targets as compared with untreated targets, and
provides a useful control that demonstrates that
higher avidity interactions are not less susceptible

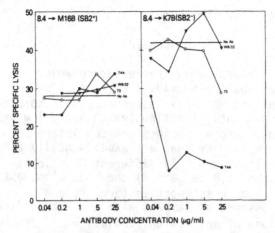

Figure 3. Comparison of susceptibility to antibody blocking of clone 8.4 assayed on SB2+ target (M16B) versus a
cross-reactive SB2- target (K7B). 8.4 was assayed on M16B
at a 1:1 E:T, and on K7B at a 40:1 E:T.

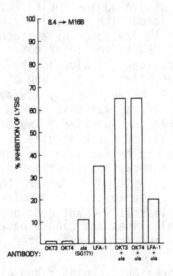

Figure 4. Susceptibility of clone 8.4 to blocking in the
presence and absence of limiting concentrations of anti-Ia
antibody. Antibody concentrations used for blocking: OKT3
and OKT4A, 25ug/ml; SG171, 1:250 ascites; LFA-1, 40ug/ml.

to blocking by any antibody.

DISCUSSION

The present report summarizes evidence which demonstrates that high avidity CTL-target cell interactions are markedly less susceptible to blocking by anti-T3 and anti-T4 antibodies than are low avidity interactions. These findings are consistant for variations in avidity that are experimentally achieved in three distinct ways: 1) different CTL clones assayed on the same target; 2) the same clone assayed on specific and cross-reactive targets; and 3) the same clone assayed on targets with and without low concentrations of anti-Ia antibodies.

The conclusion that susceptibility to blocking by anti-T4 antibodies correlates with clonal avidity is similar to conclusions drawn from studies with the murine homologue, L3T4. Marrack et al [20] reported that the ability of anti-L3T4 to inhibit secretion of IL-2 by a panel of ovalbumin-specific L3T4[+] T cell hybridomas correlated with the ability of these T cells to respond to low doses of antigen. Those T cells that responded to the lower doses of antigen were the most resistant to blocking by anti-L3T4. In addition, susceptibility to blocking of IL-2 secretion by anti-L3T4 could be enhanced by low amounts of anti-Ia antibody [20], as was observed in the present study for CTL effector function. The overall conclusion from all of these studies is that the T4 molecule is involved in facilitating low avidity CTL-target cell interactions, perhaps by binding to a non-polymorphic Ia epitope. However, the T4 molecule does not appear to be absolutely required for T cell recognition of class II MHC antigens because class II-specific T cell lines and clones have been isolated that do not bear the T4 molecule [21-23].

Results of our previous studies [6] and others [15] have also demonstrated differences in clonal susceptibility to inhibition by anti-T3 antibodies. The present results demonstrate that the inability to inhibit a particular CTL-target interaction with anti-T3 antibodies does not necessarily mean that the T3 molecule is not involved in the function of that T cell clone, because the same clone assayed on a cross-reactive target or under limiting antigen concentration can be readily inhibited by anti-T3. The function of the T3 molecular complex is probably a requirement for the triggering of all T cell clones because no functional antigen-specific T cell clone has yet been reported that does not express T3.

The observation of avidity-dependence of anti-T3 blocking may appear to be inconsistent with previous results that indicated that anti-T3 antibodies interfere with a post-binding phase of the lytic process and do not inhibit conjugate formation [24,25]. If the T3 molecular complex performs a triggering function by acting as a signal transducer subsequent to binding of antigen by the antigen-specific receptor, clones with high affinity receptors would be expected to generate more receptor-ligand interactions when conjugating with a particular target. Thus, anti-T3 blocking of high affinity clones would be more difficult to achieve because the antibody would have to interfere with a stronger signal than would be the case with low affinity clones. Alternatively, if triggering results from clustering of receptors (as has been postulated for IgE-induced mast cell degranulation [26]), triggering will then be highly dependent on the local concentration of receptor-ligand bonds. CTL-target cell interactions with high affinity clones will produce higher local concentrations of receptor-antigen bonds than will be achieved with low affinity clones. Consequently, high affinity clones will be more resistant to blocking by anti-T3 antibodies.

References

1. Meuer, S.C., Schlossman, S.F., & Reinherz, E.L. Proc. Natl. Acad. Sci. USA   79, 4395-4399 (1982).
2. Biddison, W.E., Rao, P.E., Talle, M.A., Goldstein, G., & Shaw, S. J. Exp. Med. 156, 1065-1076 (1982).
3. Krensky, A.M., Reiss, C.S., Mier, J.W., Strominger, J.L., Burakoff, S.J. Proc. Natl. Acad. Sci. USA 79, 2365-2369.
4. Engelman, E.G., Benike, C.J., Glickman, E., & Evans, R.L. J. Exp. Med. 153, 193-198 (1981).

5. Meuer, S.C., Hussey, R.E., Hodgdon, J.C., Hercend, T., Schlossman, S.F., & Reinherz, E.L. Science 218, 471-473 (1982).

6. Biddison, W.E., Rao, P.E., Talle, M.A., Goldstein, G., & Shaw, S. J. Exp. Med. 159, 783-797 (1984).

7. Biddison, W.E., & Shaw, S. in Regulation of the Immune System (eds Sercarz, E., Cantor, H., & Chess, L.) in press (Alan R. Liss, New York, 1984).

8. Reinherz, E.L., Meuer, S.C., & Schlossman, S.F. Immunology Today 4: 5-8 (1983).

9. Meuer, S.C., Acuto, O., Hussey, R.E., Hodgdon, J.C., Fitzgerald, K.A., Schlossman, S.F., & Reinherz, E.L. Nature 303, 808-810 (1983).

10. Borst, J., Alexander, S., Elder, J., & Terhorst, C. J. Biol. Chem. 258, 5135-5141 (1983).

11. van Wauwe, J.P.V., De May, J.R., Goossens, J.G., J. Immun. 124, 2708-2713 (1980).

12. Chang, T.S., Kung, P.C., Gingras, S.P., & Goldstein, G. Proc. Natl. Acad. Sci. USA. 78, 1805-1808 (1981).

13. Meuer, S.C., Hodgdon, J.C., Hussey, R.E., Protentis, J.P., Schlossman, S.F., & Reinherz, E.L. J. Exp. Med. 158, 988-993 (1983).

14. Weiss, A., Imboden, J., Shoback, D., & Stobo, J. Proc. Natl. Acad. Sci. USA 81: 4169-4173 (1984).

15. Moretta, A., Pantaleo, G., Mingari, M.C., Moretta, L., & Cerottini, J.-C. J. Exp. Med. 159, 921-934 (1984).

16. Shaw, S., Goldstein, G., Springer, T.A., & Biddison, W.E. submitted for publication.

17. Ware, C.F., Sanchez-Madrid, F., Krensky, A.M., Burakoff, S.J., Strominger, J.L., & Springer, T.A. J. Immunol. 131, 1182-1188 (1983).

18. Goyert, S.M., and Silver, J. Nature 294, 266-268 (1981).

19. Balk, S.P., & Mescher, M.F. J. Immunol. 127, 51-57 (1981).

20. Marrack, P., Endres, R., Shimon Kevitz, R., Zlotnik, A., Dialynas, D., Fitch, F., & Kappler, J. J. Exp. Med. 158, 1077-1091 (1983).

21. Ball, E.J., & Stasny, P. Immunogenetics 16, 157-169 (1982).

22. Flomenberg, N., Duffy, E., Naito, K., & Dupont, B. Immunogenetics 17, 317-324 (1983).

23. Krensky, A.M., Clayberger, C., Greenstein, J.L., Crimmins, M., & Burakoff, S.J. J. Immunol. 131, 2777-2780 (1983).
24. Landegren, U., Ranstedt, V., Axberg, I., Ullberg, M., Jondal, M., & Wigzell, H. J. Exp. Med. 155, 1579-1584 (1982).
25. Tsoukas, C.D., Carson, D.A., Fong, S., & Vaughan, J.H. J. Immunol. 129, 1421-1425 (1982).
26. Kanner, B.I., & Metzger, H. Proc. Natl. Acad. Sci. USA. 80, 5744-5748 (1983).

RECOGNITION OF HLA CLASS II MOLECULES BY FUNCTIONAL HUMAN T-LYMPHOCYTE CLONES (TLC's)

David D. Eckels

Immunogenetics Research Section, The Blood Center of Southeastern Wisconsin, 1701 West Wisconsin Avenue, Milwaulkee, WI 53233.

It is generally accepted that class II molecules are in fact Ir gene products. From a multitude of studies which began over a decade ago it can now be argued that class II molecules are somehow involved in controlling or influencing the specificity of T-cell recognition. Remaining unclear, however, is the relationship between T-cell specificity and function. That is, the question of whether particular class II gene products determine discrete immunological functions such as help or suppression has yet to be answered. Because experimental work in the mouse has so profoundly influenced immunological concepts applied to man, I would like to present first a brief overview of our current understanding of murine and human Ir gene function before framing an alternative hypothesis regarding the functional control of the human immune system by class II molecules.

Animal Models of Class II Function

Immune response (Ir) genes were first mapped to the mouse MHC by McDevitt and Chinitz[1] and later, using congenic mouse strains, to the H2-I subregion[2]. Dorf and Benacerraf[3] demonstrated that immune responses to GLØ required complementation of two I-region genes which they called alpha and beta. Possession of either component alone did not confer responsiveness; only in the presence of both alpha and beta genes could a response be generated. At the same time Cullen and co-workers[4] were able to isolate immune response associated (Ia) antigens from mur-

ine B-cells and found them to be composed of a 33K dalton
alpha chain and a 28K dalton beta chain.   In a series of
elegant studies, Rosenthal and Shevach[5] examined the ability of non-responder macrophages to present antigen to responder primed T-cells from guinea pigs. Their results suggested that it was the macrophage Ia antigen that somehow
determined whether a response was obtained[6].   Furthermore,
these studies supported the view that the antigen presenting cell (APC) and T-cell must share Ia antigens in order
to interact. Thus the concept of genetic restriction was
developed which in its simplest form requires that the T-
cell recognizes two components: antigen and "self" Ia.
Further   studies extended the notion of genetic restriction
by demonstrating that responder animals with differing Ia
antigens recognized different antigenic determinants of an
immunogen[7], a phenomenon labeled <u>determinant   selection</u>[8,9].
According to the determinant selection hypothesis, non-
responder animals would be unable to present certain antigenic determinants in association with their Ia molecules
and would thus be incapable of mounting an immune
response.

     Problems with determinant selection were identified in
the experiments of several groups[10-12]. If responder F_1
(responder x nonresponder) bone marrow cells were allowed
to differentiate in the presence of non-responder thymuses,
non-responsiveness resulted. On the other hand, if non-
responder bone marrow cells differentiated in the presence
of a responder thymus, responsive T-cells were obtained.
These and other data may have led Schwartz[13] as well as
von Boehmer, Haas and Jerne[10] to propose an alternative
theory for the mechanism of Ir gene activity. This <u>clonal
deletion theory</u> holds that during ontogeny auto-reactive T-
cells are eliminated or suppressed and implies that Ir gene
defects (a lack of response) would correspond to the absence of self cross-reactivity. A number of recent experiments support this hypothesis: Ishii and colleagues[14] reported that <u>responder</u> T-cells depleted of their alloreactivity are perfectly capable of responding to antigen presented by <u>non-responder</u> APC's; Thomas and Hoffman[15] demonstrated that <u>non-responder</u> strain 2 guinea pig APC's could
present immunogenic forms of angiotensin synthetic peptides
to F_1 <u>responder</u> primed T-cells; Clark and Shevach[16], in the
original strains of guinea pig used to advance the determinant selection theory, observed that T-cell colonies
could be generated from the <u>responder</u> strain 2 which could
recognize the GL copolymer in association with strain 13

(<u>non-responder</u>) Ia antigens; similar results have been reported using mouse T-cell clones[17]; recent results by Ishii, Klein and Nagy[18] would support the argument that not only can <u>non-responder</u> APC's present antigen to appropriately primed T-cells but they also can present the same antigenic determinants as those presented in the context of <u>responder</u> Ia antigens.

Such evidence would seem to sound the death knell for the determinant selection hypothesis. However, recent elegant studies by investigators from several different laboratories suggest that determinant selection may yet play a role in T-cell recognition.

Thomas and co-workers[19] were able to demonstrate that single amino acid differences in peptides of human fibrinopeptide B controlled immunogenicity (induction of response) and antigenicity (T-cell recognition) in strain 2 and strain 13 guinea pigs. Furthermore, substitution of different amino acid residues at different sites influenced both phenomena separately. They reasoned that two separate residues, one for T-cell receptor contact and one for Ia antigen contact, were important for T-cell activation. These results were confirmed and extended using angiotensin peptides as well[15,20]. These investigators have proposed an alternative model of T-cell recognition suggesting that it is a <u>combination</u> of Ia antigen and T-cell receptor that forms a <u>binding site</u> for relevant antigenic determinants somewhat analogous to Ig heavy and light chain interactions.

Using monoclonal T-cell hybridomas from mice immunized with cytochrome C from different species, Heber-Katz and colleagues[21] observed that distinct patterns of T-cell reactivity could be elicited depending on the source of the APC's. Thus, T-cell <u>clones</u> from responder and non-responder strains could recognize an antigenic determinant if presented in the context of an appropriate Ia epitope. These results have been extended in amino acid substitution experiments showing that a single contact residue at two disparate sites is involved in T-receptor/antigen and Ia/antigen interactions[22] and are very similar and complementary to those of Thomas and co-workers[19,20] which suggest that the T-cell recognizes very subtle features of an Ia-antigen complex.

Evidence for direct interactions between Ia antigens and synthetic polypeptide antigens has been presented by Werdelin[23] in the guinea pig where responses to DNP-poly-L-lysine (DNP-PLL) and the random copolymer L-glutamic acid, L-lysine (GL) are controlled by the same Ir gene. Primed T-cells specific for DNP-PLL were unable to respond to DNP-PLL if the presenting cells were first treated with high doses of GL. In reciprocal experiments, GL-immune T-cells were suboptimally stimulated in the presence of GL presented by APC's preincubated with DNP-PLL. Neither DNP-PLL or GL were able to inhibit responses of T-cells primed to ovalbumin, which is controlled by a different Ir gene. Binding studies with radiolabeled polypeptides revealed slight but significant loss of binding of tritiated DNP-PLL to APC's pretreated with unlabelled GL. These results and similar observations by Rock and Benacerraf[24] would support arguments in favor of direct class II molecular interactions with antigen, but they await verification in other antigen systems.

Thus, the bulk of evidence appears to favor both the determinant selection hypothesis and the clonal deletion theory: Precursor T-cells may be selected in the thymus to exclude self-reactive clones and mature further peripherally in the presence of autologous APC's and antigen. Ir gene phenomena therefore arise from "T-cell holes" in the repertoire as well as from the inability to present certain antigenic determinants in combination with self Ia. It should be pointed out that all of the above experiments concerning genetic control of immunologic responsiveness are aimed at questions of T-cell specificity and not at questions of what the T-cell does after it recognizes a viable Ia-antigen complex. Indeed, the work of Fathman[25] and others[26,27] would suggest that a given T-cell clone can express a multiplicity of functions regardless of its specificity. This last point is especially provocative in view of the experimental evidence provided by Baxevanis, Nagy and Klein[27] that in the mouse system, suppression can be restricted by the same class II molecules that also control or restrict helper responses.

Therefore, when addressing questions surrounding the function of class II molecules in humans it is important to integrate concepts gleaned from mouse studies as well. Two major considerations seem readily apparent: First, a particular T-cell is capable of exhibiting different sorts of functional behavior. Second, different functions (e.g., help and suppression) can be controlled or restricted by the same class II molecules. These two caveats are significant in view of hopes held by many immunologists working in the human system that different class II molecules

will be found to be responsible for different immunological
functions.

Class II Function in Man

An understanding of immunoregulation in man must be
tempered by concepts transferred from animal studies.
Furthermore, the development of reagents that can be used
to dissect HLA structure and function must be given high
priority. To this end, monoclonal antibodies and T-cells
have proven powerful tools for understanding human immune
responsiveness. Using such reagents it has been possible
to uncover a number of similarities and differences in the
murine and human systems.
   Complexity. Human class II molecules are coded for by
genes located in the HLA-D region on the short arm of
chromosome 6, 1-2 centiMorgans centromeric to the class I
HLA-A,B,C loci. With a variety of serological, cellular,
biochemical and molecular genetic techniques, the D-region
genes have been divided into three basic subregions termed
HLA-DR, HLA-DQ and HLA-DP. Both DP and DQ encode two alpha
and two beta chains while the DR subregion codes for at
least one alpha and up to three beta chains[28,29].
   Our progress in understanding the potential functions
of individual class II molecules was limited by the relative dearth of typing reagents capable of recognizing
specificities unique to particular molecules. However,
with the advent of monoclonal antibodies and monoclonal,
alloreactive T-cells it is now possible to begin dissecting
the relationship between class II structure and immunological function in man. By cloning T-cells from mixed
lymphocyte cultures in which class II alloantigenic differences are primarily recognized one feature became
readily apparent: Alloreactive clones recognized an ex-
ceedingly complex array of alloantigenic specificities.
While there was general correlation or inclusion within the
serologically defined antigens, most TLC's recognized subsets or "splits" of the defined specificities[30].
   We have initiated efforts at generating a large battery
of alloreactive T-cell clones against a number of HLA haplotypes and class II subregions[30-32]. As a rule, the results from these studies confirm and extend this concept
of human class II complexity (Table 1). Virtually no clone
was found which was completely correlated with a classical-
ly defined specificity. Similar observations have been

Table 1:   Complexity of HLA-D subregion haplotypes

| | Class II Specificities Studied | | | | | | | | | |
	DR1	DR2	DR3	DR4	DR5	DR6	DR7	DR8	--	DP1
# TLCs	13	11	5	8	10	6	6	7		20
# splits	11	8	5	6	3	6	4	6		4

Adapted from Rosen-Bronson and Eckels (ms in preparation)

made in other laboratories[33-35]. In general, these results are characteristic of the DR, DQ and DP subregions.
        Restriction specificity. In attempting to define the
functions of various class II molecules we have examined
the genetic restriction requirements of influenza reactive
T-cell clones (Table 2)[36-38]. Our initial studies revealed
that T-cell clones recognized a variety of viral antigens
including hemagglutinin, neuraminidase, matrix protein and
nucleoprotein. While DR-associated restriction elements
appeared to predominate in that most clones recognized antigen when presented by DR matched antigen presenting
cells, some clones were obviously restricted by non-DR interaction products[36,37]. By pursuing these studies, we
found that in addition to HLA-DR class II molecules, the
HLA-DP subregion also encoded functional restriction elements[38]. Similar genetic restriction studies in other
laboratories have demonstrated that HLA-DQ associated class
II molecules also restrict T-cell interactions with antigen
presenting cells[39]. One surprising feature of these studies was that we found no apparent correlation between clonal antigen specificity and restriction pattern. Borrowing
concepts from the mouse system, we reasoned that the reason
for this lack of correlation might be due to the complexity
of antigenic determinants found on the antigen we were currently using. In collaboration with Dr. JR Lamb the relationship between genetic restriction and antigenic fine
specificity was studied using T-cell clones specific for
influenza hemagglutinin. With synthetic peptides representing most of the amino acid sequence of the hemaglutinin
molecule, it was possible to demonstrate that a particular
immunodominant peptide or epitope was recognized by most
T-cell clones[40]. In further genetic restriction studies,
two clones recognized the same immunodominant epitope in
association with identical class II interaction elements.

Table 2:   Specificity of TLC's restricted by different
           types of class II molecules

Antigen Specificity	HLA-DP	HLA-DQ	HLA-DR
Influenza virus*	+	+	+
HSV I	+	?	+
C. trachomatis	+	+	+
*MP	?	?	+
*NP	?	?	+
*NA	+	?	+
*HA	?	+	+
*HA (aa306-329)	?	+	+

*A/Texas/1/77; MP = matrix protein; NP = nucleoprotein;
 NA = neuraminidase; HA = hemagglutinin

This result was all the more striking because the restriction pattern of the two clones could not be correlated with
any classic D-region specificity. Two other clones, each
recognizing distinct hemagglutinin determinants, displayed
characteristically unique restriction patterns as well[41].
As in the mouse system therefore, genetic restriction patterns in man correlated with the antigenic determinant recognized by the T-cell.
      Functional promiscuity. One striking feature of all
human T-cell clones studied to date is the fact that they
exhibit multiple functions. In the alloreactive system,
many clones have been decribed that proliferate in the
absence of exogenous IL-2, produce their own TCGF and can
lyse specific allogeneic targets[42]. Investigations of
the specificities of such clones determined that they recognize subclasses of both class I and class II molecules
including antigens associated with HLA-DR, DQ and DP. Further analysis of the relationship between clonal specificity and the expression of various functions revealed
that multiple functions could be activated by the same determinant[42]. Furthermore, the specificity of the clone
was maintained regardless of the functional assay used to
detect clonal activation in extensive panel testing and
blocking assays with monoclonal antibodies specific for
class II molecules.

Table 3:   TLC functions and phenotypes

TLC	GxRx	CD	Help	Ifn	TCGF	Lysis
FL1.6	DR1	3/4	+	g	-	-
FL1.37	DR1v	3/4	-	a	+	-
FL1.71	DP2	3/4	+	g	nt	nt
FL2.8	DR1v	3/4	nt	a	nt	+
FL2.20	DR3v	3/4	+	g	nt	nt
HA1.4	DQ?	3/4	+	g	-	-
HA1.7	DQ?	3/4	+	g	-	-
HA1.9	DR?	3/4	+	0	nt	nt
HA2.43	DR?	3/4	+	nt	nt	-
HA2.61	nt	3/4	+	nt	nt	+

GxRx = genetic restriction (v, variant); CD = cell surface
phenotype; Ifn = interferon (a, alpha; g, gamma); nt = not
tested. Adapted from references 43-44,48-50.

Relative to the mouse, little has been ascertained with
regard to classical immune functions expressed by T-cell
clones in man. In the influenza system, Lamb and his colleagues[43] have described multi-functional clones similar
to the alloreactive system. Characteristics such as proliferation, release of TCGF, release of gamma and alpha
interferon, cytotoxicity, release of antigen specific
helper factor and induction of B-cells to release antigen
specific antibody have been investigated to various degrees.   Results from these studies have been summarized in
Table 3.   In attempting to correlate certain functional
characteristics with clonal genetic restriction patterns no
apparent relationship could be established. As an example,
antigen specific helper factor could be elicited from
clones restricted to interaction products associated with
HLA-DR, DQ and DP. It is intriguing to note further that
two groups have described T-cell clones that exhibit both
helper and suppressor functions under different experimental conditions[44,45]. Even in clones with closely defined
peptide specificities the helper function was not confined
to clones of a particular specificity which is somewhat in
contrast to the work of Sercarz[46].

Synthesis

In summary, the Ir genes of both mouse and man control immune responses to a single antigenic determinant, probably by influencing the way in which the T-cell recognizes antigenic structures. The class II molecules appear to be responsible for selecting or proscribing T-cell specificity at two levels, minimally. First T-cells differentiate in the presence of self MHC antigens in the thymus where autoreactive clones are suppressed or removed from the T-cell repertoire. Second, there appears to be a peripheral selection or expansion of T-cells that recognize specific antigens in the presence of self Ia presented by autologous APC's. Less clear is whether, or how, class II molecules might be involved in immunoregulatory processes such as help or suppression. The work of Sercarz and some of his co-workers[46] would suggest that antigen specificities do indeed play a role in the selection of certain functional T-cell subsets. Their observations that distinct antigenic determinants are primarily recognized by helper or suppressor T-cells is powerful evidence in favor of this view.

In contrast, most of the thinking regarding the relationship of class II molecules to immunological functions in man has been decidedly one-sided in perspective. That is, most experimental questions tend to focus on the role of class II molecules in T-cell interaction with APC and neglect the role of class II molecules in T-cell/T-cell interaction. The origin of this problem may lie in the traditional perspective that murine T-cells do not express class II molecules; controversy surrounds this issue[47]. However, activated human T-cells do express high levels of class II molecules on their surfaces. That these molecules may be centrally involved in T-cell recognition has been demonstrated in the elegant experiments of Lamb and co-workers[48-50]. They observed that by incubating a T-cell clone in the presence of high concentrations of synthetic peptide antigen in the absence of any antigen presenting cell, the clone became refractory to further stimulation when co-cultured with fresh antigen and another source of APC's. Non-specific toxicity was excluded in co-culture experiments with different peptides and by showing that tolerized clones were capable of being stimulated with exogenous TCGF. Further studies revealed that treatment of the clones under tolerizing conditions resulted in a down regulation of the CD3 marker. A most interesting feature of this work is the fact that the tolerizing process as

well as CD3 modulation could be blocked by monoclonal antibodies specific for class II molecules but not by those
specific for class I molecules. Thus, in this system,
class II molecules appear to be centrally involved in an
important T-cell regulatory event. In view of the above
results, some intriguing data is available that suggest
that subsets of class II molecules may be independently
regulated on the T-cell surface (manuscript submitted).

A new explanation of how class II molecules could control immune functions must integrate three important pieces
of information. First, the reasons that T-cells express
class II molecules must be determined. Second, observations that the I-J determinant is expressed on murine
suppressor T-cells could support views that the expression
of certain of the class II subsets may correlate with T-
cell functional characteristics. Third, from the tolerance
experiments of Lamb and his colleagues[50] and other systems such as the AMLR[51], it can be seen that recognition
of antigen "presented" by T-cells may often have unexpected
regulatory consequences. I am proposing that it is at this
level that functional control may be imposed via recognition of either antigen or idiotype associated with class II
molecules. By controlling which class II antigens are expressed at any given time the T-cell modulates the sorts of
signals that may be delivered by other regulatory T-cells.

Therefore, it appears that T-cell specificity is controlled at the level of T-cell interaction with APC while
T-cell function may be controlled by some other, perhaps
subsequent, event or factor. In this regard, a fertile
area of future investigation should concern the consequence
of class II mediated, direct interactions between T-cells.
Thus, the "context" of class II recognition by T-cells may
determine the function of an individual cell during induc-
tive and later phases of an immune response.

The helpful discussions and encouragement of Dr RJ
Hartzman along with the assistance of Ms Deanna Savarese
are greatfully acknowledged. This work was supported by
grant AI 19655 from the NIAID and ONR contract No. N000-
14-83-K-0410; the opinions expressed herein are the author's and are not to be construed as those of the Department of the Navy.

1. McDevitt HO and Chinitz A. Science 163:1207 (1969).
2. McDevitt HO et al. J Exp Med 135:1259 (1972).
3. Dorf ME and Benacerraf B. PNAS 72:3671 (1975).

4. Cullen SE et al. PNAS 71:648 (1974).
5. Rosenthal AS and Shevach EM. J Exp Med 138:1194 (1973).
6. Shevach EM and Rosenthal AS. J Exp Med 138:1213 (1973).
7. Berzofsky JA. In: Biological Regulation and Develop-
    ment, vol 2, Plenum Press, New York. RF Goldberger,
    ed., p 467, (1980).
8. Benacerraf B. J Immunol 120:1809 (1978).
9. Rosenthal AS. Immunol Rev 40:135 (1978).
10. von Boehmer H, Haas W and Jerne N. PNAS (USA) 75:2439
    (1978).
11. Zinkernagle RM et al. Nature 271:251 (1978).
12. Miller JFAP et al. Scand J Immunol 9:29 (1979).
13. Schwartz RH. Scand J Immunol 7:3 (1978).
14. Ishii N et al. J Exp Med 154:978 (1981).
15. Thomas DW and Hoffman MD. J Immunol 128:780 (1982).
16. Clark RB and Shevach EM. J Exp Med 155:635 (1982).
17. Kimoto M, Krenz TJ and Fathman CG. J Exp Med 154:883
    (1981).
18. Ishii N, Nagy Z and Klein J. J Exp Med 157:998 (1983).
19. Thomas DW et al. J Exp Med 152:620 (1980).
20. Thomas DW et al. J Exp Med 153:583 (1981).
21. Heber-Katz E et al. J Exp Med 155:1086 (1982).
22. Schwartz RH. 5th Int Congress of Immunology, Kyoto,
    Japan (1983).
23. Werdelin O. J Immunol 129:1883 (1982).
24. Rock KL and Benacerraf B. J Exp Med 157:1618 (1983).
25. Fathman CG and Frelinger JG. Ann Rev Immunol 1:633
    (1983).
26. Frelinger JG et al. J Exp Med 159:704 (1984).
27. Baxevanis CN, Nagy Z and Klein J. J Immunol 131:628
    (1983).
28. Mawas C et al. Human Immunology 8:1 (1983).
29. Hurley CK, Giles RC and Capra JD. Immunology Today
    8:219 (1983).
30. Eckels DD and Hartzman RJ. Immunogenetics 16:117
    (1982).
31. Eckels DD and Hartzman RJ. Human Immunology 3:337
    (1981).
32. Eckels DD et al. In: Ir genes, past, present, and
    future, Human Press, Clifton NJ. Pierce CW et al.,
    eds., p 535 (1983).
33. Zeevi A et al. Human Immunology 6:97 (1983).
34. Pawelec G and Wernet P. Immunogenetics 11:507 (1980).
35. Reinsmoen NL and Bach FH. Human Immunology 4:249
    (1982).
36. Eckels DD et al. Human Immunology 4:313 (1982).

37. Lamb JR et al. J Immunol 128:233 (1982).
38. Eckels DD et al. Nature 301:716 (1983).
39. Qvigstad E, Digranes S and Thorsby E. Scand J Immunol (in press).
40. Lamb JR et al. Nature 300:66 (1982).
41. Eckels DD et al. Immunogenetics 19:409 (1984).
42. Zeevi A and Duquesnoy R. J Immunogenetics (in press).
43. Lamb JR et al. Immunology 50:397 (1983).
43a Jacobson S et al. 5th Int Congress of Immunology, Kyoto, Japan (1983).
44. Lamb JR et al. J Immunol 129:1465 (1982).
45. Meuer SC et al. J Immunol 131:1167 (1983).
46. Goodman JW and Sercarz EE. Ann Rev Immunol 1:465 (1983).
47. Festenstein H. personal communication.
48. Lamb JR et al. J Exp Med 157:1434 (1983).
49. Zanders ED et al. Nature 303:625 (1983).
50. Lamb JR and Feldmann M. Nature 308:72 (1984).
51. Nikaein A et al. Immunobiology 166:190 (1984).

RESTRICTION ELEMENTS ON CLASS II HLA

MOLECULES STUDIED BY CLONED HUMAN T4 CELLS

Erik Qvigstad and Erik Thorsby

Institute of Transplantation Immunology,
The National Hospital and University of
Oslo, Rikshospitalet, Oslo, Norway

Abstract

T lymphocyte clones (TLCs) specific for Chlamydia
trachomatis were obtained by the limiting dilution technique
of in vitro activated T cells from two different donors.
Most of the TLCs obtained were only able to recognize
antigen together with restriction elements on DR molecules,
expressed in the antigen-presenting cells (APC). A few TLCs
were restricted by elements on DRw53(MT3) molecules, and
one TLC by DPw4(SB4) molecules. A close relationship was
found between the restriction epitopes and those that
activate allogeneic T cells in mixed lymphocyte culture
(MLC) tests. The results of inhibition experiments using
monoclonal antibodies (Mabs) against different HLA
molecules correlated closely with the restriction
specificities of the TLCs.

HLA Class II Restriction Elements

Chlamydia-specific T lymphocyte clones (TLCs) were
generated in vitro using the limiting dilution technique,
as previously described[1,2]. Serological HLA-A,-B,-C, and
-DR typing was performed using techniques and reagents also
previously described[3]. Some of the cell donors were HLA-D
typed with a panel of homozygous typing cells (HTCs)
expressing the specificities Dw4, Dw10, Dw13, Dw14, Dw15 or
KT2[4].

All tested clones were antigen-specific and did not respond to allogeneic antigen-presenting cells (APC) without antigen. The restriction specificities of TLCs from a donor (BS) with the HLA profile HLA-A3;B7,15;DR1,4; DRw53(MT3);DPw4(SB4) have been reported[2,5]. Using APC from different allogeneic donors, we found that of 17 TLCs from BS examined extensively for HLA restriction, ten TLCs appeared to be restricted by elements on the DR1 molecules, while four TLCs were restricted by elements on DR4. In addition, two TLCs were probably restricted by elements on the DRw53 molecules, and one TLC by elements on the DPw4 molecules. TLCs specific for virus antigens may also be restricted by elements on the DRw53 or the DP molecules[6,7]. Thus, elements controlled both by the DR β1 and DR β2 chains (data from The Ninth International Histocompatibility Testing Workshop 1984), as well as present on DP class II molecules, appear able to restrict antigen-specific T cells, of which a given clone may only "use" one.

Relationship between Restriction Elements and Alloactivating Epitopes

We have previously reported that the restriction elements on DR molecules appear more closely associated with the T cell alloactivating HLA-D determinants than with those responsible for alloantibody induction, DR[5]. This was based on studies with TLCs from a donor (GR) with the HLA profile HLA-A19;B15,40;DR4,4;DRw53;DPw2, which were restimulated with antigen plus DR4-positive APC from her family donors, but not with antigen and APC from some non-related donors carrying DR4. In mixed lymphocyte culture (MLC) experiments the MLC-activating determinants on the DR4 molecule of the family donors were shown to be different from those expressed by the DR4 donors whose APC were not able to restimulate antigen-specific responses. This is in accordance with previous reports that several different HLA-D clusters may be associated with HLA-DR4[8,9]. The relationship between restriction elements and some of these DR4 associated D determinants (i.e., Dw4, Dw10, Dw13, Dw14, Dw15 and KT2) was then studied in more detail with chlamydia-specific TLCs from GR.

TLCs from GR were tested with non-T cells as APC from 20 allogeneic non-related DR4-positive individuals expressing different DR4 associated D determinants. Some representative results are given in Table 1. It can be seen

Table 1   DR4 subtype restriction of TLCs from GR

APC[a]		Ag[b]	TLCs[c]	
DR	Dw		GR14	GR15
Autologous 4,4	Dw14	−	569±54 [d]	139±26
		+	11623±689	4069±233
Allogeneic 4,0	Dw14	−	239±17	145±18
		+	8497±577	3882±211
Allogeneic 3,4	Dw14	−	330±10	180±39
		+	9969±260	3451±398
Allogeneic 4,0	Dw14	−	276±77	180±33
		+	15151±993	4901±477
Allogeneic 4,6	Dw4	−	201±54	145±16
		+	208±53	173±15
Allogeneic 4,7	Dw4	−	200±9	105±22
		+	193±10	159±36
Allogeneic 4,4	KT2	−	147±27	109±11
		+	167±16	111±18
Allogeneic 4,4	KT2	−	155±24	177±47
		+	172±9	231±91
Allogeneic 4,8	Dw13	−	371±174	107±3
		+	383±94	281±79
Allogeneic 1,4	Dw13	−	138±24	100±5
		+	195±34	149±48
Allogeneic 2,5		−	237±20	198±25
		+	332±36	288±39
Allogeneic 3,8		−	220±29	228±8
		+	254±14	212±13

a Ten thousand non-T cells as APC, irradiated 20 Gy.

b Final chlamydial antigen concentration in well
  2×10^6 IFU/ml.

c Ten thousand T lymphocyte cloned cells.

d Mean cpm ± SEM.

that autologous APC together with antigen induced strong
responses of both clones. In addition, allogeneic APC
expressing Dw14 were all able to restimulate the TLCs
together with chlamydial antigen. In contrast, APC
expressing other DR4-associated D types (Dw4, Dw13 and
KT2) were not able to restimulate the TLCs together with
antigen. The restriction elements for these TLCs seemed
therefore to be closely associated with Dw14, and less
with DR4. Thus, a very close relationship between the
alloactivating T cell determinants and those responsible
for the restriction elements is observed, as will be
published in detail elsewhere[10].

Inhibition of HLA Class II Restricted TLCs with Monoclonal Antibodies (Mabs) Against HLA Determinants

The inhibitory effect of HLA-specific Mabs on DR1-, DR4-,
DRw53-, or DPw4-restricted TLCs was studied. The TLCs were
restimulated with autologous APC plus antigen, in the
presence or absence of different dilutions of Mabs in
culture medium supplemented with 20% normal serum. Results
of two typical experiments are shown in Figs. 1 and 2,
where the effects of the Mabs on the proliferative
responses of a DR4- and a DRw53-restricted TLC are
illustrated. Mabs 7.2[11] and D-54, reactive with monomorphic DR determinants, inhibited both DR-restricted and
DRw53-restricted TLCs. In contrast, Mab 109d6[12] selectively
inhibited the DRw53-restricted TLC, without any effect on
DR-restricted TLCs. Mabs reactive with DP molecules and
Mabs reactive with class I molecules demonstrated no
inhibitory activity on any of the tested TLCs, in
accordance with the reported DRw53 specificity of this
Mab[12]. The anti-DR Mabs (7.2 and D-54) and the anti-DRw53
Mab 109d6 showed a mostly similar binding to non-T cells
from donors expressing relevant sets of restriction
elements for the clones under study[13]. These data indicate
that 7.2 and D-54 are reactive with determinants shared by
the DR (DR β1 chain) and the DRw53 (DR β2 chain) gene
products, while the epitope/molecule recognized by Mab
109d6 is separate and may be unique for the DRw53
specificity.

Antibodies directed to cell membrane components may
cause inhibition of APC-T cell interactions via several
different mechanisms. Firstly, an inhibitory effect of Mabs
may result from binding or interference with HLA molecules

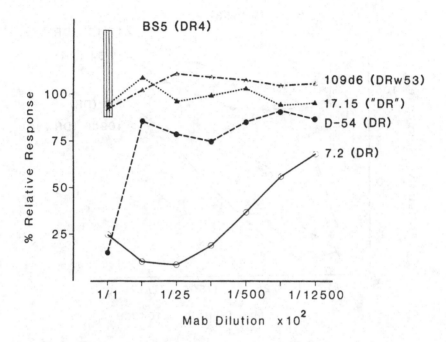

Fig. 1. Effect of monoclonal antibodies (Mabs) in
different dilutions on the proliferative response of a DR4-
restricted TLC, using antigen-pulsed monocytes as antigen-
presenting cells. The 100% cpm value (in normal serum only)
of which the % relative response was calculated, is 4522.
Final dilution of Mabs in the wells is shown on the
abscissa. The vertical column includes results using
different HLA-class I, -DQ or -DP reactive Mabs.

expressed in the membrane of the T cells. Activated
chlamydia-specific TLCs express both HLA class I and II
antigens (DR, DQ and DP; unpublished data). Since the HLA
class I specific Mabs did not inhibit the response, nor
Mabs reactive with with class II determinants not
functioning as restriction elements, binding to HLA
molecules in T cells apparently does not disturb antigen
activation in our studies. Mab 17.15 has been reported to
bind to DR determinants expressed on B lymphocytes and
activated T lymphocytes but not on monocytes[14]. Since this

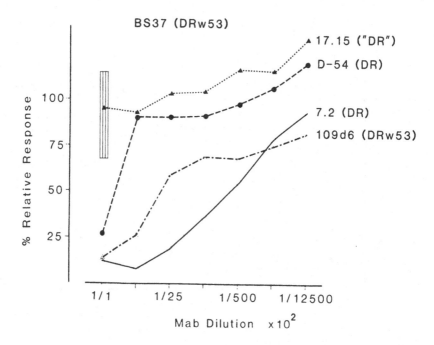

Fig. 2. Effect of Mabs on the proliferative response of
a DRw53-restricted TLC. The 100% cpm value for the TLC is
6816. Legends as for Fig. 1.

antibody also did not inhibit the responses, it provides
additional evidence that binding to DR molecules in the
T cell membrane does not in itself cause inhibition.
Secondly, inhibition could be caused by an unspecific
effect of binding of antibodies to different molecules in
the APC membrane. Again, this is unlikely for the same
reasons as given above.

   Thus, the inhibitory effects are most likely a
specific effect on the class II molecules in the APC
membrane expressing the relevant restriction elements.
Mabs directed to DR molecules (7.2 and D-54) inhibited
both DR- and DRw53-restricted clones, but not DP-restricted
TLCs. Since Mab 109d6 only inhibited the DRw53-restricted
clones, without any effect on DR-restricted clones, the
epitope recognized by this Mab may be unique for the DRw53

specificity[12]. The DPw4-restricted TLC was not inhibited
by any Mabs, including the DP-reactive Mabs, MHM4(DP)[15]
and Tü39(DR+DP)[16] (data not shown). This lack of
inhibition may be caused by insufficient avidity of the
Mabs, the Mabs may be binding to parts of the DP molecules
which are far removed from the restriction elements, or
they may react with other "DP-like" molecules.

In conclusion, our studies demonstrate that the HLA class
II molecules DR, DRw53 and DP may all express restriction
elements which are separately recognized by T lymphocytes
in conjunction with antigen. In addition, a molecule
expressing one particular DR determinant, i.e., DR4, may
express several different restriction elements, where the
restriction elements are more closely associated with the
alloactivating D determinants than with DR. Inhibition
experiments using HLA-specific monoclonal antibodies
correlated with the restriction specificities of the
clones, and the inhibitory effect was specific for the
class II molecules expressing the relevant restriction
elements.

References

1. Qvigstad, E., Digranes, S. & Thorsby, E. Scand. J.
   Immunol. 18, 291-297 (1983).
2. Qvigstad, E., Moen, T. & Thorsby, E. Immunogenetics
   19, 455-460 (1984).
3. Albrechtsen, D., Bratlie, A., Nousiainen, H., Solheim,
   B.G., Winther, N. & Thorsby, E. Immunogenetics 6,
   91-100 (1978).
4. O'Leary, J., Reinsmoen, N.L. & Yunis, E.J. in Manual
   of Clinical Immunology (eds. Rose, N.R. & Friedman, H.)
   820 (Amer. Soc. Microbiol., Washington, D.C., 1976).
5. Qvigstad, E. & Thorsby, E. Scand. J. Immunol. 18,
   299-306 (1983).
6. Ball, E.J. & Stastny, P. Immunogenetics 19, 13-26
   (1984).
7. Eckels, D.E., Lake, P., Lamb, J.R., Johnson, A.H.,
   Shaw, S., Woody, J.N. & Hartzmann, R.J. Nature 301,
   716-718 (1983).
8. Reinsmoen, N.L. & Bach, F.H. Hum. Immunol. 4, 249-258
   (1982).
9. Groner, J., Watson, A. & Bach, F.H. J. exp. Med. 157,
   1687-1691 (1983).

10. Qvigstad, E., Thorsby, E., Reinsmoen, N.L. & Bach, F.H.
    Immunogenetics in press (1984).
11. Hansen, J.A., Martin, P.J. & Nowinski, R.C.
    Immunogenetics 10, 247-260 (1980).
12. Winchester, R., Toguchi, T., Szer, I., Burmester, G.,
    Galbo, P.L., Cuttner, J., Capra, J.D. & Nunez-Roldan,
    A. Immunol. Rev. 70, 155-166 (1983).
13. Qvigstad, E., Gaudernack, G. & Thorsby, E. Hum. Immunol.
    in press (1984).
14. Torok-Storb, B., Nepom, G.T., Nepom, B.S. & Hansen,
    J.A. Nature 305, 541-543 (1983).
15. Makgoba, M.W., Hildreth, J.E.K. & McMichael, A.J.
    Immunogenetics 17, 623-635 (1983).
16. Ziegler, A. Hum. Immunol. in press (1984).

MOLECULAR AND FUNCTIONAL ANALYSIS OF HLA-CLASS II MOLECULES

RESPONSIBLE FOR THE PRIMARY MLR IN MAN

T. Sasazuki, Y. Nishimura, K. Tsukamoto,
K. Hirayama and T. Sone
Department of Human Genetics, Medical Research
Institute, Tokyo Medical and Dental University
1-5-45 Yushima, Bunkyo-ku, Tokyo 113, Japan

INTRODUCTION

HLA-D antigen is defined as a molecule responsible for
the stimulation of primary mixed lymphocyte reaction (MLR),
and nineteen specificities of HLA-D have been well established in the Ninth International Histocompatibility
Workshop (9th IHWS)[1]. The biological and biochemical
features of the HLA-D molecule have not been well understood
except the fact that they stimulate primary MLR. Polymorphic cell surface glycoproteins, on the other hand,
which are defined serologically on B cell are designated
as HLA-DR. Fourteen alleles of HLA-DR have been established
in the 9th IHWS. An HLA-D specificity shows strong correlation with a certain HLA-DR type. Furthermore, the
alloantiserum against HLA-DR can inhibit the stimulation
in MLR[2] suggesting that the DR antigen is the molecule
which stimulates MLR. However, since HLA-Dw2 and Dw12,
which are mutually stimulatory in MLR, are both defined as
HLA-DR2 in serology, we first indicated that HLA-DR epitope
is only a part of the epitopes which stimulate MLR[3]. Along
this line, it was found that Dw4, Dw10, Dw13, Dw14, Dw15
and DKT2 were correlated with DR4. It has been suggested
from these observations that HLA-D "region" consisted of
at least two "loci" including HLA-DR locus. In this paper,
we have clarified the molecular and functional differences
of HLA-DR4 associated HLA-D specificities and of HLA-DR2
associated HLA-D specificities.

HETEROGENEITY OF HLA-DR4 β CHAINS WHICH STIMULATE THE PRIMARY MLR BETWEEN HLA-Dw4, Dw15 AND DKT2

Effects of Anti HLA-Class II Monoclonal Antibodies (MoAbs) on the MLR between HLA-Dw4, Dw15 and DKT2

We have investigated the HLA-class II molecules involved in the stimulation of MLR between HLA-Dw4, Dw15 and DKT2 by using several anti HLA class II MoAbs. One way MLR was performed as described previously[4]. In blocking experiments of the MLR, ascites fluid containing anti HLA-DR framework MoAb HU-4[5] or anti HLA-DQw3 MoAb HU-18[6] was added in each culture wells at the final dilution of 1 : 1,000. Positive reaction of HU-4 and HU-18 with Dw4 or DKT2 homozygous cells at this final dilution was confirmed by staining and direct binding using ^{125}I labeled MoAbs. HU-4 also bound to Dw15 homozygous cells, whereas HU-18 did not bind to them. As a control, ascites fluid of Balb/c mouse injected intraperitoneally with murine myeloma line P3XAg8 was used at the same dilution as those containing MoAbs HU-4 or HU-18. As shown in Table I, the MLR between Dw4, Dw15 and DKT2 homozygous typing cells (HTCs) was almost completely inhibited by MoAb HU-4. Anti DQw3 MoAb HU-18, on the other hand, had no effects on the MLR. It was confirmed by the chromium release assay that MoAb HU-4 or HU-18 was not capable for causing the antibody dependent cell mediated cytotoxicity (ADCC) which will result in the complete inhibition of MLR. HLA-DR molecules

Table I. Complete inhibition of the MLR between HLA-Dw4, Dw15 and DKT2 homozygous typing cells by MoAb HU-4.

MLR		Control	MoAb HU-4	% Inhi-
resp.	stim.	(cpm)	(cpm)	bition
Dw4	Dw15	42,213	8,119	80.8
Dw15	Dw4	23,775	4,744	80.0
Dw4	DKT2	21,944	3,948	82.0
DKT2	Dw4	35,911	3,809	89.4
DKT2	Dw15	64,657	4,203	93.5
Dw15	DKT2	15,876	3,410	78.5

recognized by MoAb HU-4 are, therefore, responsible for the
primary MLR between Dw4, Dw15 and DKT2.

Biochemical Analysis of DR Molecules from HLA-Dw4, Dw15 and DKT2

Since MoAb HU-4 completely inhibited the MLR between
Dw4, Dw15 and DKT2. We have checked the molecular difference of HLA-DR molecules recognized by HU-4 from B lymphoblastoid cell lines (BLCLs) homozygous for HLA-Dw4 (ER, HA),
Dw15 (EBV-Wa, KT9) or DKT2 (KT2, KT13). BLCLs were
metabolically labeled with L-[^{35}S]-methionine for 8h or
for 30 min. Immunoprecipitates from BLCLs with MoAb HU-4
were collected by the method described by Jones et al[7].
Two dimensional polyacrylamide gel electrophoresis (2D-PAGE)
was performed by the method of O'Farrell[8] with minor
modification described elsewhere[9].

HLA-DR molecules from 8h labeled BLCLs showed serieses
of spots corresponding to the step of glycosylation of DR
molecules. In order to avoid the complex pattern of glycosylated DR molecules, 30 min pulse labeling of the BLCL was
performed and only glycosylated precursor of DR molecules
were visible as a spot by this method (Fig. 1). MoAb HU-4
precipitated a couple of DR α (32k) and DR β (28.5k) chains,
invariant chain (Ii, 31k) and actin (a, 44k) from each cell
lines. 2D-PAGE profiles of the immunoprecipitates from
independent two BLCLs of the same HLA-D specificity showed
no difference. DR α chains of all six BLCLs were identical
in 2D-PAGE profile. DR β chains of BLCLs with different
HLA-D specificities were, on the other hand, distinct. DR
β chain of Dw15 is the most basic protein and that of DKT2
is most acidic protein among three DR β chains. DR β chain
of Dw4 migrates between those of Dw4 and DKT2 in 2D-PAGE
profile. We concluded from these data that the difference
in DR4 β chain stimulated the MLR between Dw4, Dw15 and DKT2

Polymorphism of DR4 β Chains as Restriction Specificities at the Antigen Presentation to T Cell by Antigen Presenting Cell (APC)

We have already reported that the immune response of
peripheral blood lymphocytes (PBL) to streptococcal cell
wall antigen (SCW) was controlled by an HLA-linked immune
suppression gene through suppressor T cell and that the

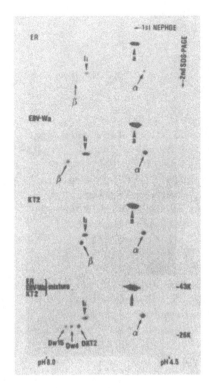

Fig. 1.   2D-PAGE profiles of immunoprecipitates with anti HLA-DR framework MoAb HU-4 from B lymphoblastoid cell lines homozygous for HLA-Dw4 (ER), Dw15 (EBV-Wa) or DKT2 (KT2).   B cell lines were metabolically labeled with L-[^{35}S]-methionine for 30 min and immunoprecipitates with HU-4 were analyzed by 2D-PAGE using non-equilibrium pH gradient electrophoresis as the first dimension and SDS-PAGE as the second dimension. a; actin, Ii; invariant chain, α; α chain, β; β chain

antigen presentation of SCW to T cell by APC was restricted by HLA-DR[10]. We used the assay system of the T cell proliferation to SCW to test the possibility of the polymorphism of DR4 β chain to be a restriction specificity at the antigen presentation.

PBL were separated from a high responder to SCW, YN (HLA-DR4,Dw4,DQw3,DPw2/DR4,DKT2,DQw3,DPw4) and the proliferative response of PBL (1x10^5) to 0.5 µg/ml of SCW was measured by the method described elsewhere[4] in the presence of anti HLA-class II MoAbs. Proliferative response of T cell to SCW was almost completely inhibited by anti HLA-DR framework MoAb HU-4. Anti HLA-DQw3 (MB3) MoAb HU-18 or anti HLA-DP (SB) MoAb MHM-4[11], on the other hand, had no effect on the immune response. HLA-DR molecule is therefore, important for the antigen presentation of SCW to T cell by APC. The same results were obtained from the blocking experiments of the proliferative response of T cell to PPD or Candida albicans.

We have, then, established the IL-2 dependent T cell

line specific to SCW from donor HG (HLA-DR4,Dw15/DRw8,D-)
and the donor KH (HLA-DR4,Dw4/DR4,DKT2), who were both high
responders to SCW, by the method described elsewhere[9]. T
cell line (1x10^4) was cultured with 5 µg/ml of SCW and
irradiated PBL (5x10^4) as APC for 60 h. The genetic
restriction between the T cell line and allogeneic APC was
tested and the strength of the immune response of the T
cell line with allogeneic APC was expressed by the percent
autologous cooperation (%AC), which was estimated by
calculating percentage of the cpm observed in a allogeneic
combination to that observed in autologous combination.
These T cell lines showed marked proliferative response in
the presence of allogeneic APC which shared DR4 associated
HLA-D specificities with the donor of the T cell lines and
immune response was completely inhibited by MoAb HU-4.
HLA-DR4 sharing but HLA-D nonsharing allogeneic APC, on the
other hand, could not present SCW to T cell lines (Fig. 2).
Receptor of the T cell lines is, therefore, able to
distinguish the heterogeneity of HLA-DR4 β chains as a
restriction specificity at the antigen presentation of SCW.

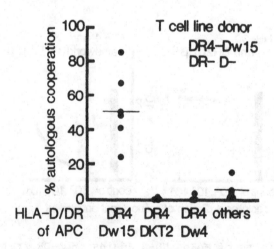

Fig. 2. Antigen presentation of allogeneic APC to the SCW
specific T cell line established from a HLA-Dw15 heterozygous high responder.

A NOVEL CLASS II MOLECULE RESPONSIBLE FOR THE PRIMARY MLR
BETWEEN HLA-Dw2 AND Dw12

Effects of Anti HLA-Class II MoAbs on the MLR between
HLA-Dw2 and Dw12

If HLA-Dw2 homozygous typing cells (HTC) were cocultured with mitomycin treated HLA-Dw12 HTC, the strong MLR
was observed. This MLR was almost completely inhibited by
anti HLA-DR framework MoAb HU-4 (Fig. 3). MoAb HU-11 [12]
against DQw1 (DC1, MB1, MT1) molecule and MoAb MHM-4 against
DP (SB) molecule had, on the other hand, no significant
effects on the MLR. These results were reproducible in the
blocking experiments of the MLR between Dw2 as a stimulator
and Dw12 as a responder. HLA-DR molecule recognized by HU-4
is, therefore, responsible for the MLR between Dw2 and Dw12
as in the case of the MLR between DR4 associated HLA-D
specificities. We have then checked the effects of anti
HLA-DR2 MoAb HU-30 [13] on the MLR between Dw2 and Dw12. To
our surprise, HU-30 could not affect the MLR suggesting
that DR2 molecule itself could not elicit the MLR between

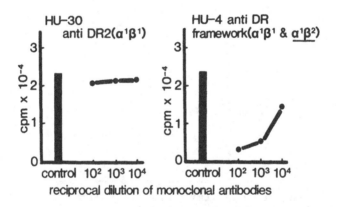

Fig. 3. Effects of MoAbs HU-4 against HLA-DR framework or
HU-30 against HLA-DR2 on the MLR between HLA-Dw2 and Dw12.
MoAbs were added in the mixed lymphocyte culture of HLA-Dw2
homozygous cell as a stimulator cell and HLA-Dw12 homozygous
cell as a responder cell.

Dw2 and Dwl2. Effects of MoAbs HU-4 or HU-30 on the MLR
between Dw2 or Dwl2 HTCs as stimulator cells and Dwl/Dwl5
heterozygous cell as a responder cell were then investigated.
In this case, HU-4 did completely and HU-30 did partially
inhibit the MLR. The range of the inhibition of MLR by
HU-4 was 85.7% to 97.2% and that by HU-30 was 33.7% to
53.0% indicating that class II molecule recognized by HU-4
or HU-30 can stimulate the MLR of this cell combination.
In order to identify the molecular difference of HLA-DR
molecule reactive with HU-4 between two HLA-D specificities,
biochemical analysis was performed.

2D-PAGE Analysis of HLA-Class II Molecules of HLA-Dw2 and Dwl2

The immunoprecipitates with HU-4 from four independent
HLA-Dw2 homozygous BLCLs, EB-CMG, PGF, Gay and EB-BY or
from two independent HLA-Dwl2 homozygous BLCLs EB-AKIBA and
EB-KT were analyzed by 2D-PAGE. Immunoprecipitates of 30
min pulse labeled Dw2 or Dwl2 homozygous BLCLs with HU-4
consisted of actin (44k), invariant chain (Ii, 31k), two
distinct β (basic β^1, 28.5k and acidic β^2, 28-28.5k) and one
α (α^1, 32k) chains of human class II molecules (Fig. 4).
Since only one α chain was observed, it is likely that the
same α chain is associated with two distinct β chains to
produce $\alpha^1\beta^1$ and $\alpha^1\beta^2$ molecules in Dw2 and Dwl2. 2D-PAGE
profiles showed no difference in the BLCLs which has the
same HLA-D specificity. α^1 and β^1 chains showed no difference among all six BLCLs, but β^2 chain of Dw2 is more
acidic than that of Dwl2. β^2 chain (28k) of Dwl2 is
slightly smaller than β^1 chains (28.5k) of both Dw2 and
Dwl2. β^2 chain (28.5k) of Dw2 has the same molecular
weight as β^1 chain of Dw2. Difference of β^2 chains between
two HLA-D specificities was confirmed by comparing the non-
glycosylated polypeptides of tunicamycin treated BLCLs.
Since Takenouchi et al.[14] found that anti HLA-DR2 MoAb
HU-30 precipitated only $\alpha^1\beta^1$ molecule from both Dw2 and
Dwl2, it is apparent that $\alpha^1\beta^1$ is the HLA-DR2 molecule.
This in turn indicates that $\alpha^1\beta^2$ molecule is distinct from
DR2 molecule.
In order to exclude the possibility that the $\alpha^1\beta^2$
molecule is a known DQwl (DC1, MB1, MT1) or FA molecule,
2D-PAGE profiles of the immunoprecipitates from PGF (Dw2)
or EB-AKIBA (Dwl2) with anti DQwl (DC1) MoAb SDR4.1 [15] or
anti FA MoAb [16] were examined. SDR4.1 precipitated DQwl

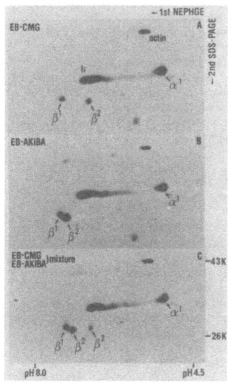

Fig. 4. 2D-PAGE profiles of
the immunoprecipitates with
MoAb HU-4 from 30 min pulse
labeled HLA-Dw2 (EB-CMG) or
Dw12 (EB-AKIBA) homozygous
B lymphoblastoid cell lines.
2D-PAGE was performed by the
same method as the legend
for Fig. 1.

molecule which was apparently distinct from $\alpha^1\beta^1$ and $\alpha^1\beta^2$
molecules in both PGF and EB-AKIBA. Both α chain and β
chain of DQw1 molecule from Dw2 were distinct from those
from Dw12. Anti FA MoAb precipitated FA β chain distinct
from β^1, β^2 and DQw1 β chains in both PGF and EB-AKIBA.
FA α chain of PGF was distinct from that of EB-AKIBA and
both α chains were indistinguishable from DQw1 α chains in
each BLCLs. FA β chain of PGF was, on the other hand,
identical with that of EB-AKIBA[9].

All these data clearly indicates that $\alpha^1\beta^2$ molecule is
a novel class II molecule responsible for the primary MLR
between Dw2 and Dw12. We tentatively designated this novel
class II molecule as DT.

Restriction Molecules for the Antigen Presentation
of SCW in Dw2 and Dw12

Effects of anti HLA class II MoAbs on the proliferative response of PBL to SCW were examined in a high responder to SCW KK (HLA-DR1,Dw1,DQw1,DPw4/DR2,Dw2,DQw1,DPw-). Anti HLA-DR framework MoAb HU-4 almost completely inhibited the immune response. MoAb HU-11 [12] against DQw1 molecule and anti DP MoAb MHM-4 did not affect the immune response of KK to SCW at all. These observations suggested that DR2 $(\alpha^1\beta^1)$ or DT $(\alpha^1\beta^2)$ molecule might be recognized by T cell as a restriction molecule in the immune response to SCW. Since anti HLA-DR2 MoAb HU-30 markedly inhibited the immune response of PBL from Dw2 or Dw12 homozygote, DR2 $(\alpha^1\beta^1)$ molecule is proved to be a restriction molecule for the antigen presentation of SCW.

In order to investigate the role of DT molecule in the proliferative response of PBL to SCW, we have generated the IL-2 dependent T cell line specific to SCW from a high responder SM (DR2,Dw12/DRw6,D-) as described elsewhere[9]. As shown in Fig. 5, the genetic restriction between the T cell line and allogeneic APC was tested and the T cell line

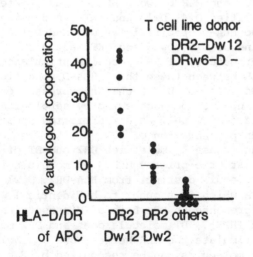

Fig. 5. Antigen presentation of allogeneic APC to the SCW specific T cell line established from a Dw12 heterozygous high responder.

showed marked immune response in the presence of APC from
seven unrelated Dwl2 positive panels without showing any
MLR and mean %AC was 32.6 ± 9.8. Decreased but apparently
positive immune response (10.0 ± 3.7 %AC) was observed when
the T cell line was cultured with APC from six unrelated
Dw2 positive panels. No immune response (1.46 ± 1.79 %AC),
on the other hand, was detected in the culture of the T
cell line with eleven unrelated DR nonsharing APC. Difference of mean %AC between DR2-Dwl2 sharing combinations and
DR2 sharing but D nonsharing combinations, or that between
the latter combinations and DR nonsharing combinations were
both statistically significant (p < 0.0005 or p < 0.002
respectively). The immune response of the T cell line
cocultured with Dwl2 heterozygous allogeneic APC was
markedly inhibited by MoAb HU-4 (60.5 to 84.0 % inhibition)
and anti HLA-DR2 MoAb HU-30 completely inhibited the immune
response of the T cell line cocultured with Dw2 heterozygous
APCs. We concluded from these observations that DT molecule
as well as DR2 molecule could be recognized as a restriction
molecule for the antigen presentation of SCW.

DISCUSSION

We have clearly identified the HLA-class II molecules
responsible for the MLR between HLA-DR4 associated three
HLA-D specificities Dw4, Dwl5 and DKT2, and between HLA-DR2
associated two HLA-D specificities Dw2 and Dwl2.
1) DR4 β chains of Dw4, Dwl5 and DKT2 are distinct and
   these heterogeneity of DR4 β chains stimulates the
   primary MLR between these three HLA-D specificities.
   This polymorphism of DR4 β chains expressed on APC,
   which have not yet been detected by serological method,
   is recognized by T cell as a restriction specificity at
   the antigen presentation of SCW.
2) Two distinct class II molecules DR2 and DT of Dw2 and
   Dwl2 stimulate the primary MLR. DT molecule is a novel
   class II molecule distinct from HLA-DR2, DQwl (DC1, MB1,
   MT1) and FA which is thought to be identical with SB
   molecule (presented by F. Bach of Minnesota University
   in the 9th IHWS). DT molecule does and DR2 molecule
   does not stimulate the MLR between Dw2 and Dwl2. Both
   DR2 and DT molecules can be recognized by T cell as a
   restriction molecule at the antigen presentation of SCW
   by APC.
       At least four class II molecules, DR[17], DQ[18], FA[16] and

DRw52 (MT2)[19] or DRw53 (MT3)[20] were identified by 2D-PAGE
in man, and molecular analysis of the HLA-D region has
revealed that at least four class II α genes existed in a
HLA-D region[21]. Recent data, furthermore, suggest the
existence of six or seven β genes (two or three DR like
genes, two DQ (DC) like genes and two DP (SB) like genes)
in a haploid (the 9th IHCWS). Important question therefore
to be answered is "what is the gene coding for DT?". Since
DRw52 (MT2) or DRw53 (MT3) like molecule has not yet been
reported so far in DR2 haplotype, it is possible that DT
might be an allele of the locus coding for DRw52 (MT2) and
DRw53 (MT3) molecules. Another possibility is that the
serologically determined DR2 may be an allele of the MT
locus such as DRw52 (MT2) and DRw53 (MT3), and that DT is
an allele of the DR locus. In this case, HLA-Dw2 and Dw12
do not share HLA-DR but share HLA-MT and it is not possible
to exclude this possibility at this stage.

In mice, two class II molecules $A_\alpha A_\beta$ and $E_\alpha E_\beta$ which
are the products of the I region of the H-2 complex, are
capable for inducing MLR[22] and for the antigen presentation
of soluble antigens to T cell. It has been estimated that
HLA-DR and DQ molecules corresponded to murine $E_\alpha E_\beta$ and $A_\alpha A_\beta$
molecules respectively by the analysis of amino acid and
base sequence[23]. However, we can not find any roles of DQ
(DC, MB) molecules on the primary MLR nor on the antigen
presentation for soluble antigens such as SCW, PPD or
Candida albicans.

We have extended the blocking experiments of MLR and
of immune response of PBL to SCW with MoAb HU-4 by using
healthy unrelated panels who were heterozygote at HLA-DR
locus. The MLR between all alleles of HLA-DR except DR3,
DR7 and DRw10 which are rare alleles in the Japanese
population was completely inhibited by HU-4. The proliferative response of PBL from these panels to SCW was also
completely inhibited by HU-4. We can, therefore, extend
our observations to conclude that HLA-class II molecules
recognized by MoAb HU-4 are responsible for the primary MLR
and for the antigen presentation of SCW to T cell by APC
in man.

ACKNOWLEDGMENTS

We are grateful to Dr. M. Aizawa of Hokkaido University
Sapporo, Japan for providing MoAbs HU-4, HU-11, HU-18 and
HU-30. We thank Dr. A.J. McMichael of University of Oxford,

England for providing MoAb MHM-4. Other MoAbs SDR4.1 and
anti FA were distributed for the 9th International Histocompatibility Workshop by Dr. W.F. Bodmer, Imperial Cancer
Research Fund Labolatories, England and Dr. F. Bach,
Minnesota University respectively. This work was supported
in part by Grants-in-Aid from the Ministry of Education,
Culture and Science, Japan.

REFERENCES

1. Albert, E.P. et al. in Histocompatibility Testing 1984
   (eds. Albert, E.D., Bauer, M.P. & Mayr, W.R.) (Springer-
   Verlag, Berlin, in the press).
2. Cresswell, P. & Geier, S.S. Nature 257, 147-149 (1975).
3. Sasazuki, T. et al. in Histocompatibility Testing 1977
   (ed. Bodmer, W.F.) 489-498 (Munksgaard, Copenhagen,
   1977).
4. Sasazuki, T., Kaneoka, H., Nishimura, Y., Kaneoka, R.,
   Hayama, M. & Ohkuni, H. J. Exp. Med. 152, 297s-313s
   (1980).
5. Koide, Y., Awashima, F., Yoshida, T.O., Takenouchi, T.,
   Wakisaka, A., Moriuchi, J. & Aizawa, M. J. Immunol.
   129, 1061-1069 (1982).
6. Kasahara, M. et al. Immunogenetics 17, 485-495 (1983).
7. Jones, P.P. in Selected Methods in Cellular Immunology
   (eds. Mishell, B.B. & Shiji, S.M.) 398-440 (W.H. Freeman
   and Company, San Fransisco 1980).
8. O'Farrell, P.Z., Goodman, H.M. & O'Farrell, P.H. Cell
   12, 1133-1142 (1977).
9. Sone, T., Tsukamoto, K., Hirayama, K., Nishimura, Y.,
   Takenouchi, T., Aizawa, M. & Sasazuki, T. (submitted).
10. Nishimura, Y. & Sasazuki, T. Nature 302, 67-69 (1983).
11. Makgoba, M.W., Hildreth, J.E.K., & McMichael, A.J.
    Immunogenetics 17, 623-635 (1983).
12. Kasahara, M., Takenouchi, T., Ikeda, H., Ogasawara, K.,
    Okuyama, T., Ishikawa, N., Wakisaka, A., Kikuchi, Y. &
    Aizawa, M. Immunogenetics 18, 525-536 (1983).
13. Kasahara, M., Ogasawara, K., Ikeda, H., Okuyama, T.,
    Ishikawa, N., Takenouchi, T., Wakisaka, A., Kikuchi, Y.
    & Aizawa, M. Tissue Antigens 21, 105-113 (1983).
14. Takenouchi, T., Hawkin, S., Kasahara, M., Ishikawa, N.,
    Ogasawara, K., Ikeda, H., Wakisaka, A., Kikuchi, Y. &
    Aizawa, M. (submitted).
15. Crumpton, M.J., Bodmer, J.G., Bodmer, W.F., Heyes, J.M.,
    Lindsay, J. & Rudd, C.E. in Histocompatibility Testing

1984 (eds. Albert, E.D., Bauer, M.P. & Mayr, W.R.) (Springer-Verlag, Berlin, in the press).

16. Watson, A.J., DeMars, R., Trowbridge, I.S. & Bach, F. Nature 304, 358-361 (1983).

17. Charron, D.J. & McDevitt, H.O. J. Exp. Med. 152, 18s-36s (1980).

18. Shackelford, D.A., Mann, D.L., van Rood, J.J., Ferrara, G.B. & Strominger, J.L. Proc. Natl. Acad. Sci. USA 78, 4566-4570 (1981).

19. Karr, R.W., Kannapell, C.C., Stein, J.A., Gebel, H.M., Mann, D.L., Duquesnoy, R.J., Fuller, T.C., Rodey, G.E. & Shwartz, B.D. J. Immunol. 128, 1809-1818 (1982).

20. Suzuki, M., Maeda, H., Mukai, R., Yabe, T. & Hamaguchi, H. Immunogenetics 18, 575-583 (1983).

21. Auffray, C., Kuo, J., DeMars, R. & Strominger, J.L. Nature 304, 174-177 (1983).

22. Murphy, D.B. in the Role of the Major Histocompatibility Complex in Immunobiology (ed. Dorf, M.E.) 1-32 (Garland STPM Press, New York, 1981).

23. Kaufman, J.F., Auffray, C., Korman, A.J., Shackelford, D.A. & Strominger, J.L. Cell 36, 1-13 (1984)

HLA-CLASS I ANTIGEN RECOGNITION BY EB VIRUS-SPECIFIC AND

ALLO-SPECIFIC CYTOTOXIC T CELLS

Lesley E. Wallace, Melanie A. Houghton and
Alan B. Rickinson
Department of Cancer Studies, University of
Birmingham Medical School, U.K. and Department
of Pathology, University of Bristol Medical
School, U.K.

It is clear that in man, just as in the mouse, virus-specific cytotoxic T cells are genetically restricted in their function, recognising a viral target antigen on the surface of infected cells not as an isolated structure but in some form of association with the polymorphic determinants of HLA class I gene products (1-3). Thus virus-specific cytotoxic T cells offer a means of probing HLA class I antigen polymorphism which is independent of that provided by allo-specific cytotoxic T cells raised in mixed lymphocyte cultures or of that afforded by serological reagents. There is now growing evidence to suggest that a divergence exists between serologically-defined and T cell-defined polymorphisms (4-7). However, relatively little is known about the relationship between those sites on HLA class I molecules recognized by virus-specific cytotoxic T cells and those recognised by allospecific cytotoxic T cells. The work reported here, seeking to distinguish between T cell restricting determinants and allo-specific T cell recognition sites on HLA class I molecules, has taken advantage of the fact that Epstein-Barr (EB) virus-transformed B cells can act as in vitro stimulators of either of EB virus-specific cytotoxic T cells (showing classical HLA class I antigen restriction) or of allo-specific cytotoxic T cells (directed against foreign HLA class I antigens) depending upon the particular in vitro responder: stimulator combination employed (8,9).

EB virus-specific T cell lines and clones

EB virus infection in man induces a strong T cell-
mediated immune response, and large numbers of virus-
specific memory cells are present in the circulating T-
cell pool of all previously infected healthy individuals
(10). These memory T cells can be reactivated in vitro by
stimulating blood mononuclear cells with X-irradiated cells
of the autologous EB-virus-transformed cell line at a
responder:stimulator ratio of 40:1, (8) and the cytotoxic
effector cells thus obtained can be expanded as interleukin
2 (IL 2) dependent T cell lines (11). Effector T cell
lines produced in this way are specifically cytotoxic
towards target cells expressing the EB virus-induced
lymphocyte-detected membrane antigen LYDMA, which they
recognise in an HLA-A and B antigen-restricted fashion.
This restriction is apparent not just from the pattern of
recognition of allogeneic EB virus-transformed target cells
(12,13), but also from the specific blocking effect which
monoclonal antibodies to framework determinants on all HLA-
A, B, and C antigens have upon the effector:target cell
interaction (14).

Effector cells from these virus-specific T cell lines
have been cloned by seeding at 0.7 cells/well into round-
bottomed microtest plate wells containing a feeder layer of
X-irradiated autologous EB virus-transformed cells and
maintained and expanded thereafter with repeated antigenic
stimulation in the presence of interleukin 2 (15).
Analysis of the first series of cytotoxic clones produced
revealed that each clone showed specificity for the viral
target antigen LYDMA in association with a single HLA
determinant. Thus the first reported clone recognised
LYDMA in the context of HLA-A11 and the second in the context of HLA-Bw35 (15).

Detailed analysis of the effector function of both
monoclonal and polyclonal populations of EB virus-specific
T cells indicated that T cell restriction may be more
precise than that expected on the basis of serologically-
defined HLA typing (6,15,16). Evidence for heterogeneity
of restriction determinants detected by EB virus-specific
T cells within a serologically defined HLA antigen has been
obtained for HLA-A2, HLA-A29, B27 and Bw35 (6,15,16,17).
The emerging biochemical information concerning the amino
acid sequences of HLA-A2 antigens (18-21) has focussed our

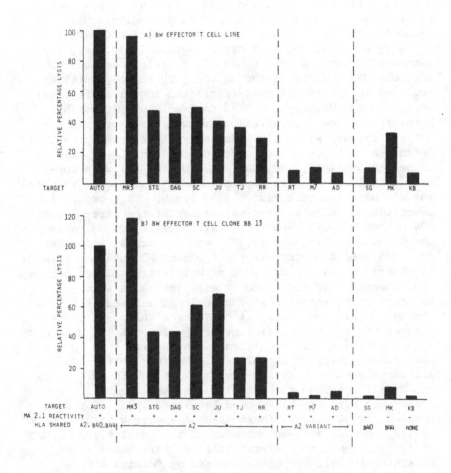

Figure 1. Cytotoxicity of a) EB virus-specific effector T cell line from EB virus-immune donor BW (HLA A2, A2, B40, B44) and of b) clone BB13 derived from that line. Results are expressed as the relative percentage lysis of the autologous target cell (BW) in the same assay at the same effector:target ratio.

present studies onto T cell-recognition of serologically
defined HLA-A2 antigens.

Fig. 1 shows an example of the ability of an EB virus-
specific effector T cell line (fig. 1a) and of a T cell
clone (fig. 1b) derived from that line to distinguish
between members of a panel of virus transformed target
cells typed as HLA-A2 both by conventional tissue typing
sera and by binding of the A2/B17 specific monoclonal
antibody MA2.1 (22). Although the polyclonal population
includes an element of Bw44-restricted function (fig. 1a)
which was not displayed by the derived clone (fig. 1b),
both effector cell preparations showed lysis of most but
not all targets with which they shared the serologically-
defined A2 antigen. Thus seven of the ten HLA-A2 bearing
targets shown (MR3, STG, DAG, SC, JU, TJ, RR) were consistently lysed by both populations at levels greater than
25% of the autologous target cell lysis. This group of
seven target cells was representative of the large majority
(24 out of 30) of A2-positive target cells tested during
the course of this work (6,23), and such cells were therefore considered to express the "common" A2 antigen. The
A2-restricted nature of these effector:target interactions
was independently confirmed in experiments in which
saturating concentrations of monoclonal antibody MA2.1
strongly inhibited the lysis of "common" A2-positive targets either by the T cell line or by clone BB 13 (data not
shown). It was very significant, therefore, that in these
same assays three of the A2-bearing target cells (RT, M7,
AD) were lysed at very low levels (<10% relative lysis by
the T cell line and <5% relative lysis by T cell clone)
comparable with the background levels of lysis of mismatched target cells. These three A2-bearing target cells
(RT, M7 and AD) are each members of the small group (6 out
of 30) of A2-positive target cells so far tested which
consistently fail to be recognized by "common A2"-
restricted EB virus-specific T cells derived from several
donors (6,23,24) and are therefore considered to express
"variant A2" antigens.

Interestingly, parallel studies in other laboratories
using polyclonal influenza virus-specific cytotoxic T cells
(4,24,25) have also identified donors RT, M7 and AD as
possessing "variant-A2" antigens. Thus in the influenza
virus system virus-infected target cells from RT, M7 and AD
were not recognized by A2-restricted cytotoxic effector

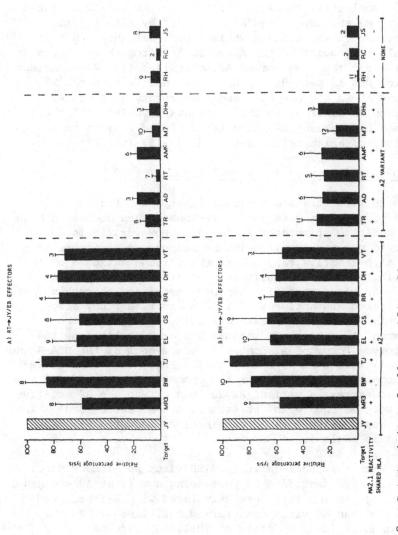

Figure 2. Cytotoxicity of allospecific effector T cell lines from EB virus-non-immune donors RT and RH.

cells raised from "common A2" donors. Furthermore, HLA-A2
restricted H-Y antigen specific cytotoxic T cells also
fail to recognise appropriate target cells from male
"variant A2" donors (26), and perhaps suggests a key
functional role for the A2-subgroup restriction determinant in its interaction with a variety of antigens.

Isoelectric focusing analysis of the HLA-A2 antigens
of RT, M7 and AD defined as "variant" by HLA-restricted
T cells such as those shown in fig. 1 has shown that the
isoelectric point of the A2 molecules from these donors is
more basic than the common A2 molecule (24). A comparison
of the HLA-A2 peptide map data obtained from donors RT,
M7 and AD on the one hand and the prototype common A2
antigen of donor JY on the other has revealed that these
common and variant A2 molecules differed only in the
regions of amino acids 36-44 and 147-157 (24).

Allo-specific cytotoxic T cell lines

EB virus-transformed cell lines are potent stimulators of allo-reactive T cell responses when used at a high
responder to stimulator ratio (9). However, it is important to use non-EB virus immune responders to ensure that
the allo-reactive response to the foreign antigens on the
EB virus-transformed stimulator cells is not accompanied
by an EB virus-specific response restricted through any of
the shared HLA antigens (27). In order to study alloreactive responses specifically directed against the
"common" A2 antigen EB virus-transformed cells from the
prototype "common" A2 donor JY (homozygous at the HLA-A and
B loci) were used as stimulators. Responder donors were
chosen who did not express the common A2 antigen (i.e. who
either express a variant A2 antigen or who are A2 negative)
but were matched with the stimulators at the B locus. The
two responder:stimulator conbinations reported here are
shown in table 1.

When responder cells from EB virus non-immune donor
RT, already identified as possessing a variant A2 antigen
(see fig. 1a and 1b), were stimulated with X-irradiated
cells of the EB virus-transformed cell line JY/EB at a
responder:stimulator ratio of 40:1, the resultant IL 2-
dependent T cell line displayed the pattern of cytotoxicity
shown in fig. 2a. It is clear that the cytotoxicity was
directed not only at the stimulator cell line (JY) but also

Table 1

Responder:Stimulator cell combinations yielding
allo-reactive T cells

		Responder cells		Stimulator cells	
	donor	HLA type		donor	HLA type
a)	RT	A2*,A3,B7,B57		JY/EB	A2,A2,B7,B7
		Cw7,DR2,DR7			Cw2,Cw7,DR4,DR6
b)	RH	Aw24,Aw26,B7,B27		JY/EB	A2,A2,B7,B7
		Cw1,Cw7,DR1			Cw2,Cw7,DR4,DR6

*variant of serologically defined HLA-A2 antigen - see text.

at all the other common A2-bearing targets tested; in contrast none of the variant A2-bearing targets or the control
A2-negative targets was significantly lysed. Preincubation
of the common A2 target cells with saturating concentrations of the anti-A2 monoclonal antibody MA2.1 was just as
effective as the anti-HLA-A,B,C monoclonal antibody W6/32
(28) at reducing the level of target cell lysis (data not
shown), indicating that it was indeed the common A2 antigen
and not some other polymorphic HLA gene product which constituted the major target for these effectors.

When cells from an A2-negative donor RH were stimulated
with X-irradiated cells of the JY/EB line, functional
analysis of the IL 2-dependent cytotoxic T cell line consistently revealed a pattern of lysis which is exemplified
by the results in fig. 2b. Again "common A2" and "variant
A2" positive target cells could be distinguished by their
differential lysis; in this situation, however, the level
of lysis of target cells with variant A2 antigens, although
always less than 50% of the lysis of the stimulating cells,
was always greater than that of the A2-negative target
cells included as controls. Moreover, as figure 3 shows,

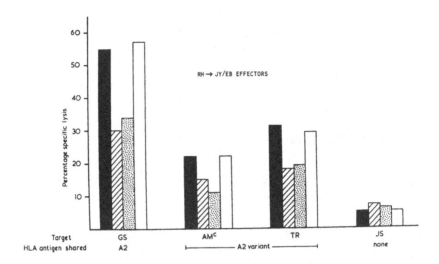

Figure 3. Effect of monoclonal antibodies on the level of
lysis of HLA-A2 positive and HLA-mismatched target cells
by allospecific effector T cells from donor RH raised
against JY/EB. Results are expressed as percentage specific
lysis in the absence of antibody (▉) and in the presence
of saturating concentrations of W6/32 (▨), MA2.1 (▦)
and MHM6 (▢).

lysis of the A2-bearing target cells, both in the "common"
and "variant" sub-groups, could be blocked by the anti-A2
monoclonal antibody MA2.1 as well as by W6/32, strongly
suggesting that within this polyclonal effector T cell line
there is a minor population of cytotoxic cells which has
been generated against a group specific determinant shared
by both "common" and "variant" A2 molecules. Unequivocal
proof of this interpretation will require detailed examination of monoclonal effector cells derived from this line;
this work is currently in progress. However, the evidence
from analysis of the polyclonal cytotoxic response suggests
that the T cell pool of an A2-negative donor has the capacity to respond to two sets of sites on the common A2
molecule: a major component of the response seems to be
directed towards regions of the A2 molecule associated with
the T cell-restricting site, whilst a minor component seems
to be directed towards other polymorphisms which, like those
detected by A2-specific allo-antibodies, are shared by all
molecules of the A2 group.

Such distinctions between T cell restricting determinants and allo-specific T cell recognition sites on
class I histocompatibility antigens have also been described in the mouse for both the H-2K^b and H-2D^d molecules
(29-31) revealing yet again the functional complexity of
the MHC both in its structure and function.

References

1. Zinkernagel, R.M. & Doherty, P.C. Nature 251, 547-548
   (1974).
2. McMichael, A.J., Ting, A., Zweerink, H.J. & Askonas,
   B.A. Nature 270, 524-526 (1977).
3. Rickinson, A.B., Wallace, L.E. & Epstein, M.A. Nature
   283, 865-867 (1980).
4. Biddison, W.E., Ward, F.E., Shearer, G.M. & Shaw, S.
   J. Immun. 124, 548-552 (1980).
5. Goulmy, E. et al. J. Exp. Med. 155, 1567-1572 (1982).
6. Gaston, J.S.H. et al. Immunogenetics 19, 475-485 (1984)
7. van der Poel, J.J., Pool, J., Goulmy, E. & van Rood,
   J.J. Immunogenetics 17, 599-608 (1983).
8. Wallace, L.E. et al. Cell. Immun. 67, 129-140 (1982).
9. Spits, H. de Vries, J.E. & Terhorst, C. Cell. Immun.
   59, 435-447 (1981).
10. Rickinson, A.B. et al. Cancer Res. 41, 4216-4221 (1981)
11. Wallace, L.E. et al. Eur. J. Immun. 12, 1012-1018
12. Moss, D.J., Wallace, L.E., Rickinson, A.B. & Epstein,
    M.A. Eur. J. Immun. 11, 686-693 (1981).
13. Misko, I.S., Moss, D.J. & Pope, J.H. Proc. Natn. Acad.
    Sci. U.S.A. 77, 4247-4250 (1980).
14. Wallace, L.E. et al. Eur. J. Immun. 11, 694-699 (1981).
15. Wallace, L.E., Rickinson, A.B., Rowe, M. & Epstein, M.A.
    Nature 297, 413-415 (1982).
16. Wallace, L.E., Rickinson, A.B. & Epstein, M.A.
    Transplant. Proc. 15, 196-199 (1983).
17. Gomard, E. et al., submitted for publication.
18. Lopez de Castro, J.A., Strominger, J.L., Strong, D.M.
    & Orr, H.T. Proc. natn. Acad. Sci. U.S.A. 79, 3813-
    3817 (1982).
19. Krangel, M.S. et al. Biochemistry 21, 6313-6321 (1982).
20. Krangel, M.S., Taketani, S., Pious, D. & Strominger,
    J.L. J. exp. Med. 157, 324-336 (1982).
21. Krangel, M.S., Biddison, W.E. & Strominger, J.L. J.
    Immun. 130, 1856-1862 (1983).
22. McMichael, A.J. Parham, P., Rust, N. & Brodsky, F.

Hum. Immun. 1, 121-129 (1980).

23. Wallace, L.E. et al., submitted for publication.
24. Gotch, F.M. et al. Immunogenetics, in press.
25. Biddison, W.E. et al. Hum. Immun. 3, 225-232 (1980).
26. Pfeffer, P.F. & Thorsby, E. Transplantation 33, 52-56 (1982).
27. Rowe, M. et al. Hum. Immun. 6, 151-165 (1983).
28. Barnstable, C.J. et al. Cell 14, 9-20 (1978).
29. Melief, C.J.M. et al. J. exp. Med. 151, 993-1013 (1980).
30. Sherman, L.A. J. Immun. 127, 1259-1260 (1981).
31. Potter, T.A., Palladino, M.A., Wilson, D.B. & Rajan, T. J. exp. Med. 158, 1061-1076 (1983).

SESSION III
Clones Recognizing Extrinsic Antigens

Chairpersons: B.R. Bloom and S. Kontiainen

This session of the meeting emphasized the hetero-geneity of T cell specificity and function. Human T cell clones with helper, proliferative or suppressor function with specificity for antigens as diverse as influenza virus, keyhole limpet haemocyanin, mycobacteria, tetanus toxoid and nickel were described. Dr Lamb analyzed cloned human helper T cells that were reactive with a 24 amino acid peptide from the carboxyl terminus of influenza haemagglutinin (HA-1). However analysis with peptide sub-fragments and structural isomers of this peptide have failed as yet to identify the epitope(s) critical in T cell antigen recognition. Dr Volkman described KLH-specific T cell clones that released multiple lymphokines (IL-2, BCDF, BCGF) and functioned as Class II restricted helper cells inducing IgG anti-KLH antibodies late after immunization. In addition he reported T cell clones specific for the parasite antigen, capable of inducing IgE production in autologous B cells.

Investigating the cellular response to mycobacterial antigens, Dr Rees reported both helper and suppressor T cell clones reactive with the same antigen (TB68). The helper T cell clone in addition to enhancing anti-mycobacterial antibody synthesis released a macrophage activating factor (MAF) which was distinct from γ-IFN. In contrast, the suppressor clone failed to secrete MAF but non specifically inhibited the proliferation of other T cells. Dr Geha working with tetanus toxoid specific T cell clones analysed antigen presentation by a variety of different cell types. It was noted that EBV transformed B cells were capable of presenting antigen to activated T cells which had no apparent dependency on interleukin-1 (IL-1) for proliferation. Similarly interferon γ induced HLA-DR+ fibroblasts were able to stimulate activated but not resting T cells. This data suggested differential activation requirements for activated and resting T cells, with the latter being best served by the monocyte/macrophage lineage.

In the final presentation in this session Dr Sinagaglia described the function and activation require-ments of T cell clones from patients with Nickel delayed type hypersensitivity. The T cell clones analyzed were of

115

the helper/inducer phenotype, secreted high levels of γIFN and induced antibody synthesis. Activation of the T cells required recognition of Nickel in association with the appropriate Class II determinants. EBV transformed B ells and Class II positive T cells were able to present Nickel to the T cell clones. This capacity of human T cell to interact directly with antigen in the absence of accessory cells is discussed in a later session (Session V).

In the experiments described in this session it is apparent that T cells are highly diverse in specificity and functional properties. As regards activation, the same is true as exemplified by the differential requirements of activated and resting T cells. However the concept that antigen is recognized in association with determinants encoded by the MHC of presenting cells appears in the majority of cases to be a general requirement (but see Session VIII). Nevertheless the physiochemical nature of this association or of the antigen component of this complex derived from "extrinsic" antigen is ill defined, and this remains an important issue in T cell receptor interactions with antigen.

ANTIGEN RECOGNITION BY HUMAN INFLUENZA VIRUS SPECIFIC

HELPER T LYMPHOCYTE CLONES

J.R. Lamb, M. Feldmann, N. Green*, R.A. Lerner*
and E.D. Zanders

Imperial Cancer Research Fund, Tumour Immunology Unit,
Department of Zoology, University College London, Gower
Street, London WC1E 6BT.

* Department of Molecular Biology, Research Institute of
Scripps Clinic, 10666 North Torrey Pines Road, La Jolla,
California 92037, U.S.A.

INTRODUCTION

T lymphocyte activation is dependent on the recognition of foreign antigen in assocation with determinants encoded by genes of the major histocompatibility complex (MHC)[1,2]. Although T cell antigen recognition is exquisitely sensitive to minor variation in antigenic structure[3,4], the precise nature of the epitope interacting with the T cell receptor is ill defined. The importance of primary amino acid sequence as opposed to the three dimensional conformation of antigen determinants in T cell recognition has been proposed based on the following experimental evidence. T cells, unlike B cells, are unable to discriminate between native and denatured proteins[5]. Furthermore, T cells reactive with small peptide antigens recognize the side chains, and single amino acid substitutions within these peptides that inhibited antibody binding had no effect on T cell responses[4,6]. More recent reports suggest that the three dimensional structure of the antigen epitope may determine T cell antigen recognition[7,8]. For example, analysis of the fine specificity of cloned insulin reactive T cell hybridomas

117

specificity of cloned insulin reactive T cell hybridomas revealed a group of clones that recognized a moiety composed of the amino acid sequence of the B chain and the A chain loop, suggesting recognition of tertiary structure[8].

The studies reported here investigate the influence of antigen tertiary conformation in the activation of human helper T lymphocytes. For this analysis we have used cloned human T lymphocytes reactive with carboxyl terminus (residues 306-329) of the Ha-1 molecule of influenza virus haemagglutinin (HA)[9].

MATERIALS AND METHODS

Peptide of the HA-1 moleucle of influenza haemagglutinin were synthesized according to the amino acid sequence of A/Hong Kong/X47[10]. The isolation and characterisation of the HA specific T cell clones has been reported in detail elsewhere[9,11].

RESULTS AND DISCUSSION

Recognition of peptides by HA induced T cell clones.

The determinants within the HA-1 molecule inducing proliferation of the HA specific T cell clones were identified using synthetic peptides. The cloned T cells were cultured with each of the peptides at concentrations ranging from 0.01 to 10 µg/ml in the presence of accessory cells. Clones HA1.4, 1.7 and 2.43 proliferated in response to stimulation with p20, but not the other peptides assayed (Table 1). All three clones also responded to the controls of HA and intact influenza virus. The T cell clone, HA2.61 responded to a determinant only present in peptide 11, failing to proliferate to the other peptides. In contrast HA3.18 while responding to HA and intact virus did not appear to recognize any of the peptides, suggesting that it may recognize a determinant either not coverd by the overlapping peptides or that resides in the HA-2 molecule (Table 1).

Using synthetic peptides of HA it has been possible to map the antigenic determinants recognized by the HA induced T cell clones, with the exception of HA3.18. Interestingly, the T cell clones (HA1.4, 1.7, 2.43 and 2.61) respond to determinants discrete from the four proposed antibody binding sites of HA[12]. For other antigens such as lysozyme[13] and myoglobin[14] T and B cells

TABLE 1

Specificity of HA induced clones for the synthetic peptides
of the HA-1 molecule

Synthetic peptides of HA-1 molecule		Antibody Binding Sites	Clone No.				
No.	Sequence		1.4	1.7	2.43	2.61	3.18
2	1-36		-	-	-	-	-
4	39-65		-	-	-	-	-
7	53-87	53-278(SiteC)	-	-	-	-	-
10	76-111		-	-	-	-	-
11	105-140		-	-	-	+	-
16	140-176	140-146(SiteA)	-	-	-	-	-
17	174-196	187-196(SiteB)	-	-	-	-	-
19	201-227	(SiteD)	-	-	-	-	-
21	266-282		-	-	-	-	-
22	282-303		-	-	-	-	-
20	306-329		+	+	+	-	-
HA			+	+	+	+	+
A/Texas			+	+	+	+	+
B/Singapore			-	-	-	-	-
Medium			-	-	-	-	-
IL-2			+	+	+	+	+

appear to recognize different determinants. It is possible
that HA3.18 may recognize the topographical B cell
determinant formed by the disulphide bond between Cys 52
and Cys 277[12], although this clone clearly cannot recognize
the other B cell sites which are covered by the peptides.

However the results reported here (Table 1) although
they distinguish between T and B cell antigen recognition,
fail to resolve whether T cell antigen recognition is
dependent on primary amino acid sequence or tertiary
structure. In an attempt to resolve this question the
response of cloned p20 reactive T cells to peptide
fragments and isomeric forms of p20 was determined.
Subunits of p20 were synthesized with the four carboxyterminal amino acids and increasing the subunit sequence
progressively by four amino acids until the intact 24 amino
acid peptide was synthesized (Fig. 1). Furthermore, larger

TABLE 2

Fine analysis of T cell antigen recognition with subunit
tetrapeptides of p20

Subunit peptides		Clone No.		
No.	Sequence	1.4	1.7	2.43
20_1	326–329	−	−	−
20_2	322–329	−	−	−
20_3	318–329	−	−	−
20_4	314–329	−	−	−
20_5	310–329	−	−	−
20	306–329	+	+	+
CNBR fragments		+	+	N.T.
CHYMO fragments		−	−	N.T.
A/Texas		+	+	+
Medium		−	−	−
IL-2		+	+	+

fragments of p20 were prepared by enzymatic cleavage with
chymotrypsin (residues 309–310) and cyanogen bromide
(residues 321–322). None of the three p20 reactive T cell
clones assayed responded to the tetrapeptide subunits of
p20 including 20_5 which lacks only the four residues at the
amino terminus. This is confirmed by the failure of
chymotrypsin fragments to induce proliferation. In
contrast the T cells of clones HA1.4 and 1.7 responded to
the cyanogen bromide fragments of p20 (Table 2). It is
also possible that amino acids at the amino terminus
determine a topographical epitope that is recognised by the
T cells. We are also unable to establish whether or not
there is an immunodominant site within p20 associated with
a particular residue such as residue 109 in sperm whale
myoglobin[14]. However the Tyr at 309 is a candidate for a
critical residue in T cell recognition in that radio-
iodinated (unlike titrated) p20 fails to bind to clone
HA1.7 or to induce a proliferative response. In addition,
neither the chymotrypsin fragments nor the subunit 20_5
stimulate proliferation. Finally within the intact HA
molecule the Tyr in p20 is an exposed residue.

The effects of optical rotation and inverted sequence on T cell antigen recognition.

If the antigenic epitopes recognized by T cells are determined predominantly by primary amino acid sequence and not by conformation it might be predicted that changing the optical rotation or inverting the amino acid sequence would have minimal effect on the immunogenicity of the antigen. To test this hypothesis the response of cloned T cells to p20 synthesized with L- or D-amino acids and with inverted sequence was investigated. The L- but not the D- form of p20 was able to induce T cells of cloned HA1.4 and 1.7 to prolfierate (Table 3). Similarly, it has been observed that the hapten azobenzenearsonate conjugated to Ficoll was only active if the peptide spacer contained one or more L-amino acids[16]. In addition neither the retro-L nor retro-D sequences of p20 were able to stimulate prolieration (Table 3). Therefore the order of residues appears to be critical and since both peptides are symmetrical with respect to lys at positions 308 and 327 (Fig. 1) it would seem that these amino acids do not determine antigne recognition for either of the T cell clones assayed. Thomas et al[17] observed that T cells primed with the fibrinopeptide Bβ7-14 failed to respond when challenged with the inverted form of the peptide.

CONCLUSION

The T cell clones induced with HA recognize determinants within the HA-1 molecule distinct from the antibody binding sites. T cell clones (HA1.4 and 1.7)

TABLE 3

Clonal specificity for Structural Isomers of p20

Isomers of p20	Clone No.	
	1.4	1.7
L amino acids	+	+
D amino acids	−	−
Retro-L-p20	−	−
Retro-D-p20	−	−

reactive with p20 (residues 306-329) were analyzed for fine specificity using enzyme cleavage fragments and tetrapeptide subunits of p20. The CNBR fragments suggested that the determinant recognized by the cloned T cells resided within the sequence 306-321, however even with the subunits the epitope could not be more precisely defined. In an attempt to distinguish whether the cloned T cells recognized primary sequence or tertiary structure the optical rotation of p20 was altered or the sequence inverted. Neither the optically roated (D-amino acis) nor the inverted peptide were able to induce proliferation suggesting that the ordering of the residues is critical. This dependency on the order of residues implies that T cells exhibit polarity in antigen recognition. This could be achieved if one sequence of the peptide associated with self MHC Class II determinants thus establishing the correct orientation of the residues recognized by the T cell.

REFERENCES

1. Zinkernagel, R.M. and Doherty, P.C. Adv. Immunol. 27, 51-77 (1968).
2. Klein, J. and Nagy, Z.A. Adv. Cancer Res. 37, 233-317 (1982).
3. Hedrick, S.M. et al. Cell. 30, 141-152 (1982).
4. Thomas, D.W., Hsieh, K.H., Schauster, J.L., Mudd, M.S. and Wilner, G.D. J. Exp. Med. 152, 620-632 (1980).
5. Chestnut, R.W., Endres, R.O. and Grey, H.M. Clin. Immunol. Immunopathol. 15, 397 (1980).
6. Thomas, D.W., Hsieh, H.H., Schwartz, J.H. and Wilner, G.D. J. Exp. Med. 153, 583-594 (1980).
7. Buchnauller, Y. and Corradin, G. Eur. J. Immunol. 12, 412-416 (1982).
8. Glimcher, L.H., Shroer, J.A., Chan, C. and Shevach, E.M. J. Immunol. 131, 2868-2874 (1983).
9. Lamb, J.R., Eckels, D.D., Lake, P., Woody, J.N. and Green, N. Nature 300, 66-69 (1982).
10. Green, N. et al. Cell 28, 477-487 (1982).
11. Lamb, J.R. and Green, N. Immunology 50, 659-667 (1983).
12. Wiley, D.C., Wilson, I.A., Skehel, J.J. Nature 289, 373-378 (1981).
13. Adorini, L., Harvey, M.A., Miller, A. and Sercarz, E.E. J. Exp. Med. 150, 293-306 (1979).

14. Berkower, I., Buckenmeyer, G.K., Gurd, F.R.N. and
     Berkofsky, J.A.   Proc. Natl. Acad. Sci. USA.
     79, 4723-7727 (1982).
15. Zanders, E.D., Feldmann, M., Green, N. and Lamb, J.R.
     Eur. J. Immunol. (in press).
16. Komatsu, T., Lawn, C.Y., Amsden, A. and Leskowitz, S.
     J. Immunol. **130**, 586-590 (1983).
17. Thomas, D.W., Hoffman, M.D. and Wilner, G.D. J. Exp.
     Med. **156**, 289-293 (1982).

FIGURE 1

Primary amino acid sequence of p20, inverted p20 and subfragments

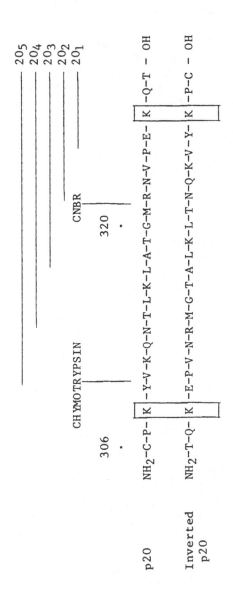

EXOGENOUS IL-2 INDEPENDENT ANTIGEN-SPECIFIC HUMAN T CELLS: ANTIGEN-SPECIFIC INDUCTION OF POLYCLONAL B CELL FACTORS

David J. Volkman, Thomas B. Nutman, Eric A. Ottesen,

and Anthony S. Fauci

National Institute of Allergy and Infectious Diseases,

National Institutes of Health, Bethesda, Maryland 20205

INTRODUCTION

The development of antigen-specific T lymphocyte lines and clones has greatly facilitated the investigation of the mechanisms by which T cells recognize foreign antigens and subsequently elaborate immuoregulatory lymphokines. Human antigen-specific helper T cell lines and clones have now been developed by the method of cyclic restimulation with antigen[1,2] which are completely independent of exogenous interleukin-2 (IL-2) for their growth. Following a narrowly restricted stimulation signal with the appropriate antigen in the context of histocompatible antigen-presenting cells (APC), these T cells can produce several polyclonal B cell factors which act on discrete subsets of B cells depending on their state of activation or receptiveness to these lymphokines.

In the present study, T cells specific for two kinds of antigen were utilized. T cells specific for the antigen keyhole limpet hemocyanin (KLH) were developed from donors immunized with this protein. Similarly, T cells specific for a microfilial parasitic antigen were developed from a patient who had recovered from naturally acquired infection[3]. The effect of the T cells themselves and of lymphokines produced by these T cells on various B cell populations was described.

125

MATERIAL AND METHODS

Antigens and immunization. Normal volunteers were
immunized with KLH with a 5 mg subcutaneous injection
followed by a 5 mg boost 2 weeks later[4]. Brugia malayi
adult antigen (BMA) was prepared as a saline extract of
adult parasites[3]. The patient from whom BMA-specific T
cells were obtained had had biopsy-proven loiasis
accompanied by angioedema, high grade eosinophilia, and
elevated levels of serum IgE. She had been successfully
treated with diethylcarbamazine prior to study.

Cell separations. Peripheral blood mononuclear cells
(MNC) were purified by Hypaque-Ficoll sedimentation.
Aliquots of cells were cryopreserved for subsequent use as
APC.

Culture and cloning procedure. The cyclic stimulation
and rest method for preparing antigen-specific T cells was
used[2]. Briefly, MNC were initially cultured with antigen at
a density of 5×10^6 per well of a 24-well cluster dish.
After 5 days of stimulation, viable cells were removed and
cultured with fresh irradiated MNC in the absence of antigen
for 10 to 12 days in a rest cycle. Alternate cycles of rest
and restimulation using fresh irradiated MNC at each step
were repeated until antigen-specific line was obtained.
Cloning was accomplished by limiting dilution. Viable T
cells were seeded at 0, 0.3, 1, 3, and 10 cells per well in
a 96-well u-bottom microtiter dish. Each well also
contained 5×10^4 irradiated MNC, antigen, and suboptimal
amounts of IL-2. Positive wells were scored at 10 to 12
days, picked, and expanded by cyclic stimulation in the
absence of exogenous IL-2. Cloning efficiencies were
usually greater than 30%.

Lymphokine assays. IL-2 was measured using the murine
IL-2 dependent T cell line HT-2. Cells were incubated with
factors for 16 hours then pulsed for 4 hours with
[3H]thymidine. B cell growth factor (BCGF) was assayed
using anti-μ stimulated human B cells as previously
described[5], and B cell differentiation factor (BCDF) was
assayed using the ability of CESS cells to respond to BCDF
by increasing IgG production[6].

ELISA for supernatant immunoglobulin. Antigen-specific
and polyclonal supernatant IgG and IgM were measured as
previously described[4] using an ELISA assay system. IgE was
measured using an avidin-biotin modified ELISA which was
highly specific for IgE, as previously described[7].

RESULTS

Antigen-specific T cell lines were developed as
described above. After several cycles of stimulation and
rest, the number of T cells was found to increase 5 to 15
times with each antigen stimulation cycle. These lines were
maintained in the complete absence of exogenous IL-2 and
were found to elaborate multiple lymphokines following
antigen stimulation. The characteristics of these
antigen-specific T cell lines are outlined in Table 1.
Without any other selection procedure except cyclic
restimulation with antigen, the lines were noted to be
composed almost exclusively of T4 positive cells. Following
4 stimulations, the lines were cloned by limiting dilution.
The characteristics of the clones were as follows: they
were greater than 90% antigen specific, they all were
capable of producing IL-2 when stimulated with antigen, and
each clone recognized antigen only in the context of
allogeneic APC sharing one or the other of the parental Ia
haplotypes.

The ability of these T cell clones to produce B cell
specific lymphokines was next investigated. One

TABLE 1
CHARACTERISTICS OF ANTIGEN-SPECIFIC T CELL LINES

1. Maintained for more than 5 months in the absence of
   exogenous IL-2.
2. Greater than 95% of cells are T4 positive.
3. Greater than 90% of cells proliferate specifically to
   antigen/Ia stimulation.
4. Each clone derived from the specific line produces
   supernatant IL-2 following antigen/Ia stimulation.
5. Each clone is restricted in its response to one or the
   other parental Ia haplotype.

KLH-specific clone, shown in Table 2, was capable of
producing significant amounts of both BCGF and BCDF in
addition to IL-2. Of note, all 3 lymphokines were produced
only in response to antigen and in the presence of APC.

The ability of these specific T cells to provide help
for antigen-specific Ig production by B cells was next
examined. Table 3 shows the results of culture specific T
cells with autologous B cells obtained from a recently
immunized individual. As few as 100 T cells stimulated IgM
anti-KLH production in the absence of antigen. Only 500
specific T cells stimulated about half the maximal anti-KLH
response seen with PWM without the marked polyclonal IgM
production seen with PWM. Almost no IgG anti-KLH synthesis
was seen at this early point. Similar anti-KLH IgM
responses could be seen using tetanus toxoid specific T
cells, or using soluble lymphokines in the complete absence
of T cells (data not shown). The data suggest that
responsive KLH-specific B cells were stimulated by small
amounts of T cell factors to progress to terminal
differentiation and KLH-specific IgM secretion without the
need of direct T-B interaction.

TABLE 2

MULTIPLE LYMPHOKINES PRODUCED BY A SINGLE
KLH-SPECIFIC T CELL CLONE

Source of supernatant	APC	KLH	Lymphokine		
			IL-2* (cpm)	BCGF† (cpm)	BCDF† (PFC)
Medium alone	+	+	493	3,053	0
T cell clone	+	-	554	2,904	20
T cell clone	+	+	40,032	16,742	546

*Aliquot of supernatant removed at day 1 for IL-2 assay.
†Supernatants assayed after 5 days for B cell factors.

TABLE 3
HELPER FUNCTION OF KLH-SPECIFIC T CELLS FOR
B CELLS FROM RECENTLY IMMUNIZED DONOR

Culture conditions*		Anti-KLH (u/ml)	Supernatant IgM Total (ng/ml)
Medium alone		6	90
KLH-specific			
T cells	10^2	18	110
	5×10^2	46	130
	10^3	51	140
10^4 autologous T cells			
+ PWM		102	5,100

*AET-treated negative autologous B cells (1.25×10^5) used
in cultures. No KLH was present.

The ability of antigen-specific T cells to provide
specific help was reevaluated 8 months following
immunization at a time when the nature of antigen-specific B
cells in the peripheral blood B cell populations had
markedly altered. The results are shown in Table 4. At
this point, cells able to produce IgG anti-KLH are
detectable. Unlike early IgM anti-KLH B cells, these IgG
cells are stimulated to produce antibody in response to
antigen-specific T cells only in the presence of small
amounts of KLH. This anti-KLH IgG production is greater
than that seen with PWM/T cell stimulation and is not
accompanied by the polyclonal Ig production seen with PWM.
Specific IgM synthesis is not stimulated by the specific T
cells, although IgM anti-KLH can still be elicited by PWM
stimulation of non-KLH specific T cell help. This system of
IgG anti-KLH induction appears similar to the in vitro human
B cell responses reported for influenza[9]. Of note, although
the induction of help in specific T cells is Ia restricted
(data not shown), the factors produced by these T cells have
proven to be polyclonal (similar to the T cell clone shown
in Table 2), having BCGF and/or BCDF activity in assays
using polyclonal B cells.

TABLE 4
HELPER FUNCTION OF KLH-SPECIFIC T CELLS FOR B CELLS
FROM DONOR IMMUNIZED 8 MONTHS PREVIOUSLY

Culture conditions*	KLH (10 ng/ml)	Anti-KLH (u/ml)		Total (ng/ml)	
		IgG	IgM	IgG	IgM
Medium alone	+	30	4	200	300
400 KLH-specific T cells	-	20	6	350	100
400 KLH-specific T cells	+	310	2	500	150
10^4 autologous T cells + PWM	-	180	105	6,000	5,700

*AET-negative autologous B cells (1.25×10^5) used in cultures.

The concept of inducing T cells with specific antigen to secrete lymphokines which act polyclonally on a distinct subset of B lymphocytes was further explored with parasite-specific T cells. As shown in Table 5, BMA-specific T cells stimulated polyclonal IgE only when stimulated with antigen in the context of autologous APC. Allogeneic APC sharing the Ia restriction element could be substituted for autologous cells. Cell free supernatants from stimulated T cells were also potent enhancers of IgE production in isolated B cells. Of note, supernatants stimulated IgE production in B cells from allogeneic donors independent of the donors' Ia tissue type or previous parasite exposure (data not shown). Once again, T cells were specifically induced to produce B cell factors that could act polyclonally on a discrete subset of B cells (IgE producers).

DISCUSSION

Human antigen-specific T cells of defined function now provide an important tool for delineating T-B interactions and for examining the mechanisms by which T cells stimulate different subsets of B cells to produce immunoglobulin.

TABLE 5
BMA-SPECIFIC T CELLS AND T CELL SUPERNATANTS
INDUCE IgE PRODUCTION IN AUTOLOGOUS B CELLS

Culture conditions*	Supernatant IgE (pg/ml)
Medium alone	< 100
BMA-specific T cells	450
BMA-specific T cells + BMA	13,800
Supernatant from stimulated BMA-specific T cells	11,450

*AET-negative B cells (1.25×10^5) were cultured as indicated.
†Supernatants were generated using 10^6 T cells, 4×10^6 APC, and BMA. Supernatant was used at 20% in B cell cultures.

These antigen-specific T cell lines and clones which produce their own IL-2 also elaborate B cell growth and differentiation factors when stimulated with antigen. The ability of various T cells to provide B cell help appears to depend on the availability of the appropriate subset of B cells.

After KLH immunization, distinct subsets of KLH-specific B cells are apparent in peripheral blood. Earliest to appear are the B cells that spontaneously secrete anti-KLH. These are followed by the preactivated B cells that need only weak T cell factors to progress to anti-KLH production. The necessary lymphokines can be provided by KLH-specific or other antigen-specific T cells or by cell-free supernatants. IgM anti-KLH is the predominant isotype seen in these earlier responses. At a later time, an antigen-specific B cell appears in the circulation which is unresponsive to lymphokines alone, but is capable of producing relatively large quantities of IgG anti-KLH when stimulated with KLH-specific T cells and small amounts of KLH. This KLH-specific help is not accompanied by polyclonal stimulation and is mediated by as few as 400 cells. Furthermore, the B cell help was HLA-Ia restricted in contrast to the early IgM anti-KLH help which could be delivered by polyclonal B cell factors.

Although the IgG anti-KLH response was dependent on both KLH-specific T cells and antigen, the T cells themselves were found to produce nonspecific polyclonal B cell factors. The ability of antigen-specific T cells to provide B cell help to the mature subset of antigen-specific B cells may well depend on the capacity to deliver B cell active lymphokines to B cells focused in close proximity by T cell recognition of antigen/Ia on B cell surfaces.

T cells specific for the parasite antigen BMA similarly act on a responsive subset of B cells, i.e., B cells which produce IgE antibodies. BMA-specific T cells obtained from a donor who was naturally infected with the related parasite and had had high levels of serum IgE, were found to secrete potent polyclonally active IgE stimulating factors when specifically induced. The factors themselves were neither antigen-specific nor HLA-restricted in their action. Factors from KLH-specific T cells did not enhance IgE production in isolated B cells.

Together these observations point to a mechanism by which T cells are highly specific in their induction but express polyclonal factors once induced. The effect of these factors depends on the character and proximity of responsive B cells.

REFERENCES

1. Kishimoto, M. & Fathman, C. G. J. exp. Med. 152, 759-770 (1982).
2. Volkman, D. J., Matis, L. A. & Fauci, A. S. Cell. Immunol. (in the press).
3. Nutman, T. B., Ottesen, E. A., Fauci, A. S. & Volkman, D. J. J. Clin. Invest. 73, 1754-1762 (1984).
4. Sredni, B., Volkman, D., Schwartz, R. H. & Fauci, A. S. Proc. natl. Acad. Sci. U.S.A. 78, 1858-1862 (1981).
5. Muraguchi, A. & Fauci, A. S. J. Immunol. 129, 1104-1108 (1982).
6. Muraguchi, A., Kishimoto, T., et al. J. Immunol. 127, 412 (1981).

7.   Nutman, T. B., Volkman, D. J., Hussain, R., Fauci,
     A. S. & Ottesen, E. A. J. Immunol. (in the press).
8.   Lamb, J. R., Woody, J. N., Hartzman, R. J. & Eckels,
     D. D. J. Immunol. 129, 1465-1470 (1982).

Probing a repertoire of T cells responding to a

mycobacterial antigen

Ann D.M. Rees, Glenda L. Knott, Paul N. Nelson, Nicola
Dobson, Ruth Mathews and Peter W. Andrew.

MRC unit for the laboratory studies of tuberculosis

Royal Postgraduate Medical School LONDON W12 OHS.

Following infection, Mycobacterium tuberculosis may often
persist in host tissues for years.   This prolonged interaction may result in a dynamic equilibrium between host
and parasite.   The situation can be disturbed with re-
activation of the infection.   Ability to clone T cells and
sustain them in long term culture allows the study of T
cells in vitro.   These studies can be used to understand
the nature of the equilibrium between host and parasite.
We have studied T cell immunity to M. tuberculosis by
using a mycobacterial antigen purified by absorbance to a
monoclonal (mab) to raise T cell clones.   The mab, TB68,
bound to antigenic determinant(s) in all strains of
M. tuberculosis and M. bovis BCG and vallee [1].   T cell
clones were generated from peripheral blood mononuclear
cells (PBMC) of a normal BCG vaccinated individual [2].
Clonality was established by sub-cloning as previously
described [3].   Clones of both helper/inducer (leu 1,3$^+$,
OKT4$^+$) and suppressor/cytotoxic (leu 1,2$^+$) phenotype were
generated and examples of both will be discussed.   All of
these clones were found to be positive for the antigen
recognised by the mab leu 8a.   The antigenic specificity
of individual clones was determined by co-culturing clone
cells with feeders and a variety of antigenic preparations, some of which are known to contain, at least in
part, determinants of the eliciting antigen [4].   The mab
TB68 also bound to PPD (Harboe, personal communication).
Table 1 shows that all clones responded vigorously to the
TB68 antigen.   Two of the clones, 68.1 and 68.7.9, also

135

Table 1.   Antigenic specificity of T cell clones.

Antigen.	Dose mg/L	Presence of TB68 antigen	Clone no		
			68.1	68.2	68.7.9
Escherichia Coli	10^{-2}	–	1946	1711	456
M. Kansasii	10^{-1}	–	1361	1083	501
M. fortuitum	10^{-1}	–	1451	975	498
TB72 antigen	10^{-1}	–	1616	1460	432
M. tuberculosis *	10^{-1}	+	15,016	12,998	9917
M. bovis BCG	10^{-1}	+	8015	881	8216
P.P.D.	10^{-1}	+	9882	1601	9362
TB68 antigen	10^{-3}	+	16,748	14,036	10,242
Medium			548	1530	412
IL2.			13,849	10,961	3026

* Strain H37Rv

10^5 T cell clones were stimulated with TB68 or other antigens at previously determined optimal concentrations. Other antigens were a similarily purified protein antigen TB72, or mycobacterial pressates4. Clone cells were tested for in vitro proliferative responses 4 days after the addition of IL2, feeders and antigen. They were then cultured with 10 antologous irradiated (3000 rads) PBMC and antigen for 48h in microterasaki plates[5]. Stimulation was by the incorporation of ^{3}H Thymidine.

responded to other antigenic preparations, but only to
those which contained determinants of the TB 68 antigen
ie PPD, M.tuberculosis H37Rv, and M.bovis BCG. Clone
68.2, on the other hand, did not respond to preparations
of M.bovis BCG or PPD, which do contain the TB68 antigen.
In addition a clone has also been described previously [2]
which proliferates to the entire range of antigenic preparations including those which do not contain the TB 68
antigen. Thus, clones were generated with specificity for
different epitopes in the TB 68 antigen. Some of these
showed similar species distribution to the determinants
identified in binding studies with the mab TB 68 (68.1 and
68.7.9); some (68.2) were more restricted; and some less.

   The effect of the products of these clones on various
target cells was determined using clone culture supernatants (s/n).   In order to avoid ambiguities introduced
by other elements in the clone culture, these were
fractionated with high performance liquid chromatography
(HPLC) [5].   Where this is not the case, a sham control
was included, consisting of all components of the clone
culture (except clone cells) with irradiated (3000 rads)
PBMC cultured for 3-5 days.
1. Macrophages.   An obvious target cell for clones with
specificity for a mycobacterial antigen is the macrophage.
Killing of intracellular organisms is the final stage of
macrophage activation [6]. Mouse macrophages activated
with a crude supernatant from PPD stimulated mouse spleen
killed M.microti [7]. This killing was probably due to
hydrogen peroxide (H_2O_2) released in increased amounts by
activated macrophages. The measurement of H_2O_2 release is
a more rapid and convenient test of macrophage activation
than microbicidal function and was, therefore, used to
observe the affect of clone s/n on macrophages.   A human
macrophage-like cell line U937, which can be
immunologically activated to express antimicrobial
immunity [8], was used as the target cell. Table 2 shows
that both of the helper/inducer clone s/n enhanced H_2O_2
production at concentrations as low as 0.3%. This
activity was not dependant on using U937 cells, as the
same enhancement was observed in macrophages matured from
peripheral blood monocytes [2]. The macrophage activating
factor(MAF) secreted by the clones has been shown to be
distinct from IFNγ [5], present at low levels in the clone
s/n, both antigenically, and by molecular weight analysis.
This indicated that there might be a number of different
MAF(s), and raised the possibility, also suggested in

Table 2 Capacity of T cell clones to secrete macrophage activating factor

Dilution of supernatant	Clone no. or preparation			
	nmol H_2O_2 per 10^6 U937 cells (mean $\pm$ SD)			
	68.1	68.2	68.7.9	Sham
30 – 50%	21.1 + 1.5	19.9 + 0.9	4.0 + 0.5	4.5 + 1.0
10	21.0 + 1.3	20.4 + 1.5	5.3 + 0.7	7.9 + 4.2
3	18.7 + 3.8	18.3 + 2.0	1.2 + 0.3	2.3 + 2.3
0.3	14.4 + 1.7	12.0 + 1.7	ND	2.6 + 1.0
0.03	2.9 + 1.0	1.3 + 0.6	ND	0

10^6 U937 cells were cultured in the presence and absence of cloned T cell supernatants, or sham control[2] (a supernatant prepared from identical cultures but in the absence of cloned T cells). Medium or supernatants were replaced at 24h intervals for 3 days. Peroxide release was determined in the presence of PMA[6]. Results are given as nMol. H_2O_2 per 10^8 U937 cells minus the values obtained for comparable cultures in the absence of supernatants.

Affect of clone s/n on IgG synthesis

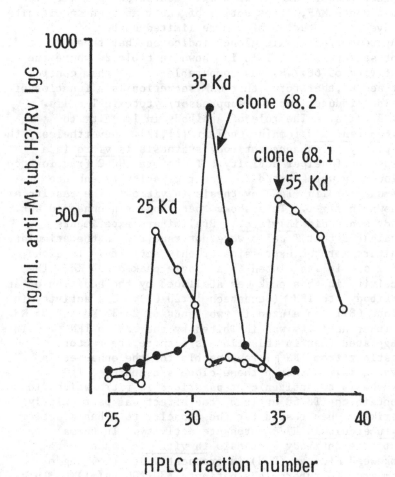

Figure 1. Human PBMC were cultured in vitro[17] with either Pokeweed Mitogen (Gibco biocult 3mg/L) or 10% of fractions of clone 68.1 (-0-) or clone 68.2 (-●-) supernatants collected from HPLC[5]. Supernatants from these cultures were assayed for anti M.tuberculosis strain H37RV expressate[5] activity using ELISA.

other work [eg 9, 10], that they might have selective
effects on macrophage activation.   Twenty-five other
helper/inducer clones were also tested and all were found
to secrete MAF, irrespective of their antigen specificity.
Conversely, studies of a more limited number of
suppressor/cytotoxic clones indicated that these cells did
not secrete MAF.   This is shown in table 2, where the
activity of 68.7.9. was comparable to the sham control.
It seems ,therefore, that MAF secretion is a function of
helper/inducer but not suppressor/cytotoxic T cells.
2. B cells.   The role of antibody in immunity to
M.tuberculosis remains unclear [11,12].   Nevertheless, the
capacity to enhance antibody synthesis in vitro is a
measure of helper activity.   Therefore, HPLC fractionated
clone s/n were tested for their capacity to enhance
immunoglobulin (IgG) synthesis in vitro.   The results are
shown in fig 1.   This shows that clone s/n enhanced antibody synthesis in vitro.   Preliminary experiments
indicated that T cells were not required in the stimulated
culture for the expression of this activity.   In clone
68.2 s/n it was eluted in a single peak of 35 Kd.   The
activity in this peak was abolished by the addition of an
antibody to IFNγ(Genentech 12:20 C8).   The activity in
clone 68.1 s/n eluted in two bands of 25-32 Kd and 55 Kd.
Neither activity was inhibited by the mab to IFNγ.   This
suggested that in this clone s/n there are factors
distinct from IFNγ, responsible for the enhanced IgG
synthesis.   Although these clone s/n enhanced IgG
synthesis to antigenic preparations in vitro which did not
contain the TB 68 antigen, the effect was particularly
striking when tested for the capacity to enhance anti-
M.tuberculosis H37RV pressate activity.   In normal
subjects antibody synthesis in vitro in response to
Pokeweed Mitogen (PWM) is frequently low (0-40 ng/ml)
compared to tuberculous patients (30-200 ng/ml).   This
suggests that in normal subjects a signal, supplied in
vitro by the clone s/n, may be absent.   This signal can
be supplied by IFN γ or other factors.   Regardless of the
nature of the factor, it does appear that these T cell
clones have helper activity.
3.   T cells. As both helper/inducer and suppressor
/cytotoxic clones were generated, it was of interest to
determine how they might affect T cell growth and,
therefore, act as regulatory cells.   In preliminary
experiments clone 68.1 s/n was found to have no affect on
either mitogen or antigen-induced proliferation in

IL2 production by T cell clones

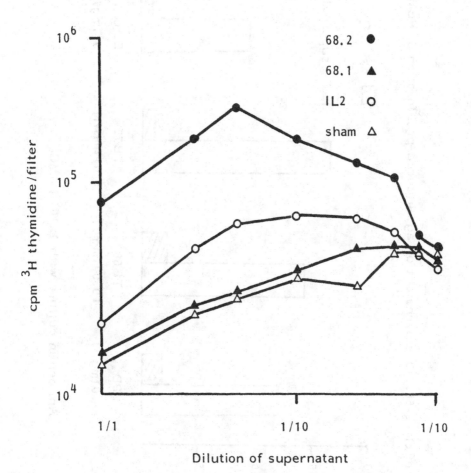

Fig 2. IL2 dependant PHA lymphoblasts were prepared as previously described [13]. They were then incubated with a range of concentrations or either clone 68.2 (●); or 68.1 (▲) supernatants; the sham control supernatant (△); or IL2 ○ (Lymphocult T lectin free Biotest folex) in microterasaki plates [14] for 24h at $37^{\circ}C$ in a 5% CO_2/O_2 incubated. After 4h stimulation was determined by [3]H Thymidine incorporation. The results are expressed as the mean cpm of triplicate cultures.

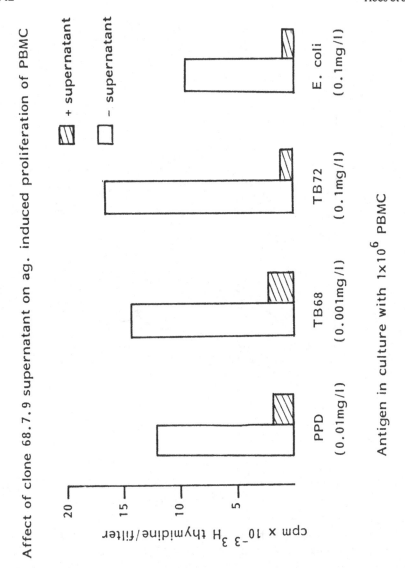

Fig 3. Supernatants from clone 68.7.9 cultures were cultured with PBMC and antigen at specified concentrations for 7 days in a microterasaki culture. ^{3}H Thymidine incorporation was then determined. The mean cpm of triplicate cultures in the presence and absence of clone cultures is shown.

heterologous PBMC.   Conversely clone 68.2 s/n
considerably enhanced both. To determine whether this
affect could be attributed to Interleukin 2 (IL2), these
clone s/n were tested on IL2 dependant lymphoblastoid cell
lines [13]. It was found (Fig 2), that the enhancement of
proliferative response by clone 68.2 s/n was due to IL2.
Clone 68.1 does not produce IL2 and had no affect on
proliferation. This differential production of IL2 was
reflected in the differing growth requirements of the two
clones, clone 68.2 requiring little exogenous IL2 for
optimal growth in contrast to clone 68.1.
In contrast, the suppressor/cytotoxic clone s/n strongly
inhibited antigen-induced proliferation (Fig 3).   This
effect was non-specific in that the response to all
antigens was similarly inhibited. This effect could also
be mediated by clone 68.7.9 cells acting on a helper
/inducer clone 68.1. As additional clone 68.1 cells
failed to have this effect, it could not be attributed to
competition for IL2. Thus the antigen specific suppressor
/cytotoxic clones had a regulatory effect on the
proliferation of helper/MAF producing T cell clones.   The
exact mechanism of this suppression remains to be
established.
In summary, 3 human T cell clones of both helper/inducer
(68.1 and 68.2) and suppressor/cytotoxic (68.7.9)
phenotype, with specificity for a mycobacterial antigen TB
68 have been described.   The helper/inducer clones can
secrete multiple lymphokines which affect different target
cells.   They enhanced B cell activity although this was
achieved by 3 different lymphokines. They secreted MAF
and one, 68.2, secreted IL2.   The suppressor/cytotoxic
clone, on the other hand, did not secrete MAF, and did not
have any affect on antibody synthesis.   The most striking
effect of this clone was on other T cells.   It non-
specifically inhibited proliferation either through the
secretion of a lymphokine or by direct interaction with a
helper/inducer clone.   It seemed, therefore, that this
clone is much more restricted in its targets than the
helper/inducer clones. Although these clones were clearly
reacting to different epitopes in the TB68 antigen, it is
of interest to note that the response to this antigen
appears to result in a regulatory network.   If the
suppressor determinants in the TB 68 antigen can be
identified then, using them as probes, we may begin to
understand the role of suppression in M.tuberculosis
infection.   This is turn might permit us to manipulate

Affect of clone 7.9 cells on clone 68.1 proliferation

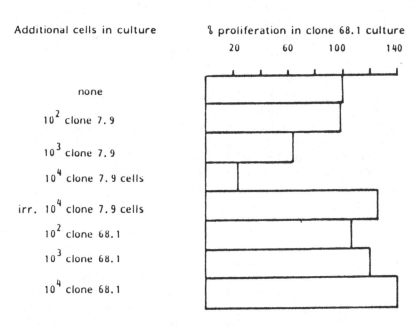

Fig 4. 10^5/ml clone 68.1 cells were cultured in a microterasaki plate[9] with 0.07 mg/L TB68 antigen and 5% irradiated autologous PBMC in the presence or absence of graded doses of clone 68.7.9 cells; irradiated (3000 rads) clone 68.7.9 cells or additional clone 68.1 cells for 24h. ^{3}H Thymidine incorporation was then determined. The results are expressed as a percentage of the proliferation in control culture (clone 68.1 cells 10^5/ml).

the immune system to preferentially generate favourable responses.

1.   Coates, A.R.M., Hewitt, J., Allen, B.W., Ivanyi, J. & Mitchison, D.A. Lancet **11**, 167-169 (1981).
2.   Mathews, R., scoging, A. & Rees, A.D.M. Immun. in press.
3.   Lamb, J. R., Eckels, D.D., Lake, P., Johnson, A.H., Hartzman, R.J. & Woody, J.N. J. Immun. **128**, 233-238 (1982).
4.   Hewitt, J., Coates, A.R.M., Mitchison, D.A. & Ivanyi, J. J.Immun. Methods **55**, 205-211 (1982).
5.   Andrew, P.W., Rees, A.D.M., Scoging, A., Dobson, N., Mathews, R., Whittal, J. T., Coates, A.R.M. & Lowrie, D.B. Eur. J. Immun. in press.
6.   Cohn, Z.A. J. Immun. **121**, 813-816 (1978).
7.   Walker, L. & Lowrie, D.B. Nature **293**, 69-71 (1981).
8.   Wing, E.J., Koren, H.S., Fischer, D.G. & Kelley, V. J. Reticuloendoth. Soc. **29**, 328-   (1982).
9.   Ratliff, T.L., Thomasson, D.L., McCool, R.E. & Catalona, W.T. Cell. Immun. **68**, 311-321 (1982).
10. Schreiber, R.D., Altman, A. & Katz, D.H. J. Exp. Med. **156**, 677-689 (1982).
11. Mackaness, G.B. J. Exp. Med. **129**, 973-992 (1969).
12, Lowrie, D.B. Trans. of the Royal Soc. of Trop. Med. **77** (5), 646-655 (1983).
13. Grimm, E.A. & Rosenburg, S.A. in Isolation, characterization utilization of T lymphocyte clones (eds. C. Garrison Fathman 7 F.W. Fitch) Academic Press, New York. pp 57-82, (1982).
14. Moir, D.J., Ghosh, A.K., Abdulaziz, Z., Knight, P.M. Mason, D.Y. Brit. J. Haem. **55**, 395-410 (1983).
15. O'Brien, J., Knight, S., Quock, N.A., Moore, E.H. & Platt, A.S. J. Immun. Methods **27**, 219-223 (1979).
16. Jackett, P.S., Andrew, P.W., Aber,V.R. & Lowrie, D.B. J. Exp. Path. **62** 419-428 (1981).
17. Callard, R.E. Nature **282**, 734-736. (1979).

ACCESSORY CELL REQUIREMENTS FOR THE PROLIFERATION OF ANTIGEN SPECIFIC HUMAN T CELLS

Raif S. Geha

Depart. of Pediatrics, Harvard Medical School

300 Longwood Avenue, Boston, MA 02115

INTRODUCTION

The availability of antigen specific human T cell clones has provided the tools to investigate the mechanisms of triggering activated T cells by antigen. In this review we will show that several types of cells e.g. monocytes, B cell lines and fibroblasts can trigger antigen specific proliferation of human T cell clones. The requirements for this triggering differ from those of freshly isolated human peripheral blood T cells particularly in regard to interleukin-1. The results presented suggest that whereas several cell types can successfully present antigen to a previously activated T cell, only certain cells such as monocytes/macrophages may be.

MATERIALS AND METHODS

Antigens and Antibodies

Tetanus toxoid (TT) and diphtheria toxoid (DT) were obtained from the Massachusetts Biological Laboratories, Boston, MA. Hybrid antibody to TT and to human IgM was described as in reference 1.

Human IL-1 and Rabbit Anti-IL-1

IL-1/LP was prepared as previously described (2). One

147

unit of activity is defined as that amounts of IL-1 required to double the proliferative response of mouse
thymocytes stimulated with 1 ug/ml of phytohemagglutinin
alone.

Rabbit antibody to human IL-1 (anti IL-1) was prepared, heat treated (56°C, 1 hour), and adsorbed with
human preipheral blood mononuclear cells (PBMC) as
described in reference 2.

Preparation of Cell Populations Monocytes Depleted PBMC

Monocytes. Adherent cells were recovered from Ficoll
Hypaque isolated PBMC by adherence over Petri dishes as
previously described (2).

T Cells. Monocyte free PBMC were rosetted with sheep
erythrocytes, the red cells were lysed and the lymphocytes
were passed over nylon wool and subsequently treated with
monoclonal anti-Ia and complement twice.

B cells. Non-adherent PBMC were passed twice through
a Sephadex G-10 column and further treated with OKM1 and
complement as described (1). They contained 90% surface
Ig cells and 0.3% OKM1+ cells.

EBV-B Cells. B cell lines transformed with EBV were
derived as described in reference 1.

Adsorption of T Cells on Monolayers of TT Pulsed Monocytes or B Cells

This was performed as described in reference 1.

Fibroblast Cultures

Fibroblast lines were derived from skin punch biopsies,
grown to confluency, trypsinized and transferred to tissue
culture flasks as previously described (3).

Preparation of T Cell Clones

TT specific lymphocyte clones were produced by
limiting dilution as described in references 1-4 for
influenza specific clones. Briefly, PBMC were stimulated
with TT (30 ug/ml, 10^6 cells/ml) for 6 days. Dividing

cells were then enriched by centrifugation over a Percoll
(Pharmacia, Uppsala, Sweden) discontinuous gradient at
1500 rpm for 45 minutes. Cells at the 30-50% interface
were cultured in RPMI 1640 at limiting dilution (0.3 cell/
well) with autologous irradiated PBMC. Cultures received
fresh IL-2 containing supernatants every 2-3 days and
irradiated PBMC (10^5/well) every 7 days.

Proliferation Assays

4 x 10^4 cloned T cells or 1 x 10^5 resting T cells
were added to triplicate cultures in 96 well flat bottomed
microtiter plates to irradiated accessory cells (fibroblasts, 3400R; transformed B cells 7500R; monocytes 2500R
or B cells 2500R). Thymidine incorporation was assessed by
pulsing with 0.8 uCi methyl ^{3}H-thymidine during the last
18 hrs of the culture (96 hr for T cell clones, 6 days for
resting T cells).

RESULTS

The capacity of EBV-B cells to present antigen to
resting T cells was studied in three donors who had no
detectable serum antibody titers against the EBV capsular
antigen. Table 1 shows that purified peripheral T cells
from these three donors did not show significant proliferation to autologous EBV-B cells. In contrast to
monocytes, EBV-B cells were unable to support the proliferation of autologous resting T cells (T_{rest}) to TT
antigen (table 1). However the EBV-B cells presented TT
antigen to TT specific autologous T cell blasts.

A possible explanation for the inability of EBV-B
cells to present antigen to resting T cells is that antigen
processing by EBV-B cells occurs only in the presence of
activated T cells. Two observations ruled out this
possibility. First, EBV-B cells pulsed with TT antigen for
18 hours then treated with paraformaldehyde to block
further antigen processing were able to present antigen to
TT-specific T cell blasts. Second, EBV-B cells pulsed
with TT in the presence of TT specific T cell blasts still
failed to present antigen to autologous resting T cells.
In this experiment, EBV-B cells were pulsed with TT for 18
hours in the presence of equal numbers of autologous TT
specific T cell blasts. The cells were then removed by

TABLE 1

Presentation of TT Antigen by Mo. and EBV-B Cells to Autologous T Cells

Responding cells	Antigen presenting cells	cpm of ^{3}H-thymidine incorporated per culture			
		Donor #1		Donor #2	
		medium	TT	medium	TT
T$_{rest}$	———	1,456	944	965	2,437
	Mo.	6,765	113,487	554	233,740
	EBV-B	1,208	1,317	2,815	2,743
T$_{bl}$	———	481	697	170	230
	Mo.	2,785	21,768	7,735	42,987
	EBV-B	2,633	24,434	2,018	34,277

lysis with OKT3, OKT11 and complement and the remaining
EBV-B cells were irradiated (7500 rads) and examined for
their capacity to present TT to autologous resting T cells.
Taken together, the above two observations suggest that the
inability of EBV-B cells to present antigen to resting T
cells is not caused by an inability to process TT.
Furthermore the failure of EBV-B cells to trigger the
proliferation of resting T cells to TT antigen was not due
to an inhibitory effect on EBV-B cells on the proliferation
of resting T cells. Addition of EBV-B cells to cultures
of autologous resting T cells and monocytes did not
suppress with the T cell proliferative response to TT
antigen.

We had previously shown that the monokine IL-1 is
necessary for the proliferation of resting human T cells
in response to antigen presented by autologous monocytes
(2). Table 2 shows that addition of 10 units/ml of IL-1
to cultures of resting T cells and EBV-B cells allowed the
T cells to proliferate to TT antigen albeit to a lesser
degree that in the presence of monocytes. These data
suggest that the inability of EBV-B cells to trigger the
proliferation of resting T cells to antigen may be due to
the inability of the EBV-B cells to secrete IL-1. Direct
examination of the capacity of EBV-B cells tc secrete IL-1
in response to a variety of stimuli which included Staph.
epidermidis and Concanavalin A revealed no biologically
active IL-1 in the cell supernatants as assessed by a
thymocyte costimulator assay.

The capacity of EBV-B cells to support the proliferation of activated T_{b1} to TT despite the failure of EBV-B
cells to secrete detectable IL-1 suggested that IL-1 may
not be required for optimal proliferation of activated T
cells to antigen. We therefore examined the effect of
anti IL-1 on Mo. dependent antigen induced proliferation of
resting T cells and of TT specific T_{b1} derived from the
same donor. Table 3 shows that the proliferative response
of resting T cells to antigen was inhibited by rabbit
antihuman IL-1, but not by normal rabbit serum (NRS) as
has been previously described (2). In contrast, the proliferative response of T cell blasts to TT presented by
monocytes or EBV-B cells was not inhibited by rabbit anti
IL-1.

Four conclusions can be derived from the above data.

TABLE 2

Effect of IL-1 on Antigen Presentation by EBV-B Cells

Antigen presenting cells	IL-1	³H-Td cpm per culture			
		Expt. #1		Expt. #2	
		—	TT	—	TT
—	—	244	209	205	145
Monocytes	—	275	81,695	328	109,630
EBV-B cells	—	1,878	3,009	1,193	1,036
EBV-B cells	10 u/ml	7,413	23,802	6,529	22,712
—	10 u/ml	317	362	269	338

TABLE 3

Effect on Rabbit Anti IL-1 on the Proliferation of Antigen
Specific Resting T Cells and T Cell Blasts

Exp. #	T cells	APC	Medium	Anti IL-1	NRS	% inhibition
1	T_{rest}	Mo	15,223	1,134	15,041	89
	T_{bl}	Mo	24,024	15,171	14,147	7
	T_{bl}	EBV-B	26,084	11,977	16,162	29
2	T_{rest}	Mo	10,793	3,830	11,939	68
	T_{bl}	Mo	61,522	34,669	34,184	0
	T_{bl}	EBV-B	50,064	25,569	29,432	13

First, EBV-B cells fail to trigger proliferation of
resting T cells in response to antigen although they
efficiently trigger the proliferation of antigen specific
T cell blasts. Second, the failure of EBV-B cells to
trigger the proliferation of resting T cells to antigen
could be reversed by exogenous IL-1. Third, EBV-B cells
fail to secrete IL-1 under conditions which result in IL-1
release by monocytes. Fourth, IL-1 is required for the
optimal proliferation of resting T cells, but not of
activated T cells to antigen.

Antigen Presentation by Resting B Cells

In contrast to EBV-B cells, highly purified peripheral
blood B cells failed to present TT antigen to either
resting T cells or T cell clones (table 1). The failure
of resting B cells to present TT was not simply due to
their poor capacity to take up antigen. When these cells
were preincubated with a hybrid antibody to TT antigen and
to IgM they took up as much $125I$ radiolabeled TT antigen
as monocytes yet failed to induce T cell proliferation
(table 4). This failure was not corrected by the addition
of interleukin 1 (data not shown). The resting B cells
were examined for their capacity to "process" antigen.
This was done by examining the capacity of monolayers of
hybrid antibody coated B cells pulsed with TT to bind TT
specific T cells. In this experiment T cells were allowed
to interact with the monolayer of B cells immobilized on
plastic via anti Ig. Non-adherent B cells were then
assessed for their proliferation to TT antigen and to the
control antibody diphtheria toxoid. Figure 1 shows that
T cells adsorbed over the B cell monolayers showed no
specific loss in their capacity to proliferate to TT.
This is in contrast to T cells adsorbed over monolayers of
TT pulsed monocytes. Thus it appears that resting B cells
may not be able to generate an immunogenic moiety of antigen plus self Ia which is recognized and bound by T cells.

Antigen Presentation by Fibroblasts

It has been previously shown that human dermal fibroblasts express HLA-DR antigens after treatment with gamma
interferon (4). We therefore examined the capacity of
IFN-γ treated fibroblasts to present antigen to T cells.

Table 5 shows that significant proliferation of cloned

TABLE 4

Antigen Presentation for TT-Specific T Cell Clones

Accessory Cells	(^{3}H) thymidine incorporated per culture		
	cpm	cpm	cpm
	Medium	TT	TT
_____	311	527	216
Monocytes	107	4,131	4,024
B cells	140	830	690
Hybrid antibody-coated B cells	178	771	593
EBV-B cells	236	4,665	4,429

TABLE 5

IFN- Treated Fibroblasts Present Antigen to Autologous TT Specific T Cell Clones

APC	Antigen	cpm of ^{3}H-thymidine incorporated per culture	
		Exp. 1 Clone G8	Exp. 2 Clone F6
None	—	103	N.D.
None	TT	139	N.D.
EBV-B cells or Mφ	—	221	1,352
EBV-B cells or Mφ	TT	30,900	42,237
Fibroblasts IFN-γ	—	181	271
Fibroblasts IFN-γ	TT	37,374	39,887
Fibroblasts	—	133	393
Fibroblasts	TT	170	4,273

T cells occurred in the presence of TT antigen and either
autologous EBV-B cells or monocytes, or with TT and autologous fibroblasts which were pretreated with IFN-γ. The
extent of T cell proliferation to IFN-γ treated fibroblasts was similar to that seen in the presence of autologous EBV-B cells or monocytes. The proliferation of
both clones F6 and G8 was antigen and accessory cell
dependent, as it did not occur in the presence of TT
alone nor in the presence of IFN-γ treated fibroblasts
alone. Untreated fibroblasts either completely failed to
present TT to the T cell clones or supported a modest
degree of T cell proliferation.

The role of HLA-DR antigens on IFN-γ pretreated
fibroblasts in T cell proliferation in response to antigen
was examined. As seen in Table 6 addition of monoclonal
anti HLA-DR (LB3.1) to the cultures abolished T cell proliferation. In contrast, monoclonal anti HLA-A,B (W6/32),
monoclonal anti-DC (Leu 10), and an irrelevant monoclonal
antibody (UPC 10) did not inhibit T cell proliferation.

We then examined the ability of fibroblasts to present
antigen to resting T cells. Peripheral blood T cells
depleted of monocytes were used. These cells failed to
proliferate in response to TT or Con A unless reconstituted
with autologous monocytes. The PHA response was also
markedly diminished ($<$90%), indicating that monocyte
depletion was nearly complete. Table 7 shows that IFN-
treated autologous fibroblasts were capable of supporting
the proliferation of these resting T cells to TT antigen
but too much lesser extent than monocytes. No proliferation was observed in the absence of antigen or when
untreated fibroblasts were used.

CONCLUSIONS

The observations discussed in this review suggest
that resting T cells differ from activated T cells in the
accessory cell requirements needed to respond to antigen
by proliferation. This is because of the following:

a) EBV-B cells present antigen to activated T cells
but not to resting T cells.
b) Interleukin 1 is needed for the activation of
resting T cells but not of activated T cells. Thus anti-

TABLE 6

Monoclonal Anti HLA-DR Inhibits Proliferation of F6 Induced by Fibroblasts

IFN- treatment of fibroblasts	TT	cpm of ^{3}H-thymidine incorporated per culture after addition of monoclonal antibody				
		media	LB3.1 (αHLA-DR)	W6/32 (αHLA-A,B)	Leu 10 (α DC)	UPC10 (control)
−	−	944	804	498	918	944
−	+	2,829	637	549	1,240	2,048
+	−	288	211	354	306	343
+	+	6,567	891	6,804	6,393	7,107
No fibroblasts	TCGF	8,120	6,864	7,297	6,312	8,828

TABLE 7

IFN-γ Treated Fibroblasts Present Antigen to Resting T Cells

APC	Antigen	cpm of ^{3}H-thymidine incorporated per culture	
		Expt. #1	Expt. #2
	—	90	155
	TT	107	261
Mφ	—	278	343
Mφ	TT	53,528	116,527
Fibroblast IFN-γ	—	399	245
Fibroblast IFN-γ	TT	12,315	8,538
Fibroblasts	—	305	376
Fibroblasts	TT	253	269

body to IL-1 inhibited the responses of but not those of
cloned T cells. In the same vein, addition of IL-1 to
EBV-B cells reverses their inability to trigger resting
T cells.

c) Fibroblasts present antigen to resting T cells much
less efficienty than to activated T cells.
Taken together these results indicate that cells of the
monocytes/macrophages series are the best triggers for
resting T cells. In addition to IL-1 factors produced by
monocytes/macrophages and/or integral to their membranes
may be necessary or more efficient triggers of T cell proliferation. For instance these cells may be better inducers of IL-2 synthesis. Our current experiments with
highly purified T cells, PHA and IL-2 suggest that high
levels of IL-2 may be needed to trigger resting T cells
which express only very few receptors for IL-2 (Katzen et
al. Unpublished observations). The lack of additional
signals in EBV-B cells may explain their less than optimal
capacity to trigger resting T cells even in the presence of
excess of IL-1. In the case of fibroblasts modest proliferation of resting T cells is seen in the absence of any
added factors. Although we need more experiments to
absolutely establish that the effect is not due to augmen-
tation by fibroblasts of residual monocytes, this is quite
unlikely because the purified T cells did not respond to
Con A and responded very poorly to PHA. If fibroblasts
turn out to truly be able to trigger resting T cells they
appear to do it rather inefficiently, again indicating that
the best accessory cells for the resting T cell is the
monocytes. This is clearly different from the situation
with activated T cells which respond equally well to monocytes, EBV-B cells and fibroblasts.

Finally it is clear that not all Ia+ cells can serve
as accessory cells because resting B cells clearly failed
to present antigen. In our experiments the B cells received 1500-2500 rads. Recently Paul and coworkers have
reported that highly irradiated (1500 rads) B cells would
present antigen (5). We have confirmed this observation
using T cell clones and are presently studying the mechanism by which irradiation prevent resting B cells from
presenting antigen. Perhaps B cells need T cell derived
activated signal to be able to present the antigen and
this signal is not transduced in irradiated B cells.

In summary resting T cells have stringent requirements

for activation which are fulfilled best if not exclusively
by monocytes/macrophages. However once activated the T
cells can be triggered by a variety of Ia+ cells. This
suggest that upon entry into the system antigen is
presented by monocytes/macrophages present in high
numbers in portals of antigen entry (skin, draining lymph
node). Later on as the T cells are activated and the
antigen disseminates several other cell types present in
target organs can interact with activated immune T cells.

REFERENCES

1. Brozek, C., Umetsu, D., Schneeberger, E., and Geha, R.S.
    "J. Immunol. 132,1144-1150 (1984).
2. Chu, E., Rosenwasser, L.J., Dinarello, C.A., Lareau, M.,
    and Geha, R.S. "J. Immunol." In press.
3. Leung, D.Y.M., Parkman, R., Feller, J., Wood, N., and
    Geha, R.S. "J. Immunol." 128,1736-1741 (1982).
4. Umetsu, D.T., Pober, J.S., Jabara, H.H., Fiers, W.,
    Yunis, E.J., Burakoff, S.J., Reiss, C.S., and Geha,
    R.S. "J. Clin. Invest." Submitted for publication.
5. Glimcher, L.H., Kim, K.J., Green, I., and Paul, W.E.
    "J. Exp. Med." 155,455-459 (1982).

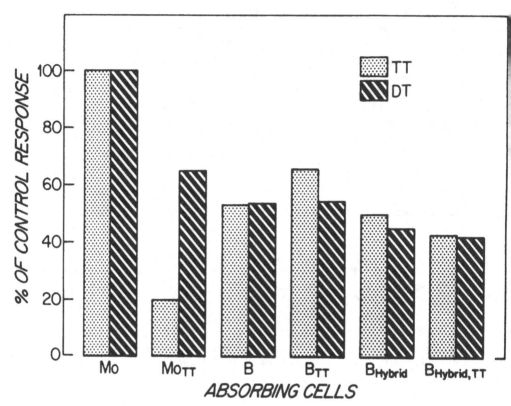

Figure 1. Effect of adsorption of peripheral blood T cells over
monolayers of autologous monocytes or B cells on the
proliferative response to antigen.   Monocytes (Mo)
were unpulsed or pulsed with TT antigen (Mo$_{TT}$).   B cells
(B) and B cells coated with hybrid antibody (B$_{Hybrid}$)
were also used unpulsed or pulsed with TT (B$_{TT}$ and B$_{Hybrid}$)
and were immobilized over anti-Fab-coated dishes.   After
2 cycles of adsorption (3 hr each) nonadherent T cells
were tested in the presence of 10% irradiated and autologous
monocytes for their proliferative response to TT and DT
antigen.   Results are expressed as the percentage of
control response that was that of T cells adsorbed over
monolayers of unpulsed monocytes.   Nonspecific loss of
T cell proliferative reactivity after passage over monolayers of unpulsed monocytes were always less than 10%.
Similar results were obtained in two experiments.

NICKEL-SPECIFIC HUMAN T CELL CLONES:

FUNCTIONAL CHARACTERIZATION AND REQUIREMENTS FOR

TRIGGERING

F. Sinigaglia, D.Scheidegger, A. Lanzavecchia*,
M. Pletscher**, R.J. Scheper*** and G. Garotta

F. Hoffmann-La Roche & Co. Ltd., Central
Research Units, Basel (Switzerland)
* Basel Institute for Immunology, Basel
(Switzerland)
** Kantonsspital Basel (Switzerland)
*** Pathology Department, Free University
Hospital, Amsterdam (Holland)

The exact nature of T cells mediating
delayed-type hypersensitivity (DTH) is still
controversial [1-3]. Investigations in both
human and animal systems suggested that T DTH
cells have the same phenotype and MHC restriction as helper T cells [4-6]. This raises
the question of whether or not helper activity
and DTH can be mediated by the same activated T
cell. In order to investigate this issue we
took advantage of a clinical situation, Ni-contact dermatitis, which is considered an expression of pure DTH reaction. Representative T
lymphocyte clones (TLC) isolated from two of
these patients show the surface phenotype and
in vitro function of T helper cells and produce
high levels of γ-interferon (IFN-γ). In
addition the simple chemical nature of this
antigen may be useful for the analysis of T
cell specificity and triggering requirements.

FUNCTIONAL CHARACTERIZATION OF Ni-SPECIFIC TLC

Peripheral blood mononuclear cells (PBM) from
patients with Ni-contact dermatitis, but not
from healthy control donors, were able to
proliferate when cultured in vitro in the
presence of $NiSO_4$ Ni-specific T cell lines
were obtained by $NiSO_4$ stimulation, expanded
in long term culture and cloned by limiting
dilution.
Table 1 shows the functional characterization
of a series of clones obtained from two
different patients. All the clones proliferated
in response to $NiSO_4$ (or $NiCl_2$) in the
presence of autologous irradiated PBM as a
source of antigen-presenting cells (APC). The
clones did not proliferate in response to other
antigens (e.g. $CrSO_4$ or alloantigens).
Furthermore the proliferative response was also
restricted, as MHC-mismatched PBM could not
serve as APC.
All the TLC were OKT3+, T4+ and T8- as
assayed by indirect immunofluorescence using
appropriate monoclonal antibodies. When the
clones were cultured with autologous B cells
and $NiSO_4$ a strong polyclonal B cell
activation was observed with production of high
levels of IgM, IgG and IgA (Table 1).
Furthermore none of the TLC was able to kill
Ni-pulsed autologous PHA blasts (data not
shown).
We also investigated the ability of Ni-specific
clones to produce lymphokines following stimulation with APC and antigen. All the clones
tested produced IL-2, at levels ranging from
9 to 62 U/ml, as measured in the 24 h culture
supernatant. Remarkably, all the clones also
produced IFN-γ and 4 out of 10 at a very high
level. These data strongly support the idea
that DTH in humans is dependent on a T cell
population of helper type that is capable of
producing high level of IFN-γ in response to
antigenic stimulation.

Clone No. [a]	^{3}H-Tdr incorporation [b] (cpm x 10^{-3})		Helper function [c] (Total Ig µg/ml)		IL-2 [d] production (U/ml)	IFN γ [e] production (U/ml)
	-	NiSO$_4$	IgM	IgG		
2/4	0.6	12	12	11	9	890
2/20	2	12	150	60	12	5000
2/24	0.9	8	1	0.6	n.d.	n.d.
2/33	0.7	6	3	1	n.d.	n.d.
2/36	1	27	n.d.	n.d.	n.d.	n.d.
3/3	4	32	n.d.	n.d.	9	1590
3/4	4	61	35	96	22	890
3/6	4	40	96	80	10	880
3/19	2	29	11	56	5	5000
3/29	2	15	n.d.	n.d.	62	900
3/35	2	34	n.d.	n.d.	19	500
3/36	4	92	256	100	n.d.	28000
3/43	2	23	5	11	n.d.	5000

n.d. = not done

Table 1: Functional characterization of
Ni-Specific T Cell Clones
a) T cell clones:
   4×10^6 PBM from patients with Ni contact
   dermatitis were cultured in 24-well Costar
   plates in the presence of 5×10^{-5} M
   NiSO$_4$ in 2 ml complete RPMI-1640 supplemented with 10% pooled AB serum (HS). After
   6 days the lymphoblasts were enriched on a
   discontinuous Percoll gradient. These blasts
   were placed in culture at a concentration of
   2×10^5/ml in RPMI-HS supplemented with 10
   U/ml of recombinant IL-2 (Roche Nutley). The
   lines were selected and maintained by a
   regime of restimulation for 7 days with
   NiSO$_4$ and antigen-presenting cells
   (irradiated autologous PBM), followed by 7
   days in culture with medium containing IL-2.
   For cloning, T blasts (Tb) cultured in IL-2

were seeded at 0.3 cell/well in 96-well flat
bottom microplates in the presence of PHA (2
µg/ml) and 1x10^5/ml allogeneic irradiated (2'500 Rad) PBM in RPMI-HS containing
10 U/ml IL-2. After 2-3 weeks cell growth
was detected microscopically and the growing
wells were expanded further using PHA,
allogeneic irradiated PBM and IL-2 until a
sufficient number of T cells was available.
13 clones from 2 patients were expanded in
IL-2 and tested for proliferative capacity
to Ni, helper activity on B cells and
lymphokine production.

b) Proliferation assay:
   2x10^4 Tb were cultured in 0.2 ml RPMI-HS
   in flat bottom microplates with 1x10^5
   irradiated autologous PBM in the presence of
   5x10^{-5} M NiSO$_4$ or medium alone. After 48
   hrs the cultures were pulsed with 1 µCi of
   3H-Tdr and the proliferative response
   determined after another 16 hours. Results
   are expressed as mean cpm of quadruplicate
   cultures.

c) Helper assay:
   5x10^3 Tb were cultured with 2x10^4
   E-rosette depleted autologous PBM in 0.2 ml
   RPMI-FCS in flat bottom microplates in the
   presence or absence of NiSO$_4$. After 8 days
   the amount of Ig produced in the supernatant
   was measured by ELISA [7]. Less than 0.2
   µg/ml of total Ig were produced in the
   absence of Ni.

d) IL-2 and IFN γ assay:
   Tb were distributed at 4x10^5 cells/well in
   2 ml of medium in Costar 24-well plates in
   the presence of the optimal concentration of
   Ni and irrradiated autologous PBM. Culture
   supernatants were usually harvested at 24 h
   for IL-2 and at 48 h for IFN determination.
   IL-2 was measured using CTLL cells as
   described [8]. IFN activity was measured

as protection of mouse L929 cells from cytopathic effect of vesicular stomatitis virus [9].

REQUIREMENTS FOR ANTIGEN PRESENTATION TO Ni-SPECIFIC TLC

As previously mentioned triggering of Ni-
specific TLC requires presentation of antigen
by appropriate antigen-presenting cells. When a
series of autologous or allogeneic PBM was
tested for the capacity to present Ni to T
cells, only autologous PBM were able to trigger
the T cell response (Fig. 1). Furthermore monomorphic anti-HLA-DR antibody, but not
anti-β_2 microglobulin, was able to inhibit
antigen presentation (data not shown). We
therefore conclude that Ni is recognised by TLC
in an MHC-restricted manner.

In order to investigate the requirement for
antigen presentation, PBM, EBV-transformed
lymphoblastoid cell lines (LCL) and activated T
cells were compared for their capacity to
present Ni to the Ni-specific TLC. Fig. 1 shows
that both autologous LCL and activated T cells
were effective in antigen presentation to TLC,
although they varied in their relative
effenciency, the LCL being on a per cell basis
almost 100 times more efficient than activated
T cells. We conclude that T cells themselves
can present Ni, provided they are Ia
(HLA-DR)-positive. This conclusion is further
supported by the fact that preincubation of T
cells with IFN-γ, a treatment that increases
their Ia expression, also increases the
efficiency of Ni presentation (data not shown).

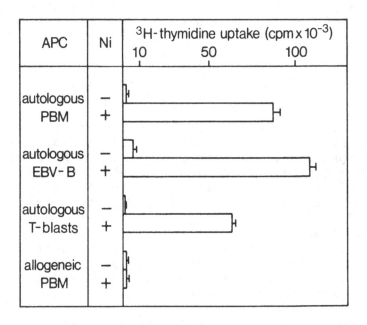

Fig. 1

Autologous Ia-positive cells can stimulate
Ni-specific TLC in the absence of macrophages

2×10^4 Tb were cultured in 0.2 ml RPMI-HS in
flat bottom microplates with irradiated autologous PBM (10^5) or LCL (10^4) or activated
T cells (5×10^5), with or without $NiSO_4$
($5 \times 10^{-5}M$). Cell proliferation was measured as
in Table 1.

It has been shown that presentation of complex
antigens to T cells requires a step of intracellular antigen processing [10]. We therefore tested the effect of glutaraldehyde
fixation on the ability of LCL to present Ni to
the Ni-specific TLC. As shown in Table 2
glutaraldehyde fixation does not affect the

Capacity of LCL to present Ni, while anti-Ia
treatment completely abrogates the proliferative response. The above data suggest that what
is recognized by TLC is indeed Ia modified by
Ni.
The alternative possibility is that Ni is bound
to cell surface molecules recognized by T cells
in association with Ia. The first hypothesis is
supported by the fact that trypsin treatment of
the antigen-presenting cells, at a concentration which removes most of the surface proteins but not Ia, does not interfere with the
antigen-presenting capability. Further experiments using purified Ia molecules in a
cell-free environment are in progress in order
to clarify this issue.

APC	NiSO$_4$	Thymidine uptake (cpm)	
	(5x10^{-5}M)	clone 3/36	clone 3/4
LCL	–	5470$\pm$ 294	4810$\pm$ 416
	+	170937$\pm$ 943	84220$\pm$ 533
LCL-Fix[a]	–	4023$\pm$ 699	3616$\pm$ 121
	+	161947$\pm$3060	97512$\pm$1552
LCL+αIa[b]	–	878$\pm$ 66	1020$\pm$ 16
	+	960$\pm$ 324	715$\pm$ 118

Table 2: Effect of fixation and anti-Ia antibody
          on the Ni-induced proliferative response
2x10^4 Tb were cultured in 0.2 ml volumes of
RPMI-HS in flat bottom microplates with 10^4
EBV-B cells in the presence or absence of
5x10^{-5}M NiSO$_4$
a) B cells were either irradiated and fixed with
   glutaraldehyde [11]
b) Anti-Ia antibody (clone EII.3/1) [12] was
   added in culture at 10 μg/ml.

REFERENCES

1. Bianchi, A.T.J., Hooijkaast, H., Benner, R., Tees, R., Nordin, A.A. and Schreier, M.H. Nature 290, 62-63 (1981)

2. Dennert, G., Weiss, S. and Warner, J.F. Proc. Natl. Acad. Sci. U.S.A. 78, 4540-4532 (1981)

3. Milan, G., Marchal, G., Seman M., Truffa-Bachi, P. and Zilberfarb, V. J. Immunol. 130, 1103-1107 (1983)

4. Miller, J.F.A.P., Vadas, M.A., Whitelaw, A. and Gamble, J. Proc. Natl. Acad. Sci. U.S.A. 72, 5095-5089 (1975)

5. Vadas, M.A., Miller, J.F.A.P., McKenzie, I.F.C., Chism, S.E., Shen, F.W., Boyse, E.A., Gamble, J.R. and Whitelaw, A.M. J. Exp. Med. 144, 10-19 (1976)

6. Platt, J.L., Grant, B.W., Eddy, A.A. and Micheal, A.F. J. Exp. Med. 158, 1227-1242 (1983)

7. Lanzavecchia, A., Ferrarini, M. and Celada, F. Eur. J. Immunol. 12, 468-474 (1982)

8. Gillis, S., Ferm, M.M., On, W. and Smith, K.A. J. Immunol. 120, 2027-2032 (1978)

9. Rubinstein, S., Familletti, P.C. and Pestka, S. J. Virol. 37, 755-758 (1981)

10. Unanue, E.R., Beller, D.I., Lu, C.Y. and Allen, P.M. J. Immunol. 132, 1 - 5 (1984)

11. Shimonkevitz, R., Kappler, J., Marrack, P. and Grey, H. J. Exp. Med. 158, 303-316 (1983)

12. Trucco, M., Garotta, G., Stocker, J., and Cepellini, R. Immunol. Rev. 47, 219-252 (1979

SESSION IV
Role of Cell Surface Molecules in T Cell Function

Chairpersons: M.J. Crumpton and A.J. McMichael

This session was very timely in that it closely followed the Second International Leucocyte Differentiation Workshop held in Boston, September 17-20, 1984. Dr Mawas in the opening presentation demonstrated by antibody inhibition studies that the CD2 and CD7 molecules are members of the lymphocyte functional antigen (LFA) molecular group, which inhibit various immune functions. In addition he described two new LFA antigens, one an early activation antigen (110K) and the second a 41Kd (CD7) molecule. Thus the LFA antigens appear to be an extensive family of molecules. Dr Burakoff analyzed the cell surface antigens involved in cytolysis mediated by human cytotoxic T lymphocytes (CTL). Data was presented that suggested that the inhibitory action of anti-T3 antibody on specific cytolysis was the result of inappropriate activation, and secondly that the T3 antigen blocks at the post adhesion stage of effector cell/target interaction. In contrast antibodies to T4, T8, LFA-1 and LFA-2 inhibit conjugate formation. The role of the T4 and T8 antigens may be to stabilize the interaction of antigen with Ti and T3 molecules and the use of such accessory structures may depend upon the affinity of Ti/Ag interaction. Similarly, it was suggested that LFA-1 may serve to stabilize the CTL-target cell conjugation. The involvement of LFA-2 and 3 in CTL target cell interactions were also discussed, although as yet their functional roles are ill defined.

This theme was continued later in the session by Dr Moretta. He described some T4$^+$ and T8$^+$ CTL clones that were not inhibited by anti-T3 antibody. In contrast anti-T11 (anti erythrocyte receptor) antibody inhibited cytolysis in all the CTL clones but not the natural killer (NK) like activity. Anti-T11 also inhibited proliferation and IL-2 release. At the end of his presentation Dr Moretta described a subclass of CTL precursors that recognized alloantigen independently of T3 or T8 molecules.

Dr Engleman discussed a regulatory circuit of antigen independent T-T interactions induced by antigen activated T cells. Amplifier and suppressor T cells are activated that are specific for the inducer T cells, thus representing an idiotypic T cell interaction. Inhibition studies with monoclonal antibodies suggested that Leu 2, Leu 4 and LFA-1

171

molecules were involved in the interaction between suppressor and inducer T cells.

Dr Crumpton reviewed the role of Ti molecules (antigen specific receptors defined by clonotypic antibodies) in the activation of T cells, and his results suggested that Ti as well as being the receptor for specific antigen was also that for PHA T3 did not bind PHA. Dr Zanders reported the biochemical events in T cells activated by anti-T3 antibody. Anti-T3 induced rapid lipid phosphorylation and an increase in cytoplasmic free Calcium, which preceded proliferation.

In conclusion the data reported in ths session suggest that a variety of cell surface molecules (T3, T4, T8, LFA) are involved in T cell function. The dependency of T cells on individual molecules for activation is hierachical, influenced by the functional subset and antigen binding receptor affinity. T3 deserves special mention in that is complexed with Ti (the antigen recognition structure) and may be associated with transduction of the activation signal across the lymphocyte membrane. Even at the end of this very exciting session one feels there is still much to learn about T cell surface molecules and their role in cellular activation.

HUMAN LYMPHOCYTE FUNCTIONAL ANTIGENS

D. OLIVE (1), D. CHARMOT (1), P. DUBREUIL
(1), A. TOUNKARA (1), M. RAGUENEAU (1), C.
MAWAS (1) and P. MANNONI (2)
1. Centre d'Immunologie INSERM-CNRS de
Marseille-Luminy, Case 906, 13288 Marseille
cédex 9 - France.
2. University of Alberta, Edmonton, Canada.

Following the extensive development of monoclonal
antibodies (mAbs) to surface membrane determinants, a
variety of surface molecules have been defined on
lymphocytes ; the expression of some of these molecules
helped to define lymphocyte subsets and/or
differentiation markers. More recently, some of these
surface molecules have acquired a "functional" status :
for many of these molecules, their "functional"
qualification came as the consequence of the "functional"
effects induced in absence of complement, in in vitro
assays, by these specific mAbs. Many authors have
restricted the qualification of Lymphocyte Functional
Antigens (LFA) (1,2) to mAbs able to block CTL lysis in
absence of complement. As will be shown, mAbs and
therefore the molecules bearing the recognized
determinants can induce a variety of agonist and/or
antagonist effects on the lymphocytes, which are not
restricted to cytolysis. At least, using the following in
vitro assays, a number of mAbs were found to interfere
with such assays as lectin stimulation, MLR, IL-2
dependent T cell growth, anti-class I or anti-class II
cell mediated lympholysis and NK lysis. Other in vitro
assays such as lymphokines secretion (IL-2, γ-IFN,
etc...), T-B cooperation, can also be studied ; we have
not used the latter assays routinely. In all cases,
however, the major issue raised by these data is the

relevance of the observed in vitro phenomenology to in
vivo physiology, and the molecular basis of its
mechanism.

MATERIALS AND METHODS
Monoclonal antibodies. Most mAbs used in this study
were derived from fusions performed either with murine or
rat spleen cells immunized by cloned T cells, IL-2
dependent T cell lines or day 4 PHA activated T cells.
Fusions were performed 76 hr after the last I.V.
injection according to published techniques (3).

In vitro assays. Most assays were performed using
standard techniques (4).

Iodination of cell surface proteins and
immunoprecipitation studies were performed as published
(3).

Cytofluorometric analysis was performed by indirect
fluorescence with F(ab') fluorescein-conjugated goat
anti-mouse or rat IgG (Cappel Laboratory, Westchester,
PA, USA), using an Epics V cell sorter (Coultronics,
Hialeah, Fl. USA).

RESULTS AND DISCUSSION
We shall review here, based on locally produced mAbs
some of the in vitro effects observed with these mAbs on
T cells function and alluded to other lymphocyte
functions when pertinent to the data or discussion.

Monoclonal antibodies to activated T cells
1. MAbs against the IL-2 receptor.
Most mAbs against the IL-2 receptor are potent
inhibitors of the IL-2 dependent growth of T cell-lines
or T cell clones. This is obvious when the screening is
itself functional, as shown in Table 1. However, not all
genuine anti-IL-2 receptors are good inhibitors as shown
in Table 1 by mAb 22 D6 11 or B1-49-9, a mAb shown to
recognize the same molecule as TAC (5) by sequential
immunoprecipitation (6). This inhibition is dose
dependent as shown in Table 2. These same mAbs are
inhibitors of primary MLR (Table 3) and their effects on
MLR parallel those on IL-2 dependent growth. As expected,
their inhibitory effects is as strong when added on day 2

Table 1 . Screening of a panel of mAb on IL-2 dependent
       growth.

MAbs used	T cell line ANT 1	T cell line ANT 2
IL-2 Rec. :		
18 E4.6	<u>1.8</u>	.5
33 B3.1	<u>1.8</u>	.8
33 B7.3	<u>9.1</u>	1.4
39 C6.5	<u>3.7</u>	2.5
22 D6.11	15.7	7.5
Others :		
39 B2.1	17.6	6.9
39 H7.3	16.8	6.8
12 E3.1	19.5	4.4
19 E3.6	17.5	4.5
39 C1.5	15.4	4.5
39 C8.18	16.3	4.2
5 B6.4	16.8	4.1
13 E1.19	18.8	6.7
Controls		
25.3 (LFA-1)	14.5	6.7
H8.109.14 (irrelevant)	18.4	7.9
B1.49.9 (IL-2 receptor)	12.4	5.3
PHA 1%	.2	1.3
W/O IL-2	.4	.7
W IL-2	22.0	7.0

mAb at 1/40 final dilution.

Table 2. Inhibition of an Il-2-dependent T cell line by anti-IL-2 receptor mAb

Dilutions of mAb	mAbs tested			
	18 E6.4	33 B3.1	33 B7.1	39 C6.5
1/40	6.0	.9	3.5	1.5
1/500	3.6	3.8	7.6	2.2
1/1000	9.5	5.8	8.1	5.1
1/2000	10.5	6.4	8.2	6.1
1/4000	14.2	12.0	12.0	12.0
1/8000	14.0	7.6	12.0	12.0
1/16,000	9.2	10.0	7.5	13.5
Controls				
W/O IL-2	.3			
W IL-2	12.0			

Table 3. Inhibition of a primary MLR by a panel of T cell specific mAbs added on day 0 or day 2.

MLR Combination	mAbs added on :		
		day 0	day 2
A alone*	NONE	.5	1.0
AB	NONE	28.5	28.0
IL-2 receptor :			
	18 E6.4	10.0	9.5
	33 B3.1	5.0	10.0
	39 C6.5	17.4	13.5
	22 D6.11	17.5	23.0
Unknown :			
	39 B2.1	3.4	7.5
	39 H7.3	4.8	13.5
	12 E3.1	5.0	15.9
	19 E3.6	5.5	15.5
	39 C1.5	5.4	18.5
	39 C8.18	10.5	15.3
	5 B6.4	7.0	18.8
	13 E1.19	6.4	13.0
Controls			
	25.3	5.0	18.3
	H8.109.14	28.0	27.2
	B1.49.9	22.6	18.5

Results are expressed as c.p.m 10^{-3}

as on day 0. However, primary CML is not abolished in
most instances, when the CTL effector generation is
obtained in the presence of anti-IL-2 receptor mAb (data
not shown). MAbs against the IL-2 receptor were not found
to interfere with CML anti-class I or class II at the
effector level. However, we have reproducibly found
(Table 4) a strong inhibition (41 and 36%) of NK lysis
(on target cells K 562) with two anti-IL-2 receptor mAbs,
i.e. 18 E6.4 and 27 E4.6 ; a lower inhibition was found
(17 to 19%) with mAbs B1-49-9, 33 B3.1, 39 C6.5, 22
D6.11. Only mAb 33 B7.3 was never able to inhibit NK
lysis. The mechanism remains unknown at present but could
be in line with reports claiming that among T PBL cells,
those expressing the IL-2 receptor have the strongest NK
activity.

Fig. 1 : Agonist effect of anti-Il-2 receptor mAb on MLR
and CML

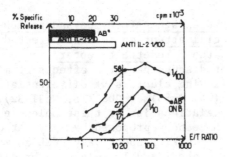

Agonist effects induced by the anti-IL-2 receptors
were first noticed when mAb dilutions were tested for
their ability to inhibit the IL-2 dependent growth of T
cell lines or clones (Table 1, mAb 18 E6.4, dilution
1/4000 to 1/8000). This was further confirmed, when a low
dilution of mAb was added to a primary MLR and day 6
proliferation measured as well as specific CTL activity
(Fig. 1). In this experiment, two different dilutions
(1/10 and 1/100, respectively) of anti-IL-2 receptor mAb
was added at the onset of the primary culture AB*.
Despite a strong inhibition of MLR by the high
concentration of mAb CML effectors were generated
although to a lesser extent than in the control culture.
With the 1/100 dilution, a strong potentiation of both
the MLR and the CTL generation is seen, suggesting an
agonistic effect potentiating the MLR help above its

control values. The precise mechanism needs to be further
analyzed.

2. MAbs against the transferrin receptor and against class II molecules.

In functional assays, both the mAbs against the
transferrin receptor BK 19 (7) or against class II
antigens were found reproducibly to interfere with the
IL-2 dependent growth of proliferative T cell lines or
clones or their restimulation by alloantigens (8) (data
not shown), an observation already reported for
anti-class II and IL-2 dependent growth of human T cell
lines by Moretta et al. (9).

Finally, many other mAbs found to react specifically
with activated T cells have not been found so far to
block T cell functions (for instance B1.19.2, reacting
against part of the T200 complex), with the exception of
mAb 46 F1.1 (see below).

Monoclonal antibodies against thymus and peripheral blood T cells with special attention to mAbs directed agaisnt the E rosette receptor

We shall not discuss here the effects of mAbs
defining the following clusters of differentiation : CD3
(T3, Gp20), CD4 (T4, Gp55) or CD8 (T8, Gp31-32). Evidence
for the spatial relationships of these molecules with the
T cell receptor have been proposed by many authors and
mAbs to these CDs block, respectively, CML as well as
proliferation to class I and II, class II or class I
mediated T cell functions (reviewed in 10). For CD3, mAbs
have also been found to strongly stimulate T cell
proliferation at low concentration or when presented by a
solid phase, and some heterogeneity in the functional
effects has been reported for the various mAbs (10). It
is important to note that many clones have been reported
not to be inhibited by mAbs directed against their
appropriate molecules and this phenomenon has been
related by most authors to the affinity of the clones for
their target (4).

We shall mainly focussed our report on the
functional effects of a family of mAbs, many of them
related to the E rosette receptor on the basis of tissue
distribution and molecular weight, but with some unusual
phenotypic characters on T PBL.

These mAbs were found upon an initial screening to have a strong reactivity on thymocytes, to label around 20–40% of unseparated T PBL and to be unreactive with B cells and monocytes. However, their reactivities were stronger on PHA blasts, compatible on these activated T cells with a pan T reactivity. Immunoprecipitation when positive gave a 55 K MW compatible with the E rosette receptor for mAb 5 B6.4, 12 E3.1, 19 E3.3, 39 C1.5 with two exceptions : 20 K for 39 C8.18 and 65 K for 39 B2.1. When tested on T cell functions, none were found inhibitory of IL-2 dependent growth of T cell lines or clones (Table 1) while all were strongly inhibitory of MLR and more so, when added on day 0 than on day 2 (Table 2). Most of them were also strongly inhibitory of CML anti-class I or class II as well as of NK lysis (Table 4).

Table 4 : Effect of mAbs on CML anti-class I and -class II and NK killing.

MAbs added :	Anti-class I clones		Anti-class II clones	NK Effectors
	PHA Blasts	EBV Targets	EBV Targets	K 562
NONE				
HB.109.14 (irrelevant)	55	45	52	86
25.3 (LFA-1)	55	52	55	85
B9.4 (T8)	24 (56)	13 (71)	20 (62)	56 (35)
BL.4 (T4)	56 (35)	NT	51	85
B1.49.9 (IL-2 receptor)	60	NT	33 (37)	82
	46 (16)	40	50	70 (19)
13 E1.19	37 (33)	23 (49)	NT	51 (41)
18 E6.4 (IL-2)	53	NT	NT	56 (35)
22 E3.2	47	27 (40)	13 (75)	55 (36)
27 E4.6 (IL-2)	48 (16)	13 (27)	51	54 (37)
39 B2.1 (67K)	39 (29)	30 (33)	20 (62)	53 (38)
39 H7.3	48	27 (40)	24 (54)	50 (42)
5 B6.4 (55K)	39 (29)	29 (36)	NT	57 (34)
33 B3.1 (IL-2)	44 (20)	NT	55	71 (17)
39 C6.5 (IL-2)	51	NT	48	70 (19)
22 D6.11 (IL-2)	45 (17)	NT	NT	70 (19)
19 E3.6 (55K)	46 (16)	NT	NT	64 (26)
39 C1.5 (55K)	42 (24)	28 (38)	19 (63)	39 (31)
39 C8.18 (20K)	48	20 (56)	21 (60)	60 (30)
41 F2.1	43 (20)	32 (29)	51	NT
46 F1.1.1	36 (35)	62	NT	NT
21 C11.14 (T8)	23 (58)	18 (60)	61	NT
25 K5.13	42 (24)	31 (31)	NT	NT
1 A3.3	51	NT	56	72 (16)
8 F3.9	46 (16)	NT	38 (27)	NT
5 B5.4	61	NT	NT	82
33 B7.3 (IL-2)	54	NT	50	NT
5 F2.14	53	NT	NT	82
15 H5.11	62	NT	NT	85

Results are expressed as percent specific ^{51}Cr release (numbers inside parenthesis represent % inhibition). Underlined results = significant inhibition.

None have been found stimulatory for T cells, using various dilutions of the mAbs. Finally, in terms of tissue distribution, 39 H7.3 and 39 C8.18 fall in a special group with unique reactivity on AML cells and mAb 13 E1.19 was the only one found negative on the T cell line RPMI 8402.

We have recently observed that (11 and manuscript submitted), upon γ-IFN treatment, the human promyelocytic leukemia cell line HL-60 differentiates towards T cells ;

by day 4 following the in vitro culture in presence of
γ-IFN, all the clusters of T cell differentiation are
expressed at the surface of 60-90% of the HL-60 treated
cells, together with the IL-2 receptor and the class II
antigens. However, among a panel of mAbs recognizing
identical molecules, only some do react with the newly
induced HL-60 T cell like molecules.

In Table 5, the molecule recognized by the mAb 9.6
(an anti-E rosette receptor kindly provided by J. Hansen,
Seattle, Wash. USA) is induced ; among the local mAbs
suspected to recognize the E rosette receptor only mAb 12
E3.1 is induced following γ-IFN treatment. The 39 C8.18
and 39 H7.3 defined molecules are both induced,
confirming their identical tissue distribution.

In conclusion, if this group of mAbs has some
similarities in tissue distribution and for some of them
for the molecule they immunoprecipitate from membrane
lysate, they are clearly belonging to discrete subgroups
despite their identical functional effects on T cell
functions. Among them, some anti-E rosette receptors are
present, confirming the qualification of LFA antigen
ascribed to this molecule (1). As for the mAbs describing
molecules different from the E rosette receptor, further
work is required to qualify them since two of them are to
our knowledge newly defined functional molecules.

Monoclonal antibodies reacting with T, B, polymorphs and monocyte cells or polymorphs and monocytes

Three mAbs were found to correspond to this class of
mAb. MAbs 25.3 and 25.5 both react with thymus T, B and
polymorphonuclear cells (PMN) or monocytes and with the
same non T leukemia lines. They both immunoprecipitate
from the solubilized membrane lysate of ^{131}I surface
labelled PHA blasts, following SDS-PAGE analysis, two
bands of 170-90 K respectively (data not shown).

These mAbs were subsequently shown to profoundly
inhibit MLR (Table 3), antigen specific proliferation of
T cell clones, more pokeweed mitogen than PHA or Con A
stimulation (data not shown) and reproducibly although
weakly (around 30%) the IL-2 dependent growth of an IL-2
dependent T cell line (Table 1). Furthermore, both mAbs
profoundly inhibit anti-class I or II CML as well as NK
lysis (K562 being used as a target)(Table 4). These mAbs
were found to alter the adhesivity to glass of PMN as
well as the phagocytosis of monocytes (data not shown).

Table 5.

mAbs used	Untreated HL-60	IFN γ-treated HL-60
39 B2.1 (67K)	8	7
39 H7.3 ?	9	70
12 E3.1 (55K, CD2)	9	40.5
19 E3.6 ?	8	8
39 C1.5 (55K, CD2)	8	7
39 C8.18 (20K)	8.5	63
5 B6.4 (55K, CD2)	8	6
13 E1.19 ?	8	80
Controls		
B9.12 (class I)	96	98.5
9.6 (E rosette recept)	10	82
39 C6.5 (I1-2 recept)	10	69
BK 19 (Transf. recept)	44	21

Cloned γ IFN (Biogen) was added to the cultures on day 0, and the phenotypic changes studied 4 days later (11).

In contrast to previous reports, mAb 25.3 although fulfilling most criteria defining so far the LFA-1 molecule[1] is able to inhibit the binding of the C3 bi complement protein to its receptor (M. Kazatchkine, personal communication), while mAb 25.5 is negative in this assay.

Finally, both mAbs were found to be absent from the surface of lymphocytes, PMN and monocytes of a young girl with recurrent bacterial infections studied by A. Fisher in Claude Griscelli's group in Paris (submitted). The PMN and monocyte functions of this patient were impaired as judged by the following tests : nylon wool adherence, cell movement, phagocytosis and opsonized particle induced oxydative response. NK activity as well as CML activity were profoundly reduced but MLR was normal as was stimulation by T cell mitogens. A profound reduction in the production of α- and γ-IFN as well as antibody to vaccinal antigens was documented, in vitro. LFA-1 molecules as well as the C3 bi receptor (CR3) and the p 150-90 molecule were absent from neutrophils, monocytes and lymphocytes as shown by IF, rosette formation with C3 bi coated erythrocytes and immunoprecipitation. Both the α and β chains of the adhesive protein complex were absent from the membrane.

The last mAb, mAb 10 G3.3, although immunoprecipitating from monocyte a 170-90 K molecular complex had a unique tissue distribution, being only strongly positive on monocytes (and weakly on polymorphs) and among the cell lines tested, only positive on AML cells. This last mAb was found to have functional activities difficult to reproduce (blocking on CML). MAbs 25.5 and 10 G3.3, in contrast to mAb 25.3 did not have any effect on the C3 bi fragment binding (M. Kazatchkine, personal communication).

Unrecognized T cell specific functional mAbs - T activated cell 46 F.1.1 (110 K).

This mAb belongs to the early T cell activated antigens (11) (peak around 9 hours) (Table 6) and its tissue distribution (Table 7) confirms this molecule as an activation antigen. It is not inducible by γ-IFN on HL-60 and its molecular weight following an SDS-PAGE analysis of the immunoprecipitate obtained from the lysate of NP 40 solubilized surface labelled PHA blasts

TABLE 6. Kinetics of the 46 F1.1 molecule on activated T cells

	Hours : 0	3	9	/ Day : 0	1	3	7
46 F1.1	12	32	46	11.2	35	20	4

Table 7. Tissue distribution of mAb 46 F1.1

	T	B	PMN	MONO	RPMI	CEM	MOLT	1301	HPB	ALL	ICHI.	HL-60	KG1	U937	AML
46 F1.1	4	3	3	18	20	5	4	7	25	4	13	5	4	5	9

is approximatively 110 K (data not shown). This mAb
blocks primary MLR, CML as well as NK lysis (Table 4).
         - Pan T mAb 8 H8.1, belonging to CD7
     This mAb, which recognizes a 41K, T cell surface
molecule (data not shown), has a tissue distribution
which correlates with the mAbs belonging to the CD7
defined during the first International Workshop on
Leukocyte Differentiation Antigens i.e. positive on T
cells, thymocytes, and acute T but also non-T.
     This mAb blocks both MLR and CML (NK not tested)
(Table 4). Such a functional effect has not yet been
reported for mAbs of similar specificity, local such as
46 B3.5 or 13 C7.4 or from colleagues (3A1, 4A).

CONCLUSIONS

     We have confirmed the functional nature of already
qualified lymphocyte functional antigens such as those
belonging to CD3 (12), CD4 (13), CD8 (4). We have further
qualify as LFA, molecules such as to the IL-2 receptor,
the transferrin receptor and class II antigens.
     We report here that through mAb dependant functional
inhibition assays, the CD2 and the CD7 molecules are LFA
antigens and that other membrane structures belong to the
LFA molecular group : i.e. those defined by mAb 39 B2.1
(67 K), 39 C1.8 (20 K) and probably mAb 39 H7.3 although
no MW has been obtained for the molecule it recognizes.
     Finally, we have described two new molecules as LFA
: an early activation antigen 46 F1.1 (110 K) and the
molecule belonging to CD7 (41K).
     We anticipate that the number of such molecules
should increase and that their nature and role should now
be looked in molecular terms. From such studies, beyond
the use of mAbs to modulate lymphocyte function, a new
class of agonist and antagonist molecules could arise by
synthesis (or screening) allowing to modulate immune
responses with agents fulfilling the criteria of
pharmacological agents.

REFERENCES

1.   Davignon, D., Martz, E., Reynolds, T., Kurzinger, K.
      and Springer, T.A. J. Immunol, 127, 590-596 (1981)
2.   Krensky, A.M. et al. J. Immunol. 131, 611-616 (1983)
3.   Olive, D., Dubreuil, P. and Mawas, C.
      Immunogenetics, in press (1984)

4. Malissen, B., Rebai, N., Liabeuf, A. and Mawas, C.
    Eur. J. Immunol. 12, 739-747 (1982)
5. Leonard, W.J., Depper, J.M., Uchiyama, T., Smith,
    K.A., Waldmann, T.A. and Greene, W.C. Nature 300,
    267-269 (1982)
6. Hemler, M.E., Malissen, B., Rebai, N., Liabeuf, A.,
    Mawas, C., Kourilsky, F.M. and Strominger, J.L.
    Human Immunol. 8, 153-159 (1983)
7. Brown, G., Kourilsky, F.M., Fisher, A., Bastin, J.
    and MacLennan, I.C.M. Human Lymphocyte
    differentiation 1, 167-182 (1981)
8. Bourgue, F., Rebai, N. and Mawas, C. Human Immunol.
    8, 33-40 (1983)
9. Moretta, A., Accolla, R. and CERROTTINI, J.C. J.
    Exp. Med. 155, 599-602, (1982)
10. Schlossman, S.F. and Reinherz, E.L. Springer Semin
    Immunopathol. 7 9-18, (1984)
11. Olive, D., Dubreuil, P., Charmot, D., Mawas, C. and
    Mannoni, P. Proceeding 16th Leucocyte Culture
    Conference, Mitchison, A. and Feldman, M. (Eds),
    Humana Press, in press (1984)
12. Platsoucas, C.D. and Good, R.A. Proc. Natl. Acad.
    Sci. USA 78, 4368-4371 (1981)
13. Biddison, N.E., Rao, P.E., Talle, M.A., Goldstein,
    G. and Shaw, S. J. Exp. Med. 156, 1065-1069 (1982)

Cell Surface Antigens Involved in Human Cytolytic

T Lymphocyte-mediated Cytolysis

Steven J. Mentzer, Julia L. Greenstein, Alan
M. Krensky, Steven J. Burakoff
Dana-Farber Cancer Institute, Harvard Medical
School, Boston, Massachusetts 02115

Cytotoxic T lymphocytes (CTL) play an important role
in host resistance to viral infections[1], some types of
tumors[2] and organ allografts.[3] The molecular mechanisms involved in the human CTL response has been the subject of
intense investigation. An important development in the
study of the lytic mechanism has been the use of monoclonal
reagents - both monoclonal antibodies (MAb) and monoclonal
CTL. Monoclonal antibodies have been used to probe the
surface of the CTL. Functionally relevant cell surface
molecules have been identified by the ability of appropriate MAb to inhibit CTL cytolysis. Cloned CTL with known
specificity and phenotype have enhanced the sensitivity of
this technique.

Using this approach, several surface structures on the
CTL have been implicated in target cell recognition. These
structures appear to be involved in a range of functions.
The T3 complex appears to be involved in activation of the
cell, while the T3-T cell receptor (Ti) complex provides a
mechanism for antigen specific activation. The T4 (Leu 3)
and T8 (Leu 2) surface structures are apparently involved
in the recognition of distinct classes of target molecules.
Through this recognition the T4 or T8 glycoprotein may
stabilize the CTL-target interaction. Other stabilizing
or "adhesion" molecules appear to be the lymphocyte func-
tion-associated (LFA-1 and LFA-2) molecules. LFA-2 is
largely restricted to T cells, whereas LFA-1 may be involved in virtually all leukocyte adhesion interactions.

187

T3 complex

The T3 antigen defines a molecular complex composed of 3 associated structures.[4] One is an unglycosylated protein of 20 kilodaltons (Kd)(termed ε by Terhorst et al); the other two are glycoproteins of 20Kd (δ) and 25Kd (γ). It is this molecular complex that is recognized by conventional T3 MAb (OKT3 and Leu4).

The T3 antigen is present on all mature T cells. T3 appears in the medullary thymus, coincident with the appearance of antigen responsiveness and antigen specificity.[5] The coordinate expression of T3 and antigen specificity in the thymus suggests a close association of T3 with the T-cell receptor.[6] The association is persistent in the peripheral lymphoid tissue as well. Biochemical evidence also exists for a T3-Ti association. It has been observed by several investigators that immunoprecipitates of the T3 complex result in the co-precipitation of two bands of larger molecular weight. The definition of the T-cell receptor has shown that these molecules are the 49Kd α chain and the 43Kd β chain of Ti. The co-precipitation of T3 and Ti has been confirmed by cross-linking studies in which the T3-Ti proteins are covalently linked to facilitate immunoprecipitation and biochemical characterization (M. Brenner, et al, submitted).

The functional association of T3 and Ti has been more difficult to investigate. A phenomenon which suggests a functional linkage is co-modulation.[6] MAb to the T3 complex induces the disappearance of the T3 antigen from the cell surface (modulation); at the same time, the Ti antigen is lost from the cell surface. The reciprocal phenomenon is also observed. MAb to Ti induces the disappearance of both T3 and Ti from the cell surface. The finding that T3 and Ti reciprocally co-modulate suggests that T3 is at least structurally associated with the antigen specific receptor. This suggestion is further supported by the finding that Ti and T3 molecules are present in equal numbers on the cell surface.[7] More relevant functional evidence for the T3-Ti association is the finding that MAb to T3 and MAb to Ti have parallel ability to inhibit antigen specific cell functions. Both MAb block specific cytolysis and antigen specific proliferation.[8]

An important observation relative to the mechanism of CTL killing is the finding that MAb to the T3 antigen

inhibits cytolysis. The inhibition of CTL lysis requires
doses of OKT3 in the range of 10 ug/ml for maximum
effect. Other effects of MAb to the T3 complex may
provide clues to the mechanism of T3 inhibition. A widely
recognized effect of MAb to the T3 antigen is non-specific
activation of the T-cell. At a range of doses, T3 MAb
stimulates mitogenesis.[9,10] The ability of T3 MAb to
trigger non-specific activation of the cell suggests an
explanation which may reconcile the apparent paradox of
CTL inhibition and T-cell mitogenesis. The observed
inhibition of lysis may be a consequence of inappropriate
or premature activation (rather than inactivation or
steric hindrance) of the CTL. Prior to engaging the target
cell in an appropriate interaction, T3 MAb might
prematurely trigger the CTL. The consequence would be, in
many cases, ineffective discharge of the lytic mechanism
and a diminution of observed cytolysis.

If T3 MAb inhibits cytolysis by inappropriate
activation of the CTL, there should be conditions in which
T3 MAb stimulates inappropriate cytolysis. Consistent
with this prediction we have recently observed that T3 MAb
stimulates non-specific killing by cloned CTL.

Using HLA-A2 or B7 specific CTL clones and T3 MAb, we
have been able to induce non-specific killing against a
variety of target cells that express neither HLA-A2 or B7.
The non-specific killing can be induced by commercially
available MAb (OKT3, Leu 4) at concentrations in the
mitogenic range; that is, concentrations as low as 10
ng/ml. Higher concentrations do not augment killing once
this threshold is reached. It is interesting that not all
target cells are killed equally well. Natural killer (NK)
targets (Eg K562 and DAUDI) as well as many murine cell
lines (Eg Ml2.4.1) appear to function better as target
cells for non-specific killing than do many B
lymphoblastoid cell lines. These results would suggest
that when the appropriate target is available,
non-specific mitogenesis and subsequent triggering of the
CTL might be inhibitory because some of the CTL would be
triggered prematurely. In contrast, when an inappropriate
target is available for lysis (i.e. against a background
of no cytolysis), non-specific activation of the CTL would
result in triggering of the lytic mechanism and killing of
the inappropriate target.

T4 and T8 Glycoproteins

MAb to T4 and T8 define glycoproteins of 62 Kd and 76

Kd respectively. The T4 and T8 antigens are co-expressed early in thymic development; the majority of cortical thymocytes are $T4^+T8^+$. Later in thymic development, the T4 and T8 antigens define mutually exclusive subpopulations. In the medulla, two thirds of thymocytes are $T4^+T8^-$ and one third is $T4^-T8^+$. The development of antigenic reactivity correlates with the expression of the mature (exclusively $T4^+T8^-$ or $T4^-T8^+$) phenotype.

It has been recognized for several years that the correlation of the mature phenotype with antigen reactivity implied an important role for the T4 and T8 molecules. Initially, the T4 and T8 phenotype appeared to correlate best with functional subsets of T cells. More recently, it has become apparent that T4 and T8 are associated with the recognition of different classes of target or restricting molecules rather than a particular T cell function. The T4 molecule has been associated with the recognition of class II molecules of the major histocompatability complex (MHC) and T8 has been associated with the recognition of class I MHC molecules.

Accumulating evidence supports the concept that T4 and T8 have a recognition-related function and are not simply markers for functional T cell subsets. Specifically, it appears that T4 is a receptor for a monomorphic determinant on class II molecules and T8 a receptor for class I molecules. This suggestion is supported by MAb blocking and evidence for $T4^+$ DR restricted CTL clones and $T8^+$ class I restricted helper T cells.[11,12,13,14,15]

The model that T4 is a receptor for class II and T8 a receptor for class I MHC antigens appeared consistent with the data until the recent description of several variant CTL clones. We have studied one such exception: a $T4^+$ CTL clone that is specific for HLA-B7, a class I target molecule. Not only is this clone phenotypically T4, but the T4 molecule appears to be involved in the lytic process. MAb to T4 significantly inhibits cytolysis by this clone. At first glance, this finding appeared to discount any direct recognition of the class II molecule.

An alternative explanation is possible. Based on work from our laboratory in the murine system, there is evidence that accessory recognition structures such as T4, or L3T4 in the mouse, need not recognize the same target molecule as the antigen specific receptor. The dissociability of the Ti and T4 (or L3T4) interactions is

illustrated by the work of Greenstein et al.[16] In this
system, a murine T-cell hybridoma with class I antigen
specificity was studied. As expected, MAb to Ti or the
class I target molecule blocked cytolysis. This hybridoma
expressed L3T4 and MAb to L3T4 also blocked function in
the presence of target cells expressing class II
molecules. An unexpected finding was that MAb to class II
target molecules blocked cytolysis as well. A plausible
interpretation for these data is that L3T4 (or T4)
receptor recognizes a class II target molecule while the
Ti receptor recognizes a class I target molecule.
Independent recognition is possible since there is no
evidence that L3T4 and Ti structures are physically
associated or required to recognize the same target
molecule. The T4 and T8 correlation with different classes
of CTL target molecules is most likely not a physical
association but an association that exists because of
developmental selection. For instance, this association
may be a reflection of intra-thymic education. Such an
early developmental selection would explain the strength
of the correlation as well as the existence of variants.
Therefore, in the case of our T4$^+$ class I restricted CTL
clone, the antigen receptor may recognize the class I
target molecule and T4 the class II molecule.

    A possible role for the T4 or T8 molecule is
stabilization of the Ti-antigen interaction. MacDonald et
al have argued that stabilization is less important if the
affinity and density of Ti is high.[17]   Conversely, a high
affinity Ti-antigen interaction may be less important if
the density of other accessory recognition structures and
their ligands are high. We can further speculate that the
"accessory" receptor interactions may play a role in the
selection of target cells; that is, the target cell range
of the CTL may be determined by the tissue distribution of
the ligand for the "accessory" receptor.

Lymphocyte Function Associated Molecules
    To define other function associated cell surface
molecules, our laboratory generated a panel of MAb and
screened them for their ability to inhibit CTL killing.
The antigens recognized by these MAb are called lymphocyte
function associated (LFA) antigens. Using this approach,
three cell surface structures have been defined.[18]

    LFA-1 is glycoprotein composed of a 177Kd α chain and
a 95 Kd β chain. It is broadly expressed on almost all
lymphocytes. MAb to LFA-1 stain almost all thymocytes,

one third of bone marrow cells, as well as monocytes and granulocytes.[19] The broad tissue distribution of LFA-1 is mirrored by functional involvement in a variety of immune processes. MAb to LFA-1 block cytolysis by class I or class II directed CTL, CTL of the OKT4 or OKT8 phenotype, and Natural killer (NK) effectors.[19] LFA-1 MAb also block a variety of proliferative responses including antigen-specific and PHA dependent mitogenesis.[19]

The importance of the LFA-1 molecule in normal immune function is highlighted by a clinical syndrome characterized by a deficiency of a 3 member glycoprotein family which includes LFA-1.[21,22] Other deficient molecules are the monocyte antigen Mol and a poorly understood molecule p150; all three molecules share the 95Kd β chain. The syndrome is manifested by life-threatening recurrent bacterial infection. Functional assessments of the affected patients have revealed impaired granulocyte phagocytosis and markedly reduced CTL lytic activity.[21,22]

A possible function for the LFA-1 molecule is stabilization of CTL-target cell conjugates. Evidence for this possibly is based on CTL-target cell binding assays. MAb to LFA-1 block conjugate formation.[23] Further, a panel of MAb recognizing different epitopes on the LFA-1 molecule have been generated.[24] The ability of MAb directed at different epitopes on the LFA-1 molecule to block cytolysis is paralleled by their ability to block conjugate formation. This is indirect evidence that the blocking of conjugate formation is the primary mechanism by which LFA-1 MAb inhibit cytolysis. The panel of MAb to at least 5 distinct epitopes on the LFA-1 molecule have been used to map functional regions on the LFA-1 molecule.[24] Four MAb recognize epitopes on the LFA-1 α chain, 1 MAb defines the β chain. The utility of this approach is illustrated by the differential ability of each of these MAb to block CTL-mediated killing. The panel of MAb define a hierarchy of inhibition which is constant regardless of the target antigen or the CTL phenotype. The same hierarchy of inhibition has recently been observed in studies of NK-mediated cytolysis (Mentzer, et al, submitted).

LFA-2 is a glycoprotein which immunoprecipitates a broad band at 49kd. Its tissue distribution is more restricted than LFA-1. MAb to LFA-2 react with almost all thymocytes, peripheral blood T cells, and a small

population of presumed NK effectors.[19] The molecular
weight and tissue distribution suggests that LFA-2 is the
molecule termed the sheep erythrocyte receptor; a molecule
also recognized by the MAb OKT11,[25] 9.6,[26] and Leu
5.[27] All of these monoclonal antibodies block cytolytic
and proliferative responses of T cells. There are,
however, functional differences. OKT11 is the only MAb
which completely modulates the molecule from the cell
surface. MAb 9.6 is unique in that it has been found to
inhibit NK cytolysis.[28] MAb to LFA-2 modulates only
50-75% (comparable to 9.6 and Leu 5) and does not block
NK-mediated cytolysis in our system.

The LFA-2 molecule has demonstrated significant
variability in its structure. It has been reported that
MAb to LFA-2 precipitates molecules of different molecular
weights from T cells at different stages of
differentiation or activation.[19] This variability may be
due to glycosylation differences or even differences in
amino acid sequence. Whether these structural changes can
be associated with functional differences remains
unanswered.

A functional property of the LFA-2 molecules is its
involvement in CTL-target cell interaction. Based on
CTL-target cell binding assays, MAb to LFA-2 have been
shown to inhibit conjugate formation.[22] This suggests
that LFA-2 may also be involved in the nonspecific
adhesion of the CTL and target cell. Meuer et al have
proposed another function for this molecule. These
workers have suggested that the molecule is involved in an
"alternative" activation pathway analogous to T3
activation.[29] Wilkinson and Morris have proposed a role
for the sheep erythrocyte receptor molecule in the
negative regulation of interferon-production.[30] More work
will be required to elucidate the function of this
molecule.

LFA-3 is a 45-65 Kd glycoprotein expressed on both T
and B lymphocytes as well as a variety of other
mesenchymal tissues.[19] Pretreatment experiments have
revealed a novel effect of the LFA-3 MAb. Unlike LFA-1 and
LFA-2, MAb to LFA-3 blocks by binding to the target cell
and not by binding to the CTL.[19] Thus, LFA-3 defines a
nonspecific CTL-target cell interaction molecule that does
not block at the level of the effector cell. Recent
studies suggest that LFA-3 may be the ligand of LFA-1.
although further studies are required to substantiate this

(Gromkowski et al, in press).

Functional Relevance

The use of MAb to probe the surface of cloned CTL has permitted the definition of several structures involved in the CTL lytic mechanism. The validity of this approach is based on the observation that, although many MAb bind to the cell surface, few of these MAb actually inhibit cytolysis. It is possible that these molecules do not directly participate in the CTL-target cell interaction. Inhibition of cytotoxicity may not always be the result of inhibiting a receptor-ligand interaction. For example, MAb to the T3 complex may prematurely or inappropriately trigger T cells. Other MAb may inhibit by an "off" signal to the T cell.

To minimize possible artifact we have employed several assays to validate the functional relevance of these surface structures. An example is the use of CTL-target cell binding assays which permit direct visualization of the CTL-target cell conjugate. The effects of MAb to T4, T8, LFA-1, LFA-2, and LFA-3 can be observed directly by their inhibition of conjugate formation. Calcium and magnesium chelators can be used to further define the relevant stage of the lytic process. The T3 antigen is the one exception in that it appears to block at a post-adhesion stage and its effects cannot be directly visualized. Perhaps not coincidentally, the T3 complex is one of the surface structures most convincingly involved in the lytic mechanism.

References

1. Burakoff, S.J., Reiss, C.S., Finberg, R., & Mescher, M.F. Rev. Infect. Dis. 2, 62-72 (1980).
2. Cerottini, J.C. & Brunner, K.T. Adv. Immunol. 18, 67-132 (1974).
3. Herberman, R.B. Adv. Cancer Res. 19, 207-263 (1974).
4. Borst, J., Prendiville, M.A., Terhorst, C., J. Immunol. 128, 1560-1565 (1982).
5. Reinherz, E.L., Schlossman, S.F. Cell 19, 821-827 (1980).
6. Reinherz, E.L., Meuer, S.C., Fitzgerald, K.A., Hussey, R.E., Schlossman, S.F. Cell 30, 735-743 (1982).
7. Meuer, S.C., Acuto, O., Hussey, R.E., Hodgdon, J.C., Fitzgerald, K.A., Schlossman, S.F., & Reinherz, E.L. Nature 303, 808-810 (1983).
8. Meuer, S.C., Fitzgerald, K.A., Hussey, R.E., Hodgdon, J.C., Schlossman, S.F., & Reinherz, E.L. J. Exp. Med. 157, 705-710 (1983).
9. Chang, T.W., Kung, P.C., Gingras, S.P., & Goldstein, G. Proc. Natl. Acad. Sci. USA 78, 1805-1808 (1981).
10. Van Wauwe, F.P., DeMay, J.R., & Goosener, J.G. J. Immunol. 124, 2708-2713 (1980).
11. Krensky, A.M., Reiss, C.S., Mier, J.W., Strominger, J.L. & Burakoff, S.J. Proc. Natl. Acad. Sci. USA 79, 2365-2369.
12. Krensky, A.M., Clayberger, C., Reiss, C.S., Strominger, J.L. & Burakoff, S.J. J. Immunol. 129, 2001-2003 (1982).
13. Meuer, S.C., Schlossman, S.F. & Reinherz, E.L. Proc. Natl. Acad. Sci. USA 79, 4395-4399 (1982).
14. Spits, H., Borst, J., Terhorst, C., & DeVries, J.F. J. Immunol. 129, 1563-1569 (1982).
15. Engleman, E.G., Benike, C.J., Grumet, F.C., and Evans, R.L. J. Immunol. 127, 2124-2129 (1981).
16. Greenstein, J.L., Kappler, J., Marrack, P., & Burakoff, S.J. J. Exp. Med. 159, 1213-1224 (1984).
17. MacDonald, H.R., Glasebrook, A.L. & Cerottini, J.-C. J. Exp. Med. 156, 1711-1722 (1982).
18. Sanchez-Madrid, F., Krensky, A.M., Ware, C.F., Robbins, E., Strominger, J.L., Burakoff, S.J. & Springer, T.A. Proc. Natl. Acad. Sci. USA 79, 7489-7493 (1982).
19. Krensky, A.M., Sanchez-Madrid, F., Robbins, E., Nagy, J., Springer, T.A. & Burakoff, S.J. J. Immunol. 131, 611-616 (1983).
20. Beatty, P.G., Ledbetter, J.A., Martin, P.J., Price, T.H. & Hansen, J.A. J. Immunol. 131, 2913-2918

(1983).

21. Crowley, C.A., Curnette, J.A., Rosin, R.E.,
    Andre-Schwartz, J. Gallin, J.I., Klempner, M.,
    Snyderman, R., Southwick, F.S., Stossel, T.P. &
    Babior, B.M. N. Eng. J. Med. 302, 1163-1171 (1980).

22. Anderson, D.C., Schmalstieg, F.C., Arnaout, M.A.,
    Kohl, S., Tosi, M.F., Dana, N., Buffone, G.J.,
    Hughes, B.J., Brinkley, B.R., Dickey, W. D.,
    Abramson, J.S., Springer, T., Boxer, L.A., Hollers,
    J.M., & Smith, C. W. J. Clin. Invest. 74, 536-551
    (1984).

23. Krensky, A.M., Robbins, E., Springer, T.A. & Burakoff,
    S.J. J. Immunol. 132, 2810-2812 (1984).

24. Ware, C.F., Sanchez-Madrid, F., Krensky, A.M.,
    Burakoff, S.J., Strominger, J.L. & Springer, T.A. J.
    Immunol. 131, 1182-1188 (1983).

25. Palacios, R. & Martinez-Maza, J. Immunol. 129,
    2479-2486 (1982).

26. Howard, F.D., Ledbetter, J.A., Wong, J., Bieber, C.P.,
    Stinson, E.B. & Herzenberg, L.A. J. Immunol. 126,
    2117-2122 (1981).

27. Kamoun, M.P., Martin, P.J., Hansen, J.A., Brown, M.A.,
    Siadak, A.W. & Nowinski, R.C. J. Exp. Med. 153,
    207-212 (1981).

28. Martin, P.J., Longton, G., Ledbetter, J.A., Newman,
    W., Braun, M.P., Beatty, P. G., and Hansen, J.A. J.
    Immunol. 131, 180-185 (1983).

29. Fitzgerald, K.a., Hodgdon, J.C., Protentis, J.,
    Schlossman, S.J. & Reinherz, E.L. Cell 36, 897-906
    (1984).

30. Wilkinson, M. & Morris, A., Eur. J. Immunol. 14,
    708-713 (1984).

MHC-RESTRICTED ANTIGEN-RECEPTOR SPECIFIC REGULATORY

T CELL CIRCUITS IN MAN

Nitin K. Damle, Dianne M. Fishwild, Nahid Mohagheghpour
and Edgar G. Engleman

From the Department of Pathology
Stanford University School of Medicine
Stanford, California 94305

INTRODUCTION

In vitro analysis of interactions among various functionally and phenotypically distinct human T and nonT lymphoid cells has been greatly facilitated by the development of monoclonal antibodies (mab) to a variety of lymphoid cell surface molecules (1). With the use of such antibodies two major sublineages of human T cells were initially defined, Leu2+/T8+ cells which mediate most cytolytic and suppressor (Tc+Ts) effects and Leu3+/T4+ cells which mediate most helper/inducer (Th+Ti) functions (2-5). Cells within these two sublineages appear to recognize antigen in association with class I major histocompatibility complex (MHC) products (HLA-A,B,C) and class II MHC (HLA-DR,DC,SB) products respectively, and this differential recognition of distinct MHC products influences the responses of cells within the two sublineages to a variety of stimuli (4,6).

Although cells within the Leu3+ subset may share a common receptor for class II MHC molecules, this population is nonetheless heterogeneous, providing helper signals that augment the differentiation of B cells into immunoglobulin secreting plasma cells as well as signals which induce Leu2+ suppressor T (Ts) cells (5,7). In order to determine whether the helper activity for B cells is mediated by a specific subpopulation of Leu3+ cells, these cells were separated into Leu3+,8- and Leu3+,8+ subpopulations using monoclonal anti-Leu8 antibody, which reacts wih 80% of circulating Leu3+ cells (7). Both Leu3+,8- and Leu3+,8+

197

subpopulations respond by proliferation to mitogens, soluble antigens, and in autologous and allogeneic MLR, and upon stimulation secrete comparable amounts of interleukin-2 (7-9). Leu3+,8- and Leu3+,8+ cells were cultured with autologous nonT cells and stimulated with either pokeweed mitogen or autologous or allogeneic nonT cells for 8 days following which Ig secreting cells were enumerated in a reverse hemolytic plaque assay. The vast majority of Ig secretion was induced by the minor Leu3+,8- subpopulation irrespective of the stimulus (7, Kansas G.S., unpublished).

Recently, analogous studies were carried out to determine if the Leu3+,8- and Leu3+,8+ subpopulations differed in their ability to induce alloantigen specific Leu2+ suppressor cells in MLR (9). In these experiments, cyclosporin A was included in MLR cultures to prevent the activation of cytolytic T cells (9). Leu3+,8- or Leu3+,8+ cells were cultured with autologous Leu2+ cells and irradiated allogeneic nonT cells in the presence of 1 ug/ml of cyclosporin, after which Leu2+ cells were recovered and examined for the ability to inhibit the fresh MLR response of autologous Leu3+ cells. Alloactivated Leu3+,8+ cells alone induced potent Leu2+ suppressor cells of the MLR, whereas alloactivated Leu3+,8- cells failed to induce suppression (9). In summary, while the Leu3+,8+ cells help B cell differentiation only weakly, this subset appears to include all or nearly all T cells capable of inducing Leu2+ suppressor T cells.

Like the Leu3+ population, the Leu2+ subset is also functionally heterogeneous, mediating both cytolytic and suppressor functions. For example, the allogeneic MLR activates Leu2+ cytolytic cells with specificity for the HLA-A or B antigens of the stimulator cell. In addition, Leu2+ cells activated in MLR suppress fresh MLR with specificity for the HLA-DR antigens of the stimulator cell (9). As described above, the induction of suppressor T cells was not affected by concentrations of cyclosporin that prevented the development of cytolytic T cells (9). Nevertheless, the question remained as to whether or not suppression and cytotoxicity are mediated by the same Leu2+ cells or by phenotypically distinguishable subpopulations. We approached this problem with monoclonal antibody 9.3 that reacts with a 44,000 dalton glycoprotein expressed on the surface of all Leu3+ cells in addition to approximaely 50% of Leu2+ cells (10). Thus, Leu2+,9.3- and Leu2+,9.3+ subpopulations were purified, cultured for 7 days with allogeneic nonT cells, reisolated, and examined for both cytolytic and suppressor effects. As reported (10), all detectable cytolytic activity was confined to the Leu2+,9.3+ subpopulation; killing by this subpopulation was specific for the class I MHC antigens of the priming cell. By contrast, suppression of proliferation in MLR was mediated predominantly by the Leu2+,9.3- cells, and the suppression by this subpopulation was specific for class II MHC antigens of the priming cell (10). The combined results suggest that Leu2+ suppressor cells are derived from a precursor pool that is phenotypically distinct from that which gives rise to Leu2+ cytolytic cells.

The studies reviewed here represent an effort to isolate the cells involved in the generation of antigen specific suppression, define the role of each cell type, and identify key cell surface molecules that mediate the function of these cells. Our findings suggest that Ts cells are activated by antigen recognition structures on Leu3+ Ti cells rather then antigen itself or antigen pulsed accessory cells.

INDUCTION OF SUPPRESSOR T CELLS BY INDUCER T CELLS
IN THE ABSENCE OF ANTIGEN

Although using bulk culture systems (9,10) we were able to detect the activation of antigen specific Ts cells, these cells could not be activated with antigen-pulsed autologous accessory cells in the absence of Leu3+ cells (8). Therefore, we examined the role of Leu3+ cells in the activation of Leu2+ Ts cells. The study described below originated from the initial observation that mitogen-activated Leu3+ cells caused activation and subsequent differentiation of fresh autologous Leu2+ cells into Ts cells that were capable of inhibiting the response of fresh Leu3+ cells to a variety of stimuli (11). This observation in an antigen nonspecific system was subsequently extended to an alloantigen-specific system. Specifically we sought to examine the functional consequences of exposing fresh Leu2+ cells to alloantigen-primed Leu3+ inducer cells (Ti) in the absence of the priming allogeneic stimulator cells. The overall experimental design for these experiments involved the activation of Leu3+ cells in MLR for 7 days followed by the isolation of Leu3+ lymphoblasts on discontinuous Percoll gradients and the use of these lymphoblasts as irradiated stimulators in 7-day cultures with fresh autologous Leu2+

cells. No allogeneic stimulator cells were present during these cultures. Leu2+ cells recovered from these cultures were irradiated to 1500 R and then examined for their suppressive effect on the proliferative response of fresh Leu3+ cells in MLR. Leu2+ cells activated with autologous alloactivated Leu3+ cells, but not those cultured with resting Leu3+ cells, suppressed the response of fresh Leu3+ cells only to the original priming allogeneic cells (12). This ability to suppress fresh MLR after activation of Leu2+ cells by alloactivated Ti cells was found to be confined to the Leu2+,9.3- subpopulation (8,12). Subpopulations of Leu3+ cells defined with anti-Leu8 antibody were examined for their ability to induce Ts cells. Thus, alloactivated Leu3+,8- and Leu3+,8+ cells were used to stimulate fresh Leu2+ cells prior to testing their suppressive effect. Alloactivated Leu3+,8+ cells but not Leu3+,8- cells induced Leu2+ Ts cells to effect suppression of fresh MLR. Therefore, the abilities to induce and effect suppression appear to be confined to Leu3+,8+ and Leu2+,9.3- subpopulations of T cells respectively (8-10,12).

These results indicate that structures either displayed on the surface of activated Ti cells or secreted by them activate precursors of Ts cells to differentiate into suppressor-effectors in the apparent absence of the priming allogeneic cells. At no point during the induction of Ts cells were cultures containing Leu2+ cells exposed directly to stimulator allogeneic cells. Thus, the mechanism of activation of these Ts cells is distinct from that involved in the activation of Leu2+ Tc cells, which require exposure to allogeneic stimulator cells in combination with signals from Leu3+ Ti cells. Other studies indicate that the inhibitory effect of these Ts cells is specific for the original allogeneic stimulus and is not due to altered kinetics of MLR or absorption by Ts cells of growth-promoting factors such as IL-2 (12). Further, suppression of MLR is observed only when Ts cells are added within 24 h of initiation of MLR cultures (12). Finally, the above described mode of activation of Ts cells is not confined to alloantigen-stimulated systems, but also applies to systems driven by soluble antigens such as purified protein derivative of tuberculin (PPD) (8). We considered the possibility that Leu2+ Ts cells might represent specialized cytolytic cells that lyse autologous antigen-activated Th/Ti cells. However, when examined directly for cytolytic activity, Ts cells failed to lyse either autologous Leu3+ blasts or the priming allogeneic nonT cells (8,12,13).

ALLOACTIVATED INDUCER T CELLS ALSO ACTIVATE
AMPLIFIER T CELLS

In addition to the induction of Leu2+ Ts cells, alloactivated Leu3+,8+ cells stimulated proliferation of fresh autologous Leu3+,8- and Leu3+,8+ cells (8,12,13). To examine the effect of such autoactivated Leu3+,8- and Leu3+,8+ cells on the development of Leu2+ Ts cells, Leu3+,8- and Leu3+,8+ cells were preactivated for 7 days with autologous alloactivated Leu3+,8+ Ti lymphoblasts and added to "suppressor induction" cultures consisting of irradiated alloactivated Leu3+,8+ Ti cells and fresh Leu2+ cells. Leu2+ cells isolated from these cultures were examined for suppression of MLR. The presence of preactivated Leu3+,8- cells in the "suppressor-induction" cultures resulted in the amplification of the suppressive effect of Leu2+ Ts cells generated in these cultures. In contrast, similarly treated Leu3+,8+ cells failed to amplify suppression (14). Thus, although both Leu3+,8- and Leu3+,8+ cells proliferate to alloactivated Leu3+,8+ Ti cells, Leu3+,8- cells alone differentiate into suppressor amplifier cells (Ta). Furthermore, the suppressor-amplifier effect of Leu3+,8- Ta cells was found to be specific for the priming alloactivated Leu3+,8+ Ti cells and thus, like Ts cells, indirectly specific for the priming allogeneic cells (14). These Leu3+,8- Ta cells do not induce Leu2+ Ts cells, but, rather, they augment the development of suppressor activity of Leu2+ Ts cells by mechanisms other than the induction of additional Leu2+ Ts cells (14).

CELL SURFACE STRUCTURES ON LEU-3+,8+ Ti CELLS
INVOLVED IN THE ACTIVATION OF Ts CELLS

Since alloantigen-specific Ts cells were activated by alloantigen-primed Ti cells in the absence of the priming allogeneic stimulus, we reasoned that molecules expressed on the surface of activated Ti cells may be recognized by and stimulate precursors of Ts cells. In an effort to block recognition of these structures by Ts cells, alloactivated Leu3+,8+ blasts were treated with monoclonal antibodies directed against molecules Leu1(p67), Leu2(p33), Leu3(p55), Leu4(p19-26), Leu5(p50), HLA-DR(p29,33), and

HLA-A,B,C(p12,45).   Thus,   alloactivated   Leu3+,8+
lymphoblasts were incubated separately with saturating
concentrations of the above monoclonal antibodies in the
absence of complement, washed extensively and examined for
their ability to induce proliferation of fresh autologous
Leu2+ cells and Leu3+ cells.   Treatment of alloactivated
Leu3+ Ti cells with anti-Leu4 antibody blocked their
ability to activate both Leu2+ and Leu3+ cells.   Similar
pretreatment of Ti cells with anti-Leu1, anti-Leu3 or
anti-Leu5 antibodies had no effect on the ability of these
cells to stimulate autologous T cell proliferation.
Interestingly, Ti cells pretreated with anti-HLA-ABC
antibody stimulated autologous Leu3+ cells but not Leu2+
cells. In contrast, activated Ti cells pretreated with
anti-HLA-DR antibody induced activation of Leu2+ cells but
not Leu3+ cells (15).   Leu2+ cells activated with
antibody-treated alloactivated Ti cells were also examined
for suppression of MLR. Activation of Leu2+ Ts cells was
blocked by pretreatment of Ti cells with either anti-Leu4
or anti-HLA-ABC antibodies, but not by antibodies to other
molecules such as Leu1, Leu3, Leu5, and HLA-DR (15). These
results suggest that the activation of Leu2+ Ts cells with
alloactivated Ti cells involves dual recognition by the
former of self class I MHC molecules and the Leu4 antigen
complex on the surface of Ti cells (15).

CELL SURFACE STRUCTURES ON LEU-2+ CELLS INVOLVED IN THE
ACTIVATION AND EFFECTOR PHASES OF SUPPRESSION

Monoclonal antibodies to various lymphoid surface
molecules were also used to probe molecules on the surface
of Leu2+ cells that participate in their activation and
suppressor function.   In addition to the antibodies
referred to above, antibodies directed against molecules
HLA-DC (p28,34), LFA-1 (p95,177), and LFA-3 (p60) were used
in this study. To assess the effects of these antibodies
on Ts activation Leu2+ cells were treated with each of the
above antibodies, washed extensively, and activated with
alloantigen-primed Leu3+ Ti cells before suppressor assay.
Pretreatment of Leu2+ cells with only anti-Leu2, anti-Leu4,
anti-Leu5, and anti-LFA-1 antibodies prevented the
development of Ts cells suggesting that these molecules are
involved in the interactions of Ts cells with Ti cells
during the differentiation of the former.   To assess the
effects of these antibodies on suppressor effector function
Leu2+ cells were activated first with alloactivated Ti

cells and then incubated with antibodies. Only anti-Leu2
and anti-LFA-1 antibodies blocked suppression. Anti-Leu5
antibody had no effect on suppression whereas anti-Leu4
antibody consistently augmented the suppressor effect of Ts
cells. These results suggest that Leu2, Leu4, and LFA-1
molecules are involved in the interaction between Leu2+ Ts
cells and Leu3+ antigen-reactive cells.

GENERAL COMMENTS

This study was an effort to examine the interactions
among various T cell subpopulations involved in an
alloantigen-specific suppressor circuit. We have shown
that alloantigen-primed Leu3+ Ti cells activate precursors
of Leu2+ Ts cells and Leu3+ Ta cells in the absence of the
priming alloantigenic stimulus (8,12-14). Although both
Leu3+,8- and Leu3+,8+ subpopulations respond to antigen and
upon activation express equivalent amounts of HLA-DR
antigens (8,9,14), only Leu3+,8+ cells induce
antigen-specific Ts cells (8,9,14). The above observations
in bulk culture systems are consistent with the reported
activation of an influenza virus specific Ts cell clone by
an influenza virus specific Th cell clone (16). More
recently, we have described an alloreactive Leu3+,8+ Ti
clone that selectively activates alloantigen-specific Leu2+
Ts cells in the absence of allogeneic stimulator cells
(13). Once activated, Ts cells are capable of inhibiting
the response of both Leu3+,8- and Leu3+,8+ cells to the
priming antigen (8,9,14). Furthermore, maximal suppression
requires the collaboration of at least three phenotypically
distinct T cells, two of which (Ta cells and Ts cells) are
activated in the absence of the priming antigen by
antigen-primed Ti cells, and are only indirectly specific
for the priming antigen (14).

These results suggest a key role for the Leu4(T3)
complex on both Leu3+ Ti cells and Leu2+ Ts cells in the
activation of the latter. Previous studies have shown that
anti-Leu4 antibodies both induce T cell proliferation and
abrogate antigen-specific proliferative and cytolytic
responses (17-21). The Leu4 structure is rapidly modulated
from the T cell surface following interaction with
anti-Leu4 antibody or antigen itself (22,23), and
antigen-specific T-cell functions require surface Leu4
expression (1,24). As shown in the present study, binding
of anti-Leu4 antibody to activated Leu3+ cells not only
blocks proliferation of Leu2+ cells but also their

subsequent differentiation into Ts cells, suggesting that recognition of the Leu4 molecule itself or an associated structure on the surface of Leu3+ blasts is involved in the activation of Leu2+ Ts cells. The structure of Leu4 is thought to be invariant (21,25) and therefore, it is difficult to envisage how recognition of this molecule alone on the surface of inducer cells could lead to antigen-specific suppression. On the other hand, a preponderance of evidence indicates that Leu4 molecules are physically associated with 90 kd clonotypic structures that form the T cell antigen receptor complex (26,27). Therefore, it is conceivable that binding of anti-Leu4 antibody to inducer cells blocks the recognition of Leu4-associated receptor structures by precursors of Ts cells. The view that Ts cells are specific for antigen-recognition structures on Leu3+ cells rather than antigen itself is compatible with the observations that the activation of Ts cells by Leu3+ blasts takes place in the absence of the priming antigen and that suppression by activated Leu2+ cells appears to be directed at Leu3+ responder cells rather than nonT stimulator cells (12). One possible explanation for these observations is that Leu4-associated antigen-recognition structures on antigen-reactive Leu3+ cells serve as both stimulus and target for Ts cells. If so, then neither the generation nor effector phase of suppression would involve direct interaction of Leu2+ cells with the priming antigen.

Treatment of Leu3+ blasts with anti-HLA-A,B,C antibody also inhibited the activation and subsequent differentiation of Leu2+ Ts cells, suggesting that class I MHC antigens as well as Leu4-associated molecules on the surface of autologous inducer Leu3+ cells are recognized by precursors of Leu2+ Ts cells as an obligatory step in their activation. Indeed, once activated, Leu2+ Ts cells inhibited the response of only those Leu3+ cells which shared at least one HLA-A or B allelic specificity with the suppressor-effector cells. Moreover, suppression was greatest when the responder Leu3+ cells shared more than one HLA-A and/or B allele with Leu2+ Ts cells (15). This raises the possibility that individual Leu3+ suppressor-inducer cells elicit activation of subpopulations of Ts cells, each restricted by a single HLA-A or B allele. Thus, while Leu2+ Ts cells may be specific for the antigen-recognition complex on inducer Leu3+ cells, their activation and effector functions are restricted by self class I MHC molecules.

The Leu2, Leu4, Leu5 (SRBC receptor, also known as
LFA-2), LFA-1 molecules on Leu2+ cells appear to be
involved in the activation and effector phases of
suppression. Antibodies to these molecules inhibit a
variety of proliferative and cytolytic responses of human
lymphoid cells (3,17-21,28-31). As these molecules are
structurally invariant, it is doubtful that they dictate
the specificity of suppression. It seems more likely that
antigen recognition structures associated with the Leu4
complex on Leu2+ cells are responsible for the observed
antigen specificity. Although the existence of such 90 kd
heterodimers on the surface of Leu2+ Ts cells has not yet
been demonstrated, recent studies suggest that the surface
expression of the Leu4 molecule is dependent on the
expression of the 90 kd heterodimer and vice versa (32,33,
Stobo J.D., unpublished). On this basis, we form the view
that the apparent specificity of Leu2+ Ts cells for the
antigen receptor on Leu3+ cells is dictated by
Leu4-associated 90 kd heterodimers on the surface of Leu2+
Ts cells. Therefore, Leu2+ Ts cells seem to utilize the
same set of molecules during their function as do Leu2+
cytolytic cells (34).

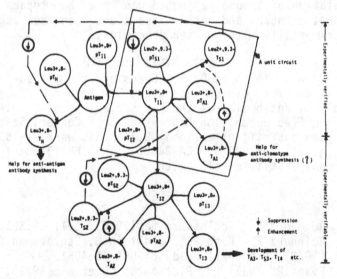

Figure 1: Immunoregulatory T-cell circuitry in man.

Incorporating the results described here with previous findings (7-14), a unified model of various regulatory T-cell interactions can be constructed as shown in Figure 1. A unique feature of this model is that it describes a complex array of antigen-independent autologous T-T interactions initiated by antigen-primed inducer T cells. Thus, upon activation with antigen, Leu3+,8+ inducer cells (Ti) stimulate Leu3+,8- amplifier (Ta) cells and Leu2+,9.3- suppressor-effector cells (Ts) both of which are only indirectly specific for the priming antigen since their specificity is dictated by inducer T cells. Amplifier T cells augment the differentiation of Ts cells, thus functionally completing the unit circuit depicted in Figure 1. It will be of particular interest to determine whether one or more of the T-T interactions described here are mediated by soluble factors and whether or not these interactions are restricted by products of genes that are localised outside the MHC in addition to those within the MHC. These issues are of paramount importance if we are to achieve success in efforts to manipulate the immune system in vivo to clinical advantage. Nonetheless, with the knowledge that several T cell subsets involved in feedback regulation of immune response can now be separated and cloned, these and other questions can be approached experimentally with greater precision.

ACKNOWLEDGEMENTS

We wish to thank Dr.R.L.Evans of the Sloan-Kettering Institute for Cancer Research, New York for his generous supply of antibodies of the Leu series, and Dr.J.A.Hansen of the Fred Hutchinson Cancer Research Center, Seattle for his generous gift of antibody 9.3. This work was supported by grants AM-32075, CA-24607, and HL-13108 from the National Institutes of Health.

REFERENCES

1. Reinherz EL, Schlossman SF (1980). Cell 19:821.
2. Reinherz EL, Kung PC, Goldstein G, Schlossman SF (1979). Proc Natl Acad Sci USA 76:4061.
3. Evans RL, Wall DW, Platsoucas CD et al (1981). Proc Natl Acad Sci USA 78:544.
4. Engleman EG, Benike CJ, Grumet CG, Evans RL (1981). J Immunol 127:2124.
5. Gatenby PA, Kotzin BL, Engleman EG (1981). J Immunol 127:2130.

6. Meuer SC, Schlossman SF, Reinherz EL (1982).
    Proc Natl Acad Sci USA 79:4395.
7. Gatenby PA, Kansas GS, Xian CY et al (1982).
    J Immunol 129:1997.
8. Damle NK, Mohagheghpour N, Engleman EG (1984).
    J Immunol 132:644.
9. Mohagheghpour N, Benike CB, Kansas GS, et al (1983).
    J Clin Invest 72:2092.
10. Damle NK, Mohagheghpour N, Hansen JA, Engleman EG
    (1983). J Immunol 131:2296.
11. Damle NK, Gupta S (1982). Scand J Immunol 16:59.
12. Damle NK, Engleman EG (1983). J Exp Med 158:159.
13. Mohagheghpour N, Damle NK, Moonka DM et al (1984).
    J Immunol 133:133.
14. Damle NK, Mohagheghpour N, Kansas GS et al (1985).
    J Immunol 134: in press.
15. Damle NK, Mohagheghpour N, Engleman EG (1984)
    J Immunol 133:1235.
16. Lamb J, Feldmann M (1982). Nature (Lond) 300:456.
17. Chang TW, Kung PC, Gingras SP, Goldstein G (1981).
    Proc Natl Acad Sci USA 78:1805.
18. Reinherz EL, Hussey RE, Schlossman SF (1980).
    Europ J Immunol 10:758.
19. Landergren U, Ramstedt U, Axberg I et al (1982).
    J Exp Med 155:1579.
20. Van Wauwe JP, Demey JP, Goosens JG (1980).
    J Immunol 124:2708.
21. Kaneoka H, Perez-Rojas G, Sasasuki T et al (1983).
    J Immunol 128:158.
22. Rinnoy Kan EA, Wang CY, Wang LC, Evans RL (1983).
    J Immunol 131:536.
23. Zanders ED, Lamb JR, Feldmann M (1983).
    Nature (Lond) 303:625.
24. Reinherz EL, Meuer SC, Fitzgerald KA et al (1982).
    Cell 30:735.
25. Borst J, Prenderville MA, Terhorst C (1982).
    J Immunol 128:1560.
26. Meuer SC, Fitzgerald KA, Hussey RE et al (1983).
    J Exp Med 157:705.
27. Meuer SC, Acuto O, Hussey RE et al (1983).
    Nature (Lond) 303:808.
28. Engleman EG, Benike CJ, Metzler C et al (1983).
    J Immunol 130:2623.
29. Damle NK, Hansen HA, Good RA, Gupta S (1981).
    Proc Natl Acad Sci USA 78:5096.

30. Palacious R, Martinez-Maza O (1982).
    J Immunol 129:2479.
31. Krensky AM, Sanchez-Madrid F, Robbins E et al
    (1983). J Immunol 131:611.
32. Weiss A, Imboden J, Shoback D, Stobo J (1984).
    Proc Natl Acad Sci USA 81:4196.
33. Weiss A, Imboden J, Wiskocil R, Stobo J (1984).
    J Clin Immunol 4:165.
34. Platsoucas CD (1984). Europ J Immunol 14:566.

EARLY BIOCHEMICAL EVENTS IN T LYMPHOCYTES ACTIVATED

BY ANTI T3

E.D. Zanders, M. Feldmann, K. O'Flynn[+], Shamshad Cockroft*
and J.R. Lamb

Imperial Cancer Research Fund, Tumour Immunology Unit,
Department of Zoology, University College London, Gower
Street, London WC1E 6BT.

[+] Department of Haematology, School of Medicine, University
College Hospital, University Street, London WC1E 6JJ

* Department of Experimental Pathology, School of Medicine,
University College Hospital, University Street,
London WC1E 6JJ

INTRODUCTION

The use of cloned T cells and monoclonal antibody
technology has resulted in a greater understanding of the
structure and function of surface molecules on human T
cells. Some of these structures have been identified as
receptors for ligands which mediate T cell growth, thus the
receptors for Il-2, antigen/MHC and an unknown ligand have
been defined by anti TAC, anti clonotypes and anti Tll
respectively (1-3). Our interest has focussed on the
antigen/MHC receptor which consists of a 90 kD disulphide
linked heterodimer in association with at least 3
polypeptides of 20,20 and 25 kD comprising the T3 antigen
system (4). The close association of T3 with the receptor
would suggest that the former is a signal transducing
mechanism which connects the initial binding of antigen/MHC
to the resulting cellular response, i.e. proliferation. We
have used the monoclonal anti T3 UCHT1 and the influenza

virus specific T cell clone HA1.7 as a system to investigate whether T3 crosslinking is required for activation. In addition we investigated two biochemical phenomena which occur within minutes of stimulation, namely calcium mobilization and phosphatidylinositol metabolism. We have found that T3 crosslinking is essential for T cell proliferation. Anti T3 under non crosslinking conditions however will give a rapid rise in intracellular free calcium and inositol tris phosphate as well as phosphorylation of inositol lipid all features of ligand activated receptor systems in other cells including transformtion by oncogenic viruses. We therefore conclude that those events, although important for activation, are insufficient to trigger T cells to divide in the abscence of receptor crosslinking.

MATERIALS AND METHODS
1. Cells

The human influenza virus specific T cell clone HA1.7 was obtained from haemagglutinin stimulated PBLs and maintained in IL-2 described previously (5). For the experiments described below, the cells were used 5-6 days after restimulation with antigen. IA3 was a human T-T hybridoma kindly supplied by D. Wallace and P.C.L. Beverley, U.C.H.

2. Antigens and antisera

Synthetic peptide antigens p17 and p20 corresponding to portions of the haemagglutinin HA.1 were kindly supplied by Dr R.A. Lerner, Scripps Clinic and Research Foundation, La Jolla, California. Antibody to T3, UCHT1, was kindly supplied by Dr P.C.L. Beverley, School of Medicine, U.C.H. The purified IgG was used throughout either in solution or coupled to cyanogen bromide activated sepharose using standard techniques. WT/31 an antibody directed against a determinant on the receptor/T3 complex (6) was kindly donated by Dr W. Tax, University of Nijmegen, Nijmegen, Netherlands. Phorbol myristic acid (PMA) was obtained from Sigma Ltd.

3. Proliferation assay

Standard proliferation assays were established using 5 x 10^3 HA1.7 in triplicate 200 μl microtiter wells with the additions indicated in the results section. After 3 days culture in RPMI 1640 containing 10% human A$^+$ serum, the cells were pulsed with 1 μCi ^{3}H thymidine for 8 hours and harvested onto glass fibre filters prior to counting. Results are expressed as mean incorporation with standard errors less than 10%.

4. Measurement of intracellular free calcium

The fluorescent indicator quin-2 (Amersham, U.K.) was used in conjunction with a recording spectrofluorimeter exactly as described by O'Flynn et al (7,8). HA1.7 at 2×10^6.ml were incubated with the indicated reagents until a stable response was obtained. Quantitation of the internal Ca^{2+} concentration was performed as described (7).

5. Labelling of HA1.7 with ^3H inositol and measurement of inositol phosphates

HA1.7 was incubated at 1×10^6 cells/ml in RPMI 1640 containing 5% FCS and 20 μCi/ml ^3H-inositol (Amersham, U.K., 10-20 mCi/mmol). After 18 hrs culture, lithium chloride was added to 10 mM to prevent resynthesis of inositol lipid and incubation continued for a further 20 minutes. The cells were then pelleted and washed in a balanced salt solution (137 mM NaCl, 2.7 mM KCl, 1 mM $MgCl_2$, 1 mM $CaCl_2$, 20 mM HEPES pH 7.4, 5.6 mM glucose, 10 mM LiCl, 1 mM myoinositol and 1 mg/ml bovine serum albumen) 10^6 cells in 400 μl of this medium were used per point with 10 μg/ml UCHT1 antibody or 100 μg PMA. After 10 minutes incubation at 37°C, 1.5 mls of acidified chloroform methanol (1:2) was added to stop the reaction followed by 1 ml of chloroform: 0.01 M HCl, 1:1. The aqueous phase was recovered, neutralized and loaded onto Dowex 1 x 8 (formate form). After washing with 10 mls water and 6 mls of 5 mM sodium tetrborate containing 60 mM sodium formate to remove inositol, and glycerophosphoinositol plus inositol 1:2 cyclic phosphate respectively, total inositol phosphates were recovered by elution with 6 mls of 0.1 M formic acid plus 1M ammonium formate. All fractions were counted directly using liquid scintillation spectometry.

6. Time course of changes in inositol lipids and phosphates

Cell labelling and measurement of inositol phosphates was as described in Section 5. Individual phosphates were eluted from the Dowex column with 0.1 M formic acid containing ammonium formate at 0.2M for IP_1, 0.4M for IP_2 and 1M for IP_3 (6 mls of each). Lipids were separated by tlc on oxalate impregnated silica gel plates using chloroform/methanol/acetone/acetic acid/water (40 : 13 : 15 : 12 : 8 by vol). Carrier lipids were added for visualisation by I_2 staining. Individual lipids were scraped from the plate eluted with methanol and counted.

RESULTS

In order to determine whether antibody to T3 would induce proliferation only under crosslinking conditions, clone HA1.7 was cultured with anti T3 either alone, with additional autologous presenting cells or with T3 covalently attached to sepharose beads. The results are shown in Table 1. It can be seen that only crosslinked anti T3 gave a proliferative response above background values of clone or presenting cells alone. Calcium mobilization was investigated using HA1.7 and soluble anti T3 under non crosslinking conditions. Figure 1 shows the increase in intracellular free calcium ions induced by UCHT1 (anti T3). It should be noted that the specific peptide antigen p20 gave no response. Another antibody against the receptor/T3 complex, WT/31 also had no effect (except when crosslinked using anti mouse Ig; data not shown). If UCHT1 was added subsequently, the response to the latter was accelerated (Figure 1, bottom graph), implying that addition of the first antibody induced a conformational change in the complex. We investigated another early event in cellular activation, namely the breakdown of phosphatidylinositides to water soluble inositol phosphates and diacylolycerol (9). Anti T3 and PMA were used in conjunction with HA1.7 and the results shown in Table 2. In this case only the anti T3 induced a measurable breakdown of membrane phospholipid to inositol phosphates. A more detailed analysis using IA3 is prevented in Figure 2 in which the individual inositol lipids and phosphates were measured over a short time course after stimulation with anti T3. Of interest was the rapid (< 1 min) formation of a phosphorylated form of phosphatidyl inositl ($PI-P_2$) from PI-P suggesting that anti T3 had rapidly induced a kinase activity. Subsequently, $PI-P_2$ was broken down to IP_3 as expected. Identical results were obtained with HA1.7 (not shown).

DISCUSSION

We have shown in this study that an IL-2 dependent antigen specific T cell clone can be induced to proliferate

TABLE 1

HA1.7	247
HA1.7 + E⁻	122
HA1.7 + T3	318
HA1.7 + p20	261
HA1.7 + E⁻ + p20	8406
HA1.7 + E⁻ + T3	5321
HA1.7 + T3-sepharose	4076
HA1.7 + E⁻ + T3-sepharose	6514
E⁻ + p20	180

HA1.7 was cultured in 96 well plates in a standard proliferation assay as described in Materials and Methods. Equal numbers of autologous irradiated E rosette negative cells (E⁻) were added as appropriate. The specific antigen p20 was used at 1 µg/ml, and approximately 10 beads of anti T3 sepharose were added per well. Results are expressed as mean cpm of triplicate responses with standard errors < 10%.

TABLE 2
Inositol Phosphate Generation in HA1.7

	Lipid	Inositol	GPI	IP$_s$
Control	66148	117299	555	923
UCHT1	67687	115717	819	4133
PMA	65424	118321	583	745

Cells were labelled with ^{3}H-inositol, treated with anti-T3 (UCHT1) and Phorbol ester (PMA). Water soluble metabolities were separated on Dowex 1 x 8 and counted by liquid scintillation spectrometry. IP$_s$ indicates total inositol phosphates (IP$_1$, IP$_2$, IP$_3$) eluted.

LEGEND TO FIGURE 1

2 x 10^6 HA1.7/ml were loaded with quin 2 as describe
(7) and incubated with 100 ug/ml p17 and p20, 3 ug/ml UCHT1
and 5 ug/ml WT/31.   Cells were stirred and maintained at
37°C.

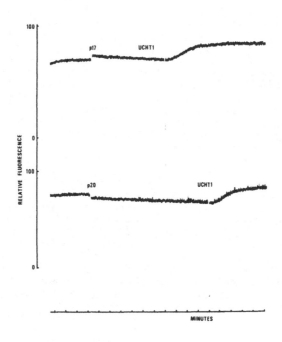

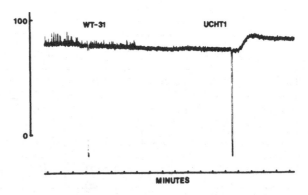

LEGEND TO FIGURE 2

IA3 cells were labelled with ^{3}H inositol and treated with or without UCHT1 over a 5 minute time course. Individual lipids were separated by tlc and counted. Individual insoitol phosphates were also analysed by stepwise elution from the Dowex column with buffer of increasing ionic strength.

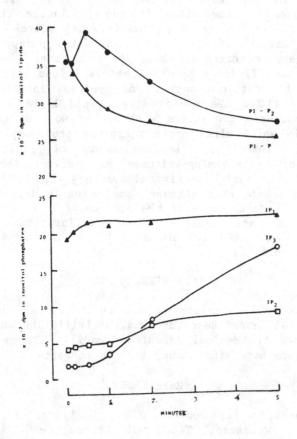

under conditions in which the T3 component of the
T3/antigen receptor complex is crosslinked using anti T3
coupled so sepharose or associated with Fc receptor bearing
presenting cells.   Because the 90 kD heterodimer is
implicated in antigen recognition per se we reasoned that
T3 molecules may be important in signal transduction and
that addition of anti T3 under non crosslinking conditions
may mimic some of these signalling phenomena.   Modern
concepts of receptor antigen in many eukaryotic cell types
recognise the importance of calcium mobilization, inositol
lipid breakdown and phosphorylation (9). We could demonstrate an increase in cytoplasmic free calcium, although it
is not clear whether this is due to influx through a
membrane channel or release from internal stores.   Breakdown of phosphatidyl inositol to inositol phosphates and
diacyglycerol occurred at about the same rate. Consistent
with previous findings, phorbol esters had no effect since
it binds to protein kinase C and bypasses inositol lipid
metabolism (10).   We could detect rapid lipid phosphorylation however which agrees with recent work on oncogenic
viruses in which viral protein kinases phosphorylate PI-P
(11,12).   Therefore, the mechanisms of proliferation
induced by transforming viruses may reflect the normal
counterpart in antigen activated lymphocytes.

     We conclude that although some clearly defined early
biochemical events occur in the absence of T3 crosslinking,
other signals are required before proliferation can occur
and that these are probably afforded by the crosslinking
process itself (8).

ACKNOWLEDGEMENTS

     We would like to acknowledge the financial support of
the Imperial Cancer Research Fund, Arthritis and Rheumatism
Council and the Medical Research Council.   Thanks are due
to those who have kindly supplied the reagents.

REFERENCES

1.   Leonard, W.J., Depper, J.M., Uchiyama, T., Smith,
     K.A., Waldmann, T.A. and Greene, W.C.   Nature
     300, 267 (1982).
2.   Meuer, S.C., Fitzgerald, K.A., Hussey, R.E., Hodgdon,
     J.C., Schlossman, S.F. and Reinherz, E.L.   J. Exp.
     Med. **157**, 705-719 (1983).

3. Meuer, S.C., Hussey, R.E., Fabbi, M., Fox, O., Acuto, O., Fitzgerald, K.A., Hodgdon, J.C., Protentis, J.P., Schlossman, S.F. and Reinherz, E.L. Cell **36**, 897-906 (1984).

4. Terhorst, C. in Receptors and Recognition (M. Greaves, ed) Chapman Hall, London (in press).

5. Lamb, J.R., Eckels, D.D., Lake, P., Woody, J.N. and Green, N. Nature **300**, 66-69 (1982).

6. Tax, W.J.M., Williams, H.W., Reekers, P.P.M., Capel, P.J.A. and Koene, R.A.P. Nature **304**, 445-447 (1983).

7. O'Flynn, K., Linch, D.C. and Fatham, P.E.R. Biochem. J. **219**, 661-666 (1984).

8. O'Flynn, K., Zanders, E.D., Lamb, J.R., Beverley, P.C.L., Wallace, D.L., Fatham, P.E.R., Tax, W.J. and Linch, D.C. Eur. J. Immunol. (in press).

9. Beveridge, M.J. Biochem. J. **220**, 345-360 (1984).

10. Nishizaka, Y. Nature **308**, 693-697 (1984).

11. Macaro, I.G., Movinett, G.V. and Baluygi, P.C. Proc. Natl. Acad. Sci. (1984).

12. Sugimoto, Y., Whitman, M., Cantley, L.C. and Erikson, R.L. Proc. Natl. Acad. Sci. **81**, 2117-2121 (1984).

SURFACE STRUCTURES INVOLVED IN HUMAN CYTOLYTIC

T LYMPHOCYTE FUNCTION

Alessandro Moretta and Giuseppe Pantaleo

Ludwig Institute for Cancer Research

Lausanne Branch, 1066 Epalinges, Switzerland

INTRODUCTION

The recent availability of monoclonal antibodies (mAbs) directed against surface antigens expressed by human T lymphocytes has resulted in rapid advances towards understanding of the nature of the molecules involved in cytolytic T lymphocytes (CTL)-target cell interaction (1). Mabs against T3 and T8 molecules have been shown to inhibit the cytolytic activity of alloactivated MLC T lymphocytes against target cells bearing the sensitizing alloantigens. Recent studies at the clonal level have indicated that a clonal heterogeneity exists in the requirement for T8 and T4 molecules (2,3) in CTL-target cell interaction; thus, although anti-T8 or anti-T4 mAbs inhibited the specific cytolytic activity of 50-85% CTL clones expressing the T4 or T8 surface antigens, the remaining specific CTL clones were resistant to inhibition even when the relevant antibody was added in large excess. More importantly, up to 30% MLC-derived CTL clones with specific cytolytic activity were found to be resistant to the inhibitory effect of anti-T3 mAb (2). These results were of particular interest in view of the fact that a physical association has been described between T3 molecules and molecules carrying clonotypic determinants; they would suggest that T3 molecules and molecules serving as antigen receptors are not necessarily functionally and physically linked on the CTL surface. It should be also stressed that anti-T3 and anti-T8-resistant CTL clones were found to be largely overlapping (2); since the proportion of alloreactive CTLs resistant to anti-T8 inhibition were found to be more than 80% in clones derived from alloimmune donors, it is possible that T3-independent CTL may as well occur frequently in vivo. In view of these findings, it was of interest to investigate whether other non-clonotypic surface structures were involved in the specific CTL activity of T3/T8-resistant clones. Along this line we have recently selected a series of mAbs on the basis of their ability to inhibit the specific cytolytic activity of a T3/T8-resistant CTL clone used for immunization. Interestingly enough, all the selected mAbs, that were not directed against clonotypic structures were found to recognize the T-specific 50 Kd sheep erythrocyte (E) receptor associated molecule (T11).

INVOLVEMENT OF T11 MOLECULES IN SPECIFIC CTL FUNCTION

It is noteworthy that anti-T11 mAbs, similarly to anti-T8 and anti-T3, were previously shown to inhibit the specific CTL activity of MLC populations (4); in addition, Meuer et al (5) recently reported that mAbs recognizing different epitopes of the T11 molecules acted sinergistically to promote T cell proliferation and lymphokine release. Both of these findings are consistent with the idea that T11 molecules may be functionally linked to the antigen receptor of T cells. In an attempt to further clarify this point, we analyzed a large number of MLC-derived CTL clones for their susceptibility to inhibition by the 3 anti-T11 mAbs proven to be inhibitory on the immunizing clone. Such specific CTL clones were analyzed for their cytolytic activity in the presence or in the absence of anti-T11 or anti-T3 mAbs. As shown in fig. 1, 2 out of 11 T4+ clones and 4 out of 16 T8+ clones were unaffected by anti-T3 mAb, in contrast, all the clones were strongly inhibited by addition of anti-T11 mAb, independent upon their T8/T4 phenotype. In addition, no correlation was observed between the degree of anti-T11-induced inhibition and the resistance to anti-T3 mAb. Similar results were obtained in two additional experiments, moreover, all 3 anti-T11 mAbs showed a comparable inhibitory activity on all CTL clones tested. In order to gain further information on the physical and functional link existing between T11

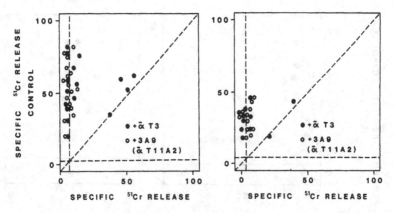

Fig 1   Effect of UCHT1 (anti-T3) (●) and 3A9 (anti-T11)
(○) mAbs on the specific cytolytic activity of T8+ (left
panel) or T4+ (right panel) CTL clones. Each point
represents the control vs. the "inhibited" cytotoxicity
values of an individual clone. Note that 4 out of 16 T8+
clones and 2 out of 11 T4+ clones were resistant to
inhibition by anti-T3 whereas all the clones were
inhibited by anti-T11 mAb.

molecules, T3 molecules and molecules serving as the
specific receptor for (allo)antigens, we investigated the
effect of modulation of T3 molecules in CTL clones
resistant to anti-T3 inhibition. We showed previously
that such clones maintain their ability to specifically
lyse target cells even after complete removal of T3
surface molecules induced by the interaction with anti-T3
mAb (2). We found that T3 modulation did not affect the
T11 antigen expression in all T3-resistant clones
analyzed; more importantly, the cytolytic activity of all
such clones (that was not affected by T3 modulation) was
strongly inhibited by anti T11 mAb (not shown).

ANTI-T11 mAbs DO NOT INHIBIT NK-LIKE ACTIVITY

Inhibition of CTL effector function by anti-T11 mAbs
could be secondary to a generalized inhibitory activity
on cytolytic cell functions, rather than result from a
selective inhibition on specific target cell killing. To
evaluate this possibility we selected several
allospecific CTL clones that simultaneously displayed
NK-like activity. We have recently shown that such

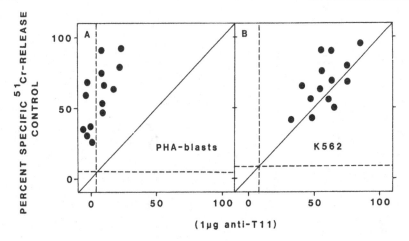

(1µg anti-T11)

Fig 2 Differential effect of 3A9 (anti-T11) mAb on lytic activity of clones with "dual" (specific and NK-like) cytolytic activity. Each clone was tested for specific (A) or NK-like (B) cytolytic activity in the presence or absence of 3A9 mAb. Each point represents the control vs. the "inhibited" cytotoxicity values of an individual clone; uninhibited clones would thus be expected to fall close to the 45° line.

clones are relatively frequent among CTL clones derived from primary MLC, moreover we demonstrated that specific CTL activity, but not NK activity, was inhibited by anti-T8 mAbs (6). 14 clones with dual cytolytic activity were tested against PHA-activated specific lymphoblasts or K562 cells in the presence or in the absence of 1 ug anti-T11 mAb. As shown in fig. 2, while specific CTL activity was strongly inhibited in all clones, the NK activity was not affected or only minimally inhibited.

ANTI-T11 Mabs INHIBIT CELL PROLIFERATION AND IL-2 RELEASE
INDUCED BY ALLOSPECIFIC STIMULATION

Our data argue in favor of the possibility that T11 molecules may be involved in the specific T cell receptor function. To further investigate this possibility we studied whether anti-T11 antibodies had any effect on other T cell specific responses analyzed at the clonal level. Several MLC-derived clones were selected according to their ability to release IL-2 (and proliferate) following interaction with the specific allogeneic stimulating cells (7). Out of 11 clones so selected, 3 were T4-/T8+/T3+ and the remaining were T4+/T8-/T3+. As little as 10 ng/microwell (50 ng/ml) of anti-T11 mAb were sufficient to sharply inhibit both proliferation and IL-2 release of all these clones. In contrast, addition of anti-T3 mAbs in large excess (to avoid the mitogenic effect of the antibody itself) led to a clonal heterogeneity in the susceptibility to inhibition of IL-2 release and cell proliferation, thus providing further evidence of heterogeneity in the requirement for T3 molecules in T cell receptor activity.

A SUBCLASS OF CTL-PRECURSORS DO NOT REQUIRE T3 OR T8 MOLECULES FOR ALLOANTIGEN RECOGNITION

As mentioned above, the finding that a marked clonal heterogeneity exists in the requirement for molecules such as T3, T4 and T8 may be particularly important for those CTL generated during alloimmunization in vivo. Indeed, as shown by Malissen et al (8) less than 20% of CTL clones derived from an alloimmune donor were susceptible to anti-T8 inhibition: these findings are in striking agreement with data by Mac Donald et al (9) showing that only a minor proportion of CTLs generated in alloimmunized mice were susceptible to anti-Lyt-2 inhibition. Given these data, it is possible that T8 (or Lyt-2)-independent CTLs may actually represent the class of CTL which play a major role during response to allografts in vivo; in contrast, T8-dependent CTLs may consist of cells equipped with low affinity receptors that may play a marginal role during in vivo alloimmunization. The latter cells, however, would easily undergo proliferation in vitro in MLC, since under these condition, any cell expressing IL-2 receptors (either as a consequence of cell activation by alloantigens in vitro or because being already activated in vivo) would proliferate independently upon the actual affinity of the receptor for antigen. Thus, no particular selection of high affinity clones would occur under in vitro conditions.
If indeed T3, T4 or T8-independent CTLs represent a different class of effector cells which can be distinguished on the basis of the affinity of their receptors for antigen, the precursors of these cells

should exist among unprimed T lymphocytes. As an
alternative possibility, all CTL-P may require T3, T4 or
T8 molecules during the induction phase initiated by the
interaction with alloantigens, however some CTL would
lose such dependancy during clonal expansion. It has
been shown that both anti-T3 and anti-T8 mAbs strongly
inhibit the generation of cytolytic effector cells when
added at the initiation of MLC, however, it should be
stressed that such studies at the bulk culture level may
be difficult to interpret in view of the heterogeneity of
the responding population and of possible interactions
occurring among cells and/or soluble factors. In
addition, they do not provide any information on the
actual proportion of CTL-P inhibited by the mAb. In
order to obtain precise information on whether T3,
T8-independent CTL-P indeed exist among unprimed
peripheral blood lymphocytes, we used a sensitive
limiting dilution microculture system recently applied in
our laboratory to the study of the frequency and subset
distribution of allospecific CTL-P in human peripheral
blood (10). In these experiments, anti-T3 or anti-T8
mAbs were added to micro-MLC containing limiting numbers
of peripheral blood T cells as responding cells and an
exogenous source of IL-2. In the presence of the
inhibiting mAb, a 70-80% reduction of the frequency of
specific CTL-P undergoing clonal proliferation was
observed; perhaps more importantly, the cytolytic
activity of those CTL-P that underwent clonal expansion
in the presence of anti-T3 or anti-T8 mAbs (and were thus
T3, T8-independent during their induction phase) was not
inhibited by the corresponding mAb. Moreover, most of
the cytolytic microcultures resistant to anti-T8 mAb were
also unaffected by anti-T3 mAb. Thus it appears that
most, if not all, CTL-P growing under these conditions
are both T3 and T8 independent and are likely to
represent the precursors of the T3, T8-independent CTL
detected in our studies at the clonal level.

In order to gain more precise information on the actual
stage of CTL-P activation affected by the two mAbs, we
further compared the effect of anti-T3 and anti-T8 mAbs
on resting peripheral blood CTL-P and on MLC-activated
(operationally defined) CTL-P (10). Limiting numbers of
cells of each population were cultured in the presence of
irradiated allogeneic cells, an exogenous source of IL-2
and either anti-T8 or anti-T3 mAbs. While, as discussed

above, the CTL-P frequency was sharply reduced in the
presence of the inhibitory mAb in unprimed peripheral
blood T cells, no inhibitory effect was observed in
MLC-activated T cells. A likely interpretation of these
results is that, due to the presence of IL-2 receptor on
MLC-activated T cells, the only limiting factor for
proliferative responses of these cells is represented by
the exogenous source of IL-2 added to the assay. On the
contrary, peripheral blood CTL-P would require a first
activation signal in order to express IL-2 receptors and
only in a second stage exogenous IL-2 would promote cell
proliferation. Therefore, anti-T8 or anti-T3 mAbs will
interfere only with those peripheral blood CTL-P that
require T3 or T8 molecules for antigen recognition (and
IL-2 receptor expression). The remaining CTL-P recognize
the antigen also in the presence of anti-T3 or T8 mAb and
give rise to cytolytic effector cells that are T3 and/or
T8 independent as well. It seems important to recall
that these cells most likely represent the type of CTL
which is primarily generated during alloimmunization
in vivo.

REFERENCES

1) Meuer, S.C., Hussey, R.E., Hodgton, J.C.,
   Hercend, T., Schlossman, S.F. and Reinherz, E.L.
   Science (Wash.D.C.) 218-417 (1982)
2) Moretta, A., Pantaleo, G., Mingari, M.C., Moretta, L
   and Cerottini, J.C. J.Exp.Med. 159, 921 (1984).
3) Biddison, W.E., Rao, P.E., Talle, M.A., Goldstein, G.
   and Shaw, S. J.Exp.Med. 159,783 (1984).
4) Krensky, A.M., Sanchez-Madrid, F., Robbins, E., Nagy,
   J.A., Springer, T.A., and Burakoff, S.J. J.Immunol.
   131, 611 (1983)
5) Meuer, S.C., Hussey, R.E., Fabbi, M., Fox, D., Acuto,
   O., Fitzgerald, K.A., Hodgdon, J.C., Protentis, J.P.,
   Schlossman, S.F. and Reinherz, E.L. Cell 36, 897
   (1984).
6) Moretta, A., Pantaleo, G., Mingari, M.C.,
   Melioli, G., Moretta, L. and Cerottini, J.C.
   Eur.J.Immunol. 14,212 (1984).
7) Moretta, A. Eur.J.Immunol. in press (1984)
8) Malissen, B., Rabai, N., Liabeuf, A. and Mawas, C.
   Eur.J.Immunol. 12,739 (1982).
9) MacDonald, H.R., Thiernesse, N. and Cerottini, J.C.
   J.Immunol. 126,1671 (1981).
10) Moretta, A., Pantaleo, G., Moretta, L., Mingari, M.C.
   and Cerottini, J.C. J.Exp.Med 158,571 (1983)

SESSION V
T Cell Clones and the Analysis of Disease

Chairpersons: I. Roitt and R.N. Maini

T cells, with their involvement in the early events of humoral and cell mediated immunity, and in the subsequent stages of the latter would be expected to be intimately involved in all types of diseases involving the immune system. Thus analysis of many diseases involving auto-immunity, immune deficiency and retro viral malignancy using T cell clones has begun, and this session reviewed progress in this field.

Dr Londei reviewed the in vitro analysis of human autoimmune hyperthyroidism (Graves' disease). Because of the relative ease of access of tissue at operation, this is a very good model for analysis. By cloning T cells activated in vivo, using mitogen free IL-2, 3 types of clones were isolated: one group recognizing autologous, thyroid epithelium but not blood or heterologous thyroid. Another group recognized autologous thyroid and blood, and presumably any DR$^+$ cells. The majority of cells did not proliferate in response to autologous thyroid or blood, and their specificity remains unknown. Further analysis of the thyroid specific cells was reported: all clones were of T4 (helper) phenotype, cells bound avidly to autologous (DR$^+$) thyroid epithelial monolayers and grew on their surface. These epithelial cells were not killed by contact over 2-3 days with cloned T cells, so these were not killer cells. However, they caused increased HLA-DR expression but reduced expression of microsomal/microvillar antigens indicating some direct pathogenic effects of these T cells; confirming the expectation that the cloning approach would yield an in vitro model of the disease.

Dr Cohen reviewed his work with rat models of autoimmune diseases. Despite possible reservations concerning the relevance of rodent models to clinical diseases, certain aspects of the work do point to future possibilities, especially the capacity of irradiated T cell lines to modulate of "vaccinate" against the infection or maintenance of the appropriate disease. At the moment the mechanism of the protective effect is not fully understood, but one possibility of anti receptor suppressor cells, has already been documented in a human system (Lamb and Feldmann, Nature **300,** 456, 1982). Further analysis and substantiation of the protective effects in other structures is clearly essential.

227

    Bone   marrow   transplantation   is   a   procecdure   of
increasing clinical relevance for a variety of conditions
including   severe   combined   immunodeficiency,   often
abbreviated as SCID.   The fate of the engrafted marrow
cells   in   patients   of   this   type   and   discussed   the
differentiation and self tolerance induction which occurs
during repopulation of the lymphoid system was discussed.
    Dr Gallo described his group's discovery of the HTLV
family of human retroviruses, a series of studies which,
'en passant', led to the discovery of 'T cell growth
factor' and IL-2.   The mechanism by which HTLV-1 causes T
cell leukaemia is unknown but it is intriguing that these
cells express very high levels of receptors for IL-2.   In
vitro infection with HTLV-1 rapidly yields analogous cells,
but also causes various dysregulation of T cell function.
These   may   be   of   significance   in   the   consequent
leukaemogenesis.   The identification of HTLV-III (also
termed LAV by others) as the etiological agent of AIDS was
reviewed.

MANIPULATION OF AUTOIMMUNE DISEASES USING AUTOIMMUNE T LYMPHOCYTES

Irun R. Cohen, M.D. Department of Cell Biology, The Weizmann Institute of Science P.O. Box 26, Rehovot, 76100, ISRAEL.

The object of this report is to summarize some of the work done by myself and my colleagues on experimental autoimmunity using lines and clones of T lymphocytes. The justification for discussing rodent experiments in a conference on "Human T cell Clones" is that the rodent experiments can serve as sign posts pointing out profitable directions for efforts in human studies. Therefore, after briefly describing our animal models, I shall relate the results to two issues of clinical interest: (1) The development of functional clones despite ignorance of the target self-epitope; and 2) manipulation of autoimmunity, the possibility of treating ongoing disease with lines.

MODEL DISEASES

We have used lines and clones to study experimental autoimmune encephalomyelitis (EAE) in rats (1,2), experimental autoimmune thyroiditis (EAT) in mice (3) and adjuvant arthritis (AA) in rats (4). Active EAE is inducible by immunizing MHC-gene susceptible strains of rats with the basic protein of myelin (BP) or the major encephalitogenic fragment of BP (amino acids 68-88) in a suitable adjuvant such as complete Freund's adjuvant (CFA;5). After an incubation period of about 11-13 days, the immunized rats develop severe paralysis and pathologic evidence of mononuclear cell infiltration in the white matter of the central nervous system. EAT can be induced

229

actively in MHC-genetically susceptible strains of mice by
immunizing them with mouse thyroglobulin (Tg) in CFA (6).
The incubation period of EAT is about a month and the
disease is characterized by mononuclear cell infiltration
of the thyroid gland.

AA, unlike EAE and EAT, is induced, not by
immunization with a defined self-antigen, but by
immunization with antigens of Mycobacterium tuberculosis
(MT) in oil, that is CFA (7). Chronic polyarthritis,
chiefly of the extremities, develops about 11-13 days after
immunization. Histologic examination of inflamed joints
shows cellular infiltration and thickening of the synovium
and invasion into the cartilage. Active inflammation can
last for weeks to months. Disease is probably induced by
some antigenic cross-reactivity between MT and joints (8).
For each of these three models we have succeeded in
isolating T cell lines and clones that can mediate the
specific disease in recipient animals within a few days.
Moreover, each of the diseases can be prevented by
administering specific line cells under conditions in which
they do not induce disease, a type of vaccination
(3,4,9,10). What have we learned that could be applied to
human diseases?

ISOLATION OF FUNCTIONAL CLONES

Diseases such as multiple sclerosis, type I diabetes
mellitus, or rheumatoid arthritis are believed to be caused
by autoimmune processes. In contrast to EAE and EAT,
however, the target self-antigens in these and other
diseases have not yet been identified. Can we hope to
isolate the specifically pathogenic T lymphocytes from
patients if the specific antigen is unknown?

The antigen is important because procedures for
raising lines of antigen-specific T lymphocytes usually
make use of the antigen to provide a selective advantage in
culture to the desired lymphocytes. For example, anti-BP T
lymphocyte lines were raised from the draining lymph nodes
of rats that had been incubated with BP and CFA (2). These
lymph nodes contained T lymphocytes specific for the
purified protein derivative (PPD) antigen of MT as well as
T lymphocytes specific for BP, and probably for many other
antigens. The strategy for selecting specific anti-BP or
anti-PPD lines was to grow the lymph node cells in the

presence of BP or PPD. Receptor-bearing T lymphocytes that
see their specific antigen are stimulated to grow at the
expense of the other lymphocytes in the culture which
consequently die. In a few generations, the selected
antigen-specific T lymphocytes predominate in the culture
and the entire population becomes composed of T lymphocytes
of the desired specificity. Thus, when we grew the lymph
node cells in the presence of BP, we derived a line of
anti-BP T lymphocytes that mediated EAE in vivo and did not
respond to PPD or to any other antigen. However, when we
grew a portion of the same lymph node cells in the presence
of PPD, the emergent line was anti-PPD and could not
respond to BP or cause EAE (2). Hence, the presence of the
specific antigen was central. Furthermore, even if one
were to have the antigen in hand, could there be any
guarantee that a T cell line arising in culture would be
directed to the functionally relevant epitopes? Assuming
that a T cell line could be developed from the blood or
lymph nodes of a patient, what are the chances that it
would have any relationship to his or her disease? Our
experience with the AA and EAE models sheds some light on
these questions.

    One of the virtues of the AA model was that the
critical antigen was unknown and, therefore, the attempt to
raise an arthritogenic T cell line constituted a test of
the issue. We reasoned that, although we scientists were
ignorant of the antigen of MT critical for arthritis, the
arthritogenic lymphocytes were outfitted with receptors for
that antigen. Therefore, we decided to offer the
lymphcoytes all of the antigens of MT and allow them to
identify and react to the critical epitopes on their own.
We simply grew the lymphocytes in the presence of whole,
ground MT, which probably contained the critical epitopes,
together with MT antigens to which the rat probably had
been immunized but which had nothing to do with AA. We
found that lines regularly emerged that were able to cause
arthritis in irradiated syngeneic rats (4). When we
selected lines using a non-arthritogenic antigen of MT such
as PPD, we developed only an anti-PPD line that was not
arthritogenic. Thus, AA relevant lines were derived using
a very crude mixture of perhaps hundreds of antigens, while
irrelevant lines could be isolated from a similar
population of cells using a more purified, but irrelevant
antigen.

We interpret these results in the following way: as
the donor rat suffered from arthritis, arthritogenic T
lymphocytes must have been present, activated,and in
relatively large numbers. These factors may have allowed
the arthritogenic lymphocytes to compete successfully with
the other, irrelevant anti-PPD lymphocytes which also saw
their antigen in the crude MT mixture. The anti-PPD
lymphocytes grew into lines only when the culture was
confronted with PPD alone. In other words, if an
individual suffers from an autoimmune disease, it is not
unlikely that the disease-specific lymphocytes are in
ascendency in vivo and can also predominate in vitro in
Darwinian competition for antigen, space, and ATP (11).
This form of laissez faire competition can be thwarted by
offering the lymphocyte population selected antigens.

The results of the AA studies indicate that it might
be possible, without knowing the critical auto-antigen, to
raise functionally specific lines from patients using
extracts of target organ; crude white matter in multiple
sclerosis, beta cell membrane preparations in type I
diabetes, joint cartilage extracts in rheumatoid arthritis,
and so forth. Once lines emerge the critical antigens
might be identified by testing the fine specificity of the
lines themselves. For example we have used crude MT to
derive an arthritogenic clone (8) that reponds to
particular fragments of MT and cross-reacts with
proteoglycans of joint cartilage (unpublished). This by
itself implies that proteoglycan - MT cross-reactivity is
responsible for induction of AA and that a proteoglycan
epitope is the target of disease. Thus, the lymphocyte
clones that reveal themselves in vitro can be consulted for
important information about the disease. Note however,
that the T lymphocytes should be cloned only after they
have demonstrated their fitness in competition. Avoid
pampering undesirable lymphocytes with antigens that may
have been so "purified" that the critical, but unknown
epitopes are lost.

The fidelity of lymphocyte lines for critical epitopes
has been demonstrated in recent studies of EAE which our
group has carried out with Drs. Arthur Vandenbark, Halina
Offner and Robert Fritz (in preparation). We tested the
fine specificity to defined fragments of BP of numerous
lines and clones obtained from 4 different strains of rats.
Whole BP was used to immunize the rats and to select the

lines and clones. Nevertheless, all the lines and clones
derived from Lewis, PVG (Weizmann) and F344 rats reacted
specifically with the major encephalitogenic 68-88 peptide
of BP. There was no reactivity to any of the other
peptides. In contrast, two different lines obtained from
BN rats resistant to EAE did not respond to the 68-88
fragment,but did respond to the 47-67 fragment. Thus,
there seems to be genetic control of which epitopes are
dominant, and the lines reflect this dominance. However,
it is also possible to obtain lines to "minor" epitopes of
BP if they are used for immunization and selection in vitro
(12).

        Obviously, T lymphocytes derived from patients cannot
be assayed for their pathogenic potential using transfer
experiments. An alternative is to develop in vitro tests
of organ specific virulence. For instance, we have
discovered that T cells capable of causing EAE in vivo can
paralyze nerve transmission in vitro (13). In addition,
comparisons between lines obtained from patients with
different diseases and from healthy persons may uncover
epitope specificities or other properties characteristic of
particular diseases.

        The message then, is that when allowed to express
their preferences, populations of T lymphocytes can tell us
much about key elements in autoimmune disease.

MANIPULATION OF AUTOIMMUNE DISEASE

        In each of the three experimental autoimmune diseases
- EAE, EAT and AA - we have shown that it is possible to
induce resistance to the particular disease using specific
autoimmune line cells as agents of vaccination (10). In
the EAE and EAT models, vaccines were prepared by
irradiating (1500R) specific line cells, or by inhibiting
their synthesis of DNA chemically (3,9,12,14). Such
treated cells could not mediate disease, but animals
receiving a single inoculation of 10^6-10^7 specific anti-BP
or anti-Tg line cells acquired marked resistance to active
induction of EAE or EAT respectively. Resistance to AA
without arthritis could be achieved without irradiating the
line cells because the expression of disease required heavy
irradiation (750R) of the recipients (4). Thus,
vaccination against AA involved inoculating non-irradiated
rats with non-irradiated line cells.

    It appears that vaccination, as well as mediation of
disease by line cells requires their "activation" by
contact with specific antigen or T cell mitogen before
inoculation (15). Activation results in a number of
changes in line cells: increased proliferation, expression
of peanut agglutinin receptors on the cell membranes (15),
migration to thymus (16) or to target organs in vivo (15),
expression of specific enzymes (17), pathogenic potential,
in vitro (3) and in vivo (15), as well as the ability to
induce resistance to active disease.

    We have not investigated all of these properties in
all the disease models and I expect that we will find
exceptional T cell lines that will not require activation
to mediate their functions.

    Resistance in the EAT model is effective equally
against active disease and line-mediated disease (13). In
EAE, resistance is more marked against active disease than
it is against line mediated disease (14), although
resistance to line mediated EAE can also be induced (not
published). Because of the requirement for irradiation to
express line mediated arthritis, we have only studied
protection against active AA (4,8).

    Lately it has become clear that not all lines that can
cause disease can protect. We have studied 8 clones
derived from anti-BP lines. Although the parent lines both
mediate EAE and can vaccinate against EAE, most of the
clones cause disease, but do not induce resistance to EAE
(unpublished). Cloning of the A2 line in the AA model has
led to isolation of two clones: the A2b clone that only
causes arthritis but does not induce resistance (8) and a
second clone that only induces resistance but does not
appear to be arthritogenic (unpublished). Thus, different
cells may be responsible for disease and protection.

    How can we explain the diverse effects of these T
cells? All the T cell lines and clones we have derived
from rats or mice bear the markers of T helper/delayed
hypersensitivity cells. Regardless of whether they mediate
disease or protection or both, all the cells are negative
for the OX8 (rat) or Lyt2 (mouse) markers of T
suppressor/cytotoxic cells (2,3,8). It is possible that
the protecting lines include suppressor-inducer T cells,
but as yet we have no evidence in this regard.

The fine specificity of the cells has also failed, thus far, to pin-point critical differences. Anti-BP lines that mediate both disease and protection show the same specificity for the 66-88 major encephalitogenic peptide as do the clones that cause disease but do not induce resistance (unpublished). Certainly there may be more than one epitope in the 68-88 sequence and a suppressor epitope may be found (18). For example the arthritogenic A2b clone does seem to recognize a different epitope on MT than does the protecting clone. Therefore there may exist critical suppressor epitopes on self-antigens. Nevertheless, once we succeed in identifying such a suppressor epitope we shall yet have to explain how disease is shut off by T cells that recognize it.

Along with the possibility of suppressor epitopes, there exists the possibility that resistance to disease could be based on anti-receptor or anti-idiotypic immunity. There is a hint that such a mechanism might exist. We have studied two lines of anti-BP T cells that both mediate EAE and protection (12). These lines each recognize different epitopes on the BP molecule and each induces protection only against EAE produced in response to its own epitope. Thus, the fine specificity of the T cell receptor seems to determine the fine specificity of protection, a finding compatible with anti-receptor immunity.

In summary, our working hypothesis is that T cell lines might induce protection by two mechanisms, either separately or in concert; anti-receptor immunity and suppression triggered by suppressor epitopes. The term vaccination should probably be reserved for anti-receptor immunity while the other putative mechanism could be called suppression. Whatever the protective mechanisms turn out to be, they are clearly effective and long-lasting. Rats have been protected against EAE, EAT or AA for at least 6 months after a single inoculation of line cells (unpublished). Moreover, we have been able to passively transfer protection to AA to naive rats using thymocytes, but not serum of line-protected rats (submitted for publication). Thus, the protective mechanism is probably immune.

In addition to preventing a future exacerbation of disease, it would be desirable clinically to terminate ongoing disease. We therefore have begun to study the effects of administering line cells to rats in which we have induced active AA. We chose AA to study treatment because of its chronicity. Rats were immunized with MT in adjuvant and then given line or protective clone cells at various times before or after the onset of overt arthritis 11 days later. We found that treatment of arthritis on day 16 led to a rapid remission of arthritis (submitted for publication). However, administering line cells before appearance of clinical signs did not appear to prevent disease. Therefore, line cells were effective in preventing disease before the induction of arthritis and in treating overt arthritis, but they were not effective when administered during the latent period between induction and clinical expression of disease. These findings indicate that manipulation of disease by line cells can be complicated by processes evolving within the host. Be that as it may, it is a source of hope to observe prevention and treatment of illness by cultured cells (10,19).

REFERENCES:

1. Ben-Nun, A., Wekerle, H. and Cohen, I.R. Eur. J. Immunol. 11: 195-199 (1981).

2. Ben-Nun, A. and Cohen, I.R. J. Immunol. 129: 303-308 (1982).

3. Maron, R., Zerubavel, R. Friedman, A. and Cohen, I.R. J. Immunol. 131: 2316-2322 (1983).

4. Holoshitz, J. Naparstek, Y., Ben-Nun, A. and Cohen, I.R. Science, 219: 56-58 (1983).

5. Paterson, P.Y. In: 'Autoimmunity: Genetics, Immunology, Virology and Clinical Aspects'. (Ed. Talal, N.) 643-692 (Academic Press, New York, 1977).

6. Maron, R. and Cohen, I.R. J. Exp. Med. 152: 1115-1120 (1980).

7. Pearson, C.M. Arth. Rheum. 7: 80-86 (1964).

8. Holoshitz, J., Matitiau, A. and Cohen, I.R. J. Clin. Invest. 73: 211-215 (1984).

9. Ben-Nun, A., Wekerle, H. and Cohen, I.R. Nature 292: 60-61 (1981).

10. Cohen, I.R., Ben-Nun, A., Holoshitz, J., Maron, R. and Zerubavel, R. Immunol. Today. 4: 227-230 (1983).

11. Grossman, Z. and Cohen, I.R. Eur. J. Immunol. 10: 633-640 (1980).

12. Holoshitz, J., Frenkel, A., Ben-Nun, A. and Cohen, I.R. J. Immunol. 131: 2810-2813 (1983).

13. Yarom, Y., Naparstek, Y., Holoshitz, J., Ben-Nun, A. and Cohen, I.R. Nature 303: 246-247 (1983).

14. Ben-Nun, A. and Cohen, I.R. Eur. J. Immunol. 11: 949-952 (1981).

15. Naparstek, Y. et al. Eur. J. Immunol. 13: 418-423 (1983).

16. Naparstek, Y. et al. Nature 300: 262-263 (1982).

17. Naparstek, Y., Cohen, I.R., Fuks, Z. and Vlodavsky, I. Nature 310: 241-244 (1984).

18. Swierkosz, J.E. and Swanborg, R.H. J. Immunol. 119: 1501-1508 (1977).

19. Cohen, I.R. Adv. Int. Med. 29: 147-165 (1984).

ACKNOWLEDGEMENTS

The author is the incumbent of the Mauerberger Professorial Chair in Immunology. Parts of the research described here were supported by NIH grants AM 32192 and NS 18168.

CLONING OF AUTOIMMUNE T CELLS: IMPLICATIONS FOR

PATHOGENESIS AND THERAPY

Marco Londei, G. Franco Bottazzo* and Marc Feldmann

Imperial Cancer Research Fund, Tumour Immunology Unit,
Department of Zoology, University College London,
Gower Street, London WC1E 6BT.
* Department of Immunology, Middlesex Hospital, London

In autoimmune diseases there is a functional lack of
tolerance and an "autoantigen" is recognized by the immune
system leading to the development of pathological
conditions. A broad spectrum of diseases are included in
this definition, and they are often subdivided into non-
organ specific diseases such as systemic lupus erythe-
matosus (SLE), and organ specific diseases, such as Graves'
and Hashimoto's diseases (reviewed 1). In all these
diseases autoantibodies, mainly IgG, are detected, to
different "autoantigens". In a few circumstances the
nature of these autoantigens has been defined. Often these
are cell surface receptors for hormones, such as TSH in
Graves' disease (2) or for neurotransmitters, as in
myasthenia gravis (3).
Although humoral immunity has played the major role in
the definition of the autoimmune nature of these diseases,
an involvement of the T cell compartment has been recently
shown, and would be expected from our knowledge of T cell
helper function in antibody production. Thus imbalances of
the T lymphocyte subpopulations in the peripheral blood
(4), the presence of activated T lymphocytes during the
acute phase of the disease (5) and conspicuous infiltration
by T lymphocytes of the afflicted tissue (6) are common
features in autoimmune conditions. These findings indicate
that a better understanding of the autoimmune disorders
could be obtained by studying the nature of T lymphocytic
populations. It has become apparent that T cell cloning

239

has provided the most refined approach to analyze the immune system as a homogeneous population of cells can be analyzed repeatedly. Analysis of T cell clones in human and mouse experimental models recognizing peptides (7), bacteria (8), and cell surface markers (9) has been performed, and clones with the characteristics of helper, cytotoxic and suppressor cells (10,11,12) have all been isolated, indicating that practically all types of T lymphocytes can be cloned (13) but with different efficiencies.

Although T cell cloning is a well established technique several problems arise when we try to apply it in humans especially with autoimmune disorders, and for this reason different strategies can be used to obtain T cell lines from the patients afflicted by autoimmune diseases. We can use a purified source of the "putative" autoantigen to stimulate PBL (e.g. acetylcholine receptor in Myasthenia Gravis (14)); or expand the in vivo "activated" T lymphocytes using a source of mitogen free IL-2 since activated T lymphocytes are present during the acute phase of the diseases (4,5,6).

We preferred to expand already in vivo activated T lymphocytes obtained from the tissue, as this represents a closer approximation to the relevant patho-physiological condition. Thus among the autoimmune diseases we had to find one in which "the target tissue" was heavily infiltrated by lymphocytes, and moreover was obtainable in reasonable quantity, as it was both as a source of lymphocytes and of target cells.

The disorders which best fit these conditions are the autoimmune diseases of the thyroid gland. It is well established that these glands are infiltrated by T lymphocytes (15) and noteworthy that some of these are "activated" T lymphocytes (6). Currently, surgical treatment of these conditions, particularly Graves' disease, is relatively common.

MATERIALS AND METHODS

The thyroid tissue, obtained after surgical removal, was treated in two different ways:
One part was digested with collagenase type IV (Worthington) 5 mg/ml for 3 h at 37°C in the absence of any serum to release the epithelial cells, then stored in liquid nitrogen as previously described (16), while the other part was diced and pushed through a 200 μm mesh in

the presence of cold BSS to release the mononuclear cells infiltrating the tissue. These cells were then purified using a Ficoll- Hypaque gradient (15).

As some of the mononuclear cells express the receptor for IL-2, as assessed by the anti Tac monoclonal (17), we cultured these cells in the presence of a source of mitogen free IL-2 (18) to allow the expansion of already in vivo activated T lymphocytes. From previous experiments we know that such a source of IL-2 cannot allow the growth of resting lymphocytes. After one week of expansion these cells were put onto a Ficoll-Hypaque gradient to isolate the blasts, which were seeded at 0.3 per well in Terasaki plates, in the presence of autologous feeder cells (5 x 10^5/ml) and IL-2 produced from PBL stimulated by mitogen as previously described (19) or recombinant IL-2 (Sandoz). This procedure allowed us to obtain many clones (20).

RESULTS AND DISCUSSION

The specificity of the growing clones was tested using the autologous thyrocytes which had been previously stored in liquid nitrogen. It was assumed that the autoantigen(s) to be recognized by the T lymphocytes should be expressed on the surface of the thyrocytes, which in pathological conditions also express MHC class II molecules (6), essential elements in the induction of any immunological response (21), and suggesting that those thyroid cells may act as antigen presenting cells (22).

To test this hypothesis we used a T helper cell clone which recognizes Influenza A virus, and specifically proliferates, in the presence of histocompatible antigen presenting cells, using various preparation of the virus (19) as well as a short 24 amino acid peptide (residues 306-329) of the haemagglutinin molecule, termed p20 (7). When the usual antigen presenting cells (PBMNC) were substituted with irradiated (3000 Rad) HLA-DR[+] thyrocytes from a histocompatible Graves' patient we induced a proliferative response of clone HA 1.7 only when p20 was used as antigen, but not in the presence of the intact virus (Table 1). These results indicate that the HLA-DR[+] thyrocytes may act as antigen presenting cells for small "processed" peptides, but that they cannot process the whole virus, unlike the thyroid donor's PBMNC. Furthermore, this latter finding excludes a contamination of the cultures by APC(s) present in the blood. However to avoid any risk of contamination by other APC, such as dendritic cells possibly present in the thyrocyte preparation, the cultures were extensively washed 24 h after their initiation, and then used for the proliferative experiment as after this time the only adherent cells detected in the culture are thyrocytes (as judged using monoclonals to macrophages, and antibodies to thyrocytes).

In this way all the non adherent cells such as B lymphocytes, or T lymphocytes that in certain conditions can present antigen were removed; including dendritic cells which are often powerful antigen presenting cells (23), are adherent in the first hours of incubation but are not adherent after 18 hours of culture (24).

TABLE 1

Antigen	HA1.7 + PBL	HA1.7 + thyrocytes 10^4	HA1.7 thyrocytes 10^3
p20			
01	51939 ± 3943	6758 ± 1376	2100 ± 413
1	137169 ± 5917	29361 ± 5152	15572 ± 5139
10	94180 ± 26086	35434 ± 320	21991 ± 4546
A/Texas			
0.5	5809 ± 2655	1250 ± 714	799 ± 193
5	50345 ± 6387	1602 ± 927	667 ± 608
50	106906 ± 25458	1012 ± 349	320 ± 298
A/Bank			
0.5	–	752 ± 127	134 ± 50
5	–	1149 ± 210	308 ± 92
50	–	1184 ± 679	236 ± 102

Proliferative response of clone HA1.7 to different preparations of Influenza virus in presence of PBMNC from the thyroid donor 2.10^4/well and DR^+ thyrocytes 10^4 or 10^3/well.

The results are expressed as arithmetic mean cpm ± standard deviation; – not done.

HA1.7 only, 392 ± 259; HA1.7 ± IL-2 33417 ± 7839, thyrocytres (10^4) alone 142 ± 26, thyrocytes (10^3) alone 328 ± 100.

Peptide concentration expressed in µg/ml, virus concentrations expressed in HAU/ml.

The immunological nature of the proliferative response
was confirmed by blocking it with monoclonal antibody to
the class II molecules of the MHC, e.g. HIG 78 (25), that
specifically inhibits the response of clone HA 1.7 when
challenged with the specific antigen and histocompatible
APC. Moreover peptide RB6B4 (residues 314-329) from the
haemagglutinin molecule which is not recognised by clone
HA1.7 was unable to stimulate its proliferative response
(Table 2).   These data clearly indicate that the
proliferative response was not due to a non specific
release of hormones by the thyrocytes under these
experimental conditions (e.g. the presence of viral
peptides) but was due to capacity of the HLA DR$^+$ thyrocytes
to present the appropriate antigen.   The results
demonstrate that thyrocytes may act as APC in some
particular conditions and suggest that autoantigens present
on the surface of these cells may be effectively presented
to autoreactive T lymphocytes.

TABLE 2

Cells	Antigen	Antibody	Response (cpm ± sd)
HA1.7	–	–	114 ± 77
"	IL-2	–	40,813 ± 4,930
" thyrocytes	RB6B4	–	1,110 ± 571
" "	p20	–	75,041 ± 14,844
" "	"	Anti class II	3,460 ± 610
"	–	"	1,112 ± 90
–	"	–	142 ± 26

Cloned T cells (10^4/well) were cultured with MHC Class
II$^+$ irradiated (3000 Rad) thyrocytes (10^4/well) in the
presence of p20 or RB6B4 (1 µg/ml).   Anti-HLA class II
ascites (HIG78)[25] which is known to block the response of
HA1.7 was included at the initiation of the cultures at a
dilution of 1/200 and left in for the duration of the
experiments.   Proliferation was determined as described in
the legend to Figure 1.   Control responses of HA1.7 alone
or with added IL-2 are shown.

Results reproduced, with permission from Londei, M.,
Lamb, J.R., Bottazzo, G.F. and Feldmann, M. Nature 312,
639 (1984).

When we challenged the growing T cell clones with the autologous thyrocytes, many of them (about 10%) reacted specifically with these cells, but not with any of the controls used: autologous peripheral blood mononuclear cells or unrelated HLA DR$^+$ thyrocytes from other thyrotoxic patients. A clone with this particular behaviour was clone 17 (Table 3). Once again to confirm the nature of the proliferative response we performed blocking experiments using monoclonals antibodies to the HLA-D region of HLA. The results expressed in Table 4 indicate that inhibition of the proliferative response was obtained by these monoclonal antibodies but not by the appropriate controls.

Other clones yielded different patterns of response, some such clone 15 (Table 3) which did not proliferate against any of the targets used, but only in the presence of IL-2. The specificity of these clones remains obscure

TABLE 3

Clone	Response to Stimulus (cpm ± sd)			
	Autologous		Unrelated	IL-2
	Thyrocytes	PBMNC	TEC	
15	1160 ± 320	1110 ± 468	990 ± 502	18598 ± 242 [b]
51	5791 ± 2369	5541 ± 3224	2688 ± 3108	18973 ± 7774 [a]
17	5144 ± 674	605 ± 118	1838 ± 473	30640 ± 3351 [a]

Clone 15 does not respond to thyroid or blood cells, only to IL-2. Clone 51 is an autologous MLR clone, responding equally to autologous thyroid and peripheral blood mononuclear cells (pbmnc). Clone 17 thyrocyte is specific. It proliferated when challenged to autologous thyrocytes. All the experiments were performed in triplicate in a 72 hr proliferative assay. Cultures were pulsed with 1 µCi of ^{3}HTdR (NEN) during the last 10 hours. Incorporation was measured by liquid scintillation spectroscopy. Results expressed as mean cpm ± standard deviation (sd).

10^4 T cell and 10^4 thyrocytes or peripheral blood cell per well were used.

Incorporation of isotope by autologous TEC and unrelated TEC were:
Expt a autologous 821 ± 705, unrelated TEC 1869 ± 1393
Expt b autologous 606 ± 407, unrelated TEC 228 ± 160.

TABLE 4

Response of:	Proliferation (cpm ± sd)	
	Exp 1	Exp 2
Clone 17		845 ± 185
" + TEC	5144 ± 674	3718 ± 1580
	(821 ± 705)	(1050 ± 197)
" + allo TEC	1839 ± 473	686 ± 200
	(1869 ± 1393)	(597 ± 224)
" + TEC + anti II	815 ± 187[a]	772 ± 96[b]
" + TEC + anti II	−	1080 ± 135[c]
" + TEC + anti T p67[d]	−	3503 ± 1533
" + TEC + anti Bp32[e]	−	3855 ± 158
" + PBL	605 ± 118	−
" + IL-2	30640 ± 3351	3051 ± 52

Clone 17 (10^4/well) was stimulated with $\sim 10^4$ autologous (DR 2,3) or unrelated (DR1,10) thyrocytes in 96 well flat bottom culture plates for 3 days, in tripliate. Cultures were pulsed with 1 µCi of ^{3}HTdR (NEN), and incorporation measured by liquid scintillation spectroscopy. Results expressed as arithmetic mean cpm ± standard deviation, − not done.
Antibodies used, in range 10-20 µg/ml:

(a) Mixture of anti DR, anti DQ anti DP (DA2[32], HIG78[25], DA 6.231[33])
(b) anti DR and DP (DA 6.231)
(c) anti DR (19.26.1[33])
(d) anti T cell p67 (G19-3.2 Tl antigen)
(e) anti B cell p32 (TH7, Bl antigen)

Figures in brackets indicate the incorporation of thyrocytes alone (background).

TEC   - autologous thyrocytes (DR 2,3).
alloTEC - allogeneic thyrocytes (DR 1,10)
PBL   - peripheral blood lymphoid cells.

but they could be T killer cells or T suppressor cells.
Other clones responded like clone 15 (Table 3) which
proliferated in the presence of both autologous thyrocytes
and PBMNC, behaving as an "autologous mixed lymphocyte
response cell" suggesting that the specificity recognized
by these cells is the HLA-D region of HLA expressed on the
two different types of cells. The relevance of these cells
in autoimmune diseases is not clear, but they have been
postulated to be a major source of lymphokines (26,27).

Using monoclonal antibodies we could analyze the
phenotype of the clones so far analyzed. All of them were
positive when stained with UCHT1 (28), and Leu 3a (Fig. 2)
but not when stained with UCHT4 (29) indicating that they
are of the helper/inducer phenotype, bearing the CD3 and
CD4 antigens but not CD8.

The autoreactive clones also adhered to and grew in
direct contact with the autologous thyrocytes (Fig. 1-3).
Although these cells are of the helper phenotype and do not
effectively kill the thyrocytes reduced expression of the
microsomal/microvillar antigen was observed when the
thyrocytes were cultured in the presence of autoreactive

FIGURE 1

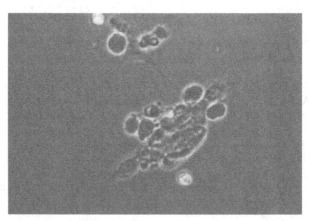

Phase contrast showing adherence of autoreactive T
cell clone to the thyroid epithelial cells.
Cells were plated onto a coverslip in a Linbro 24 well
plate at a ratio of 1:1. After 2 days the coverslip was
washed to remove unattached cells.

clones compared to thyrocytes cultures in absence of autoreactive clones. Data not shown (20).

The demonstration of human autoreactive T cell clones provides an _in vitro_ model of the initiation of a human autoimmune disease, and closer analysis of these clones will permit us to define in detail the mechanisms underlying the pathogenesis of this disease, e.g. the nature of the mediators involved in triggering B cells, the moieties inducing MHC Class II expression, and the MHC Class II specificities recognized. In the same way as it has been suggested that B cell receptors and the idiotype network (30) may be involved in autoimmunity, we have now the means of directly determining whether T cell receptors and a receptor network are of importance in the generation of organ specific autoimmune diseases. As shown in animal

FIGURE 2

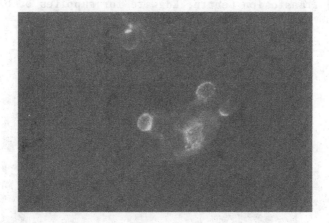

Photomicrograph of same cells as in Fig. 1.

The preparation was incubated with monoclonal antibody Leu3a (CD4 antigen) and stained with fluoresceinated rabbit anti mouse Ig (green) antiserum. At the end of the staining procedure the coverslip was fixed in acetone, mounted and viewed under a Zeiss type III microscope equipped with epi-illuminations. Note that only T cells are brightly stained. Their helper phenotype was demonstrated by similar experiments using UCHT1 (CD3) and UCHT4 (CD8). The T lymphocytes were stained by the UCHT1 but not by UCHT4. Data not shown.

models (31), the use of such clones should provide clues as to the possible means of abrogating undesirable autoimmune responses, either specifically or non specifically.

In conclusion, autoreactive T cells of the helper phenotype are present in thyroid affected by autoimmune diseases, are driven in vitro by DR$^+$ thyrocytes acting as antigen presenting cells, appear to cause reduced expression of the microsomal/microvillar antigens, may provide help for autoantibody production, and may be a prime target for selectively abrogating undesirable autoimmunity.

ACKNOWLEDGEMENTS

We thank Dr J.R. Lamb and Ms J. Johnson for their help, Drs Beverley, Bodmers and Van Heyningen for gifts of antibodies, Dr J. Skehel and R. Lerner for gifts of antigen, Dr M. Contreras and her colleagues at the National Blood Transfusion Centre, Edgware for supplies of blood and serum, and Dr E. Liehl (Sandoz) for gift of IL-2.

FIGURE 3

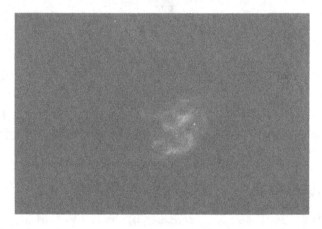

Same preparations as in Fig. 1 and Fig. 2, stained by double immunofluorescent technique with a serum from a patient with Hashimoto's thyroiditis (diluted 1/10) known to contain autoantibodies to microvillar/microsomal thyroid antigens as previously described. The reaction was revealed with rabbit anti human Ig, rhodamine conjugate (red dye). The T cells are negative and only thyrocytes are stained, indicating no cross reactivity among reagents obtained from different species.

REFERENCES

1. Essential Immunology.   Ed. I. Roitt.   Blackwell
    Publications, London, 1984.
2. Rees Smith, B.   Receptor regulation, series B
    'Receptors and recognition' (Ed, R.J. Lefkowitz) Vol
    13. Chapman and Hall, London (1981) p 217.
3. Toyka, K.V., Drachman, D.B., Pestronk, A. and Kao, I.
    Science 190, 397-399 (1975).
4. Canonica, G.W., Bagnasco, M., Corte, G., Ferrini, S.,
    Ferrini, O., Giordano, G.   Clin. Immunol and
    Immunopathol. 23, 616-625 (1982).
5. Hayward, A.R. and M. Herberger.   Diabetes 33,
    319-333 (1984).
6. Hanafusa, T., Pujol-Borrell, R., Chiovato, L.,
    Russell, R.C.G., Doniach, D. and Bottazzo, G.F.
    Lancet ii, 1111-1115 (1983).
7. Lamb, J.R., Eckels, D.D., Lake, P., Woody, J.N. and
    Green, N. Nature 300, 66-69 (1982).
8. Matthews, R., Scoging, A. and Rees, A. Immunology
    54, 17-23 (1985).
9. Braciale, T.J., Andrew, M.E. and Braciale, V.L.   J.
    Exp. Med. 153, 910-923 (1981).
10. Moller, G. (ed) Immunol. Rev. 51, (1980).
11. Moller, G. (ed) Immunol. Rev. 54, (1981).
12. Lamb, J.R. and Feldmann, M.   Nature 300, 456-458
    (1982).
13. Moretta, A., Pantaleo, G., Moretta, L., Cerottini,
    J.C. and Mingari, M.C. J. Exp. Med. 157, 743-754
    (1983).
14. Hohlfeld, R., Toyka, K.V., Heininger, K., Grosse-
    Wilde, H. and Kalies, I. Nature 310, 244-246 (1984).
15. McLachlan, S.M., Dickinson, A.M., Malcolm, A.,
    Farndon, J.R., Young, E., Proctor, S.J., Rees Smith,
    B. Clin. Exp. Immunol. 52, 45-53 (1983).
16. Khoury, E.L., Hammond, L.J., Bottazzo, G.F., Doniach,
    D. Clin. Exp. Immunol. 45, 316-328 (1981).
17. Leonard, W., Depper, J.M., Uchiyama, T., Smith, K.A.,
    Waldmann, T.A. and Green, W.C. Nature 300, 267-269
    (1982).
18. Rabin, H., Hopkins, R.F., Ruscetti, F.W., Neubauer,
    R.H., Braun, R.L. and Tawakami, T.G.   J. Immunol.
    127, 1852-1856 (1981).
19. Lamb, J.R., Eckels, D.D., Phelan, M., Lake, P., Woody,
    J.N. J. Immunology 128, 1428-1432 (1982).

20. Londei, M., Bottazzo, G.F. and Feldmann, M. Science (1985) in press.

21. Erb, P. and Feldmann, M. Nature 254, 352-354 (1975).

22. Bottazzo, G.F., Pujol-Borrell, R., Hanafusa, T. and Feldmann, M. Lancet ii, 1115-1119 (1983).

23. Inaba, K., Steinman, R.M., Van Voorhuis, W.C. and Maramatsu, S. Proc. Natl. Acad. Sci. USA 80, 6041-6045 (1983).

24. Kuntz-Crow, M. and Kunkel, H.G. Clin. Exp. Immunol. 49, 338-346 (1982).

25. Guy, K., Van Heyningen, V., Dewar, E. and Steel, C.M. Eur. J. Immunol. 13, 156-159 (1983).

26. Smith, J.R. and Talal, N. Scand J. Immunol. 16, 269-278 (1982).

27. Rosenberg, Y., Steinberg, A.D. and Santoro, T.J. Immunol. Today 5, 64-67 (1984).

28. Beverley, P.C.L. and Callard, R.E. Eur. J. Immunol. 11, 329-334 (1981).

29. Guarnotta, G., Campbell, M.A., Hart, A., Overton, T.G., Banga, J.P., Beverley, P.C.L., Lydyard, P.M. and Roitt, I.M. In: 'Leucocyte Typing' (Eds. Bernard, A., Boumsell, L., Dausett, H., Milstein, C. and Schlossman, S.F.) Springer-Verlag, Berlin, p312 (1984).

30. Cooke, A., Lydyard, P.M. and Roitt, I.M. Immunol. Today 4, 170-175 (1983).

31. Cohen, I.R., Ben-Nun, A., Holoshitz, J., Maron, R. and Zerubavel, R. Immunol. Today 4, 227-230 (1983).

SELF EDUCATION AFTER MISMATCHED HLA HAPLOIDENTICAL BONE MARROW TRANSPLANTATION

JP De VILLARTAY, A FISCHER, C GRISCELLI

Unité d'Immuno Hématologie - Hôpital des
Enfants Malades - INSERM U 132
149 Rue de Sèvres - 75 015 PARIS (FRANCE)

Animal models of major histocompatibility complex (MHC)
incompatible bone marrow transplantation have gained considerable insight into the understanding of self education
mechanism. It has been shown that the Ia molecules expressed
on intrathymic cells inprint the self recognition pattern of
engrafted MHC incompatible T cells and thus tolerance to
host cells (1,2,3). The origin of the Ia positive cells
present into the thymus is only dependent from the dose of
irradiation delivered to the host (4,5). In the thymus of
900 rads-irradiated mice, one finds host-derived Ia^+ cells
resulting in self tolerance to host Ia antigen by engrafted
T cells whereas in the thymus of 1,200 rads-irradiated mice
there are firstly host Ia bearing cells, then bone marrow
derived, donor type Ia^+ cells which dictate both host and
donor Ia to be viewed as self (4,5). The precise mechanisms
of education or selection of self Ia recognition by engrafted T cells remain unknown. We would like to present
data obtained in an human model of HLA haploincompatible
bone marrow transplantation (BMT) which appears to have
unique characteristics. The patients who received these
transplants are naturally devoid of T lymphocytes because
they have inherited severe combined immunodeficiency (SCID)
(6). All of them do have normal numbers of Ia positive cells
(B lymphocytes and monocytes). Finally, most of these patients do not receive any immunosuppression prior to BMT because of their natural and profond inability to develop
immune response. It is thus possible to study in these patients, after the transplantation of HLA haploidentical

251

bone marrow harvested from one of the parents, the role of self/non self and of HLA-restricted T cell mediated immune responses. No such a model could be experimentally reproduced since in these patients one may observe either the differentiation of T lymphocytes from donor origin or the differentiation of T plus B cell and monocyte from donor origin (table I) while in all experimental models immunosuppression of the host always results in the differentiation of all types of bone marrow derived cells from the donor.

In order to avoid a fatal graft versus host reaction (GVHr) due to major differences in HLA class I and II antigens, mature T cells were revoved from harvested bone marrow by E rosetting (7) resulting in a 2 log order T cells depletion. Furthermore, patients received cyclosporin A for two months post transplant.

Results and Comments

1) Five patients have been successfully transplanted 550 to 200 days ago. All of them are doing well in the absence of therapy except for immunoglobulin administration in one of them. No significant GVHr has been observed in any of them. As indicated on table I, four patients have experienced the development of full T and B cell immune functions. In these patients, there is a mixed chimerism since T cells are of donor origin, B cells and monocytes are of both donor and host origin as determined by HLA typing on separated cells and sometimes Y chromosome fluorescence by quinacrine if there was a sex difference between donor and recipient. In one patient, T cells are of donor origin but B cells and monocytes remain exclusively of host origin. This patient has not developped full T cell functions since antigen-induced T lymphocyte proliferation, delayed type hypersensitivity and cytotoxic T cell responses are subnormal and variable . Furthermore, an agammaglobulinemia is persisting.

Table I

Chimerism and immune functions post HLA haploidentical BMT in 5 patients with SCID

Patients	Origin	of	Immune functions	
	T lymphocytes	B lymphocytes monocytes	T	B
1,2,3,4	D	D+R	++++	++++
5	D	R	++	0

D = donor   R = recipient

Table II
Tolerance of engrafted T lymphocytes to recipient HLA antigens

Responder PBM	Stimulatory cells (4000 rads irradiated)	^{3}H Thymidine (Δ cpm) $\pm$ 1 S.E.M
Donor	Recipient PBM	47,900 $\pm$ 300
Donor ⟶ Recipient	Recipient PBM	1,200 $\pm$ 200
Donor ⟶ Recipient	Unrelated PBM	90,700 $\pm$ 6100
Donor ⟶ Recipient Donor ＋ (1=1 ratio)	Recipient PBM	38,500 $\pm$ 4900

2) Tolerance towards host cells
As shown on table II engrafted T cells were not reactive to
recipient peripheral blood mononuclear cells (PBM) in a conventional mixed leukocyte reaction assay whereas prior to
BMT donor PBM reacted strongly to recipient PBM. This observation has been made in the five patients tested and was a
constant feature throughout the follow up post transplant.
Similar data have been obtained in other groups of patients
who received HLA haploidentical BMT (8,9). Several mechanisms
can be proposed to account for this tolerance to the host.It
could be due to the presence of specific suppressor T cells
blocking the alloreactivity to host antigens as seen in some
animal models (10,11). Such a phenomenon has been observed
only once and transiently in a patient who was still treated
with cyclosporin A a drug known to preserve the induction of
specific suppressor cells in MLR (fig. 1)(12).The usual absence of suppression could indicate that suppression is not
involved in this tolerance or that suppressor cells play a
transient role leading to a clonal reduction of alloreactive
T cells. It might be that T cells alloreactive to host antigens are eliminated into the thymus according to the clonal
deletion hypothesis. Finally alloreactive T cells could be still
present but tolerized by the continuous presence of high
doses of host class II antigens (13).
3) Tolerance towards donor cells. Engrafted T lymphocytes
have never been shown to react to donor cells in any experimental model studied. To our surprise we have observed in
all cases that PBM isolated post transplant from the recipient were significantly reactive to irradiated donor PBM as
shown in table III. This reactivity was found early post
transplant and was shown to be mediated by T lymphocytes of
donor origin since blasts cells were T_3^+, T_{11}^+ and expressed
donor HLA antigens. Moreover patients never had any detec-

Figure 1
Specific suppressor T cell activity of engrafted T lymphocytes (T(D——→R)) for Donor (D) / Recipient (R) MLR

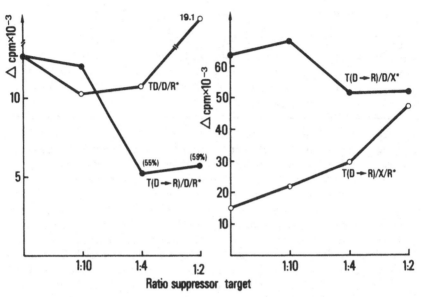

Ratio suppressor target

* = 4000 rads-irradiation
TD = T of donor origin
X = unrelated cells

Table III
Auto and alloreactivity of engrafted T lymphocytes

Responder PBM	Stimulatory PBM (4000 rads-irradiated)	^{3}H thymidine cpm $\pm$ SEM	
Donor——→Recipient	Recipient	1,500	$\pm$ 300
Donor——→Recipient	Donor	32,700	$\pm$ 2,800
Donor——→Recipient	X	24,400	$\pm$ 3,600
Donor	Recipient	19,500	$\pm$ 4,900
Donor	Donor	1,200	$\pm$ 400
Donor	X	19,500	$\pm$ 5,800

X is an unrelated subject.

table T lymphocytes prior to BMT because of their disease.
This autoreactivity progressively disappeared 6 months post
transplant in the same time as i) T and B cell functions developped and ii) Donor derived Ia+ cells (B lymphocytes and
monocytes) were first detected in recipients'blood. In one
patient this autoreactivity was found to be more intense
and above all persisting over one year post transplant. As
shown on table I two characteristics distinguish this patient from the others. His immune system does function poorly and no donor-derived Ia+ cells could be detected in his
blood. Furthermore, by weekly stimulation with irradiated
donor PBM, it was possible to grow an IL2-dependent T cell
line from recipient's blood which specifically proliferated
in the presence of donor's PBM. As shown on fig 2 a low number of these T cells were able to block the allogeneic reactivity of donor cells to unrelated cells. This blocking activity was restricted to the donor since third party cells
that did not share HLA class II antigens were not inhibited.

Figure 2
Inhibitory activity of (D R) T cell line specific for D
cells on D lymphocyte response in MLR (patient 5)

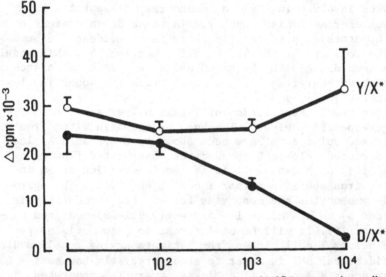

Number of (D⟶R) T cells added to 1×10⁵ responder cells

(D⟶R) T cells = engrafted T cells
D = Donor
X,Y= unrelated third party cells which are HLA class II in-
     compatible with D and R.

This inhibitory activity was not mediated by a cytotoxic
effect since these cells were not able to kill donor's cells
in a conventional 51Cr release cytotoxic assay. By family
study and reactivity to Dw homozygous cells, the specificity of these autoreactive cells was ascribed to HLA class
II antigens and not to idiotypes. The precise HLA class II
specificity (ies) recognized by these cells is under study.
These observations led to a model of self tolerance education that could be used as a working hypothesis for further
studies. The assumption is made that immature T cells have
a full potential repertoire to class II antigens. In an
early period post BMT host Ia+ cells only, are present (into
the thymus and are dictating, by an unknown mechanism the
elimination of cells with high affinity to host Ia antigens
Later, at least two months post transplant in the mouse, Ia +
cells derived from the donor do appear and allow the elimination of T lymphocytes reactive to donor Ia antigens leading eventually to tolerance to donor cells. If, for any
reason like in patient n°5, there is no differenciation of
donor derived Ia positive cells, a reactivity to donor (but
not to host) cells will persist. These T lymphocytes could
impair the normal reactivity of Ia$^+$ activated donor T lymphocytes involved in a given immune response putatively by
a suppressor mechanism. Much remain to be demonstrated in
this hypothesis, particularly there is no evidence in humans
for the role of the thymus in self education, but this model
is in accordance with the known animal experimental systems
in which an engraftment of Ia$^+$ cells from the donor is always achieved (1,5).
4) HLA class II restriction of T cell helper activity.
Antigen-specific helper T lymphocytes grown in vitro from
sensitized volunteers have been shown to exert an HLA class
II-restricted help to B lymphocytes unseparated from monocytes (14). As shown on table IV the interaction of an influenza virus specific helper T cell clone with both separated B lymphocytes and monocytes for antibody production is
governed by an HLA class II (presently HLA-DR)-mediated restriction (15). It will be of interest to grow antigen-specific helper T cell clones from patients having received HLA
haploidentical BMT in order to study precisely how host
and/or donor HLA class II antigens govern T-B-monocytes
interactions.Chu et al have shown that antigen specific T
cell lines obtained from such patients can proliferate with
the relevant antigen presented either by host- or donor HLA
class II antigens-expressing monocytes (16). We have shown
with uncloned cells that post transplant, engrafted T

Table IV
HLA class II restriction of cell interactions between an
antigen-specific helper T cell clone (L2), B lymphocytes
and monocytes (M) for antiinfluenza antibody production.

Cells in culture			IgG to influenza virus (ng/ml) (A/H3N2)
L2 (DR1)	B (DR1+)	M (DR1+)	17. 5
L2 (DR1)	B (DR1-)	M (DR1+)	. 6
L2 (DR1)	B (DR1+)	M (DR1-)	1. 0
L2 (DR1)	B (DR1-)	M (DR1-)	1. 2
L2 (DR1)	B (DR1-)	M (DR1-,DR1+)	1. 4
	B (DR1+)	M (DR1+)	1. 7

Antibody concentration to influenza virus A/H3N2 is measured
by an Elisa on culture supernatants of 12-day cultures (14,
15), L2 is a IL-2 dependent T cell clone grown from an
influenza-sensitized healthy donor (15).

lymphocytes were able to help not only donor B lymphocytes
(unseparated from monocytes) but also B lymphocytes expressing host HLA class II antigens for in vitro antibody
production to influenza virus. These T lymphocytes did not
help B lymphocytes that are HLA class II incompatible to the
host and the donor (table V).These preliminary data have to be
repeated in several patients and confirmed with cloned helper
T cells. They do however suggest that T lymphocytes able to
recognize antigen plus either host or donor Ia antigens are
selected, may be in a parallel way as tolerance to both donor
and host Ia is indicted (see chap 3). This is in accordance
with the model build from experimental data with MHC incompatible BMT (1-5).
5) HLA class I restriction of cytotoxic T cells post HLA
haploidentical BMT. In the same way as HLA class II restriction of helper T cells has been studied, we have investigated the HLA class I restriction of cytotoxic T cells to
influenza-infected targets. The first results are suggestive
of a recognition by engrafted cytotoxic T cells of both host
and donor HLA class I antigens. Indeed, engrafted T cells
like donor T cells (from the father) could kill donor target
cells evaluated in a classical ^{51}Cr release assay but they
were also able to kill cells expressing class I antigens of
the host not shared with the donor (from the mother)(table
VI). This would be the first indication that HLA class I
recognition could be learned by T cells according to a similar pattern as for HLA class II antigens. Murine models of
H2 incompatible BMT have   rather suggested a distinct

pattern for MHC class II (intrathymic) and MHC class I
(extrathymic) restriction education (17).

Table V

HLA class II restriction after haploidentical BMT in vitro
antibody response to influenza virus Bangkok (A/H3N2)
(specific IgG - O.D u./ml)

Source of T lymphocytes	Source of B lymphocytes + monocytes		
	D DR 1,2	A DR 4,6	B DR 3,5
D (DR 1,2)	. 300	. 000	. 040
D ⟶ R (DR1,2) (DR1,4)	. 325	. 230	. 010

D = donor   A, B = unrelated subjects
R = recipient
Antibody concentration is measured by an Elisa on culture
supernatants of 12-day cell cultures (14,15).
Donor and patients have been vaccinated with killed virus
1 month prior blood collection.

Table VI

HLA class I restriction, after HLA haploidentical BMT, T cell
cytotoxicity to influenza virus (Bangkok A/H3N2) infected
cells.

Effector cells	Target cells	Cytotoxic index [x](%)	
		Ratio effector = target	
		50 = 1	25 = 1
D	D	24	18
D ⟶ R	D	16	17
D	mother	8	3.5
D ⟶ R	mother	20	5
D	X	15	4
D ⟶ R	X	15	9

D = donor HLA class I haplotypes = b,c
D ⟶ R : engrafted cells into recipient (HLA class I haplotypes of the recipient = a,b).
mother   : HLA class I haplotypes = a,d
X   : unrelated subject. HLA class I haplotypes c,x
  cytotoxic index: % index (infected target cells) − % index
(non infected target cells).

CONCLUSION

The data we obtained in the patients having received mismatched HLA-haploidentical BMT, dealing both with tolerance
and restriction of T cell responses point to the central role of the presence in the host of HLA class II-expressing,
bone-marrow derived donor cells together with HLA class II
expressing-host cells (table VII). The peculiarity of this
model of HLA mismatched BMT led to the observation of an
autoreactivity to donor antigens which disappears in the
same time as donor HLA class II + cells are first detected.
Although these results are strongly suggestive of the role
of HLA class II + cells in self tolerance education one
should envisage a possible role for the short term administration of cyclosporin A in these patients. Cyclosporin A
(Cy A) when given to irradiated, syngeneically transplanted
mice or rats led to a diminished expression of Ia antigens
within the medulla of the thymus and the development of
autoreactive T cells and of a severe GVHr when Cy A administration is stopped (18). However if such a phenomenon would be
involved in this human model, then a reactivity to host HLA
class II antigens (+GVHr)   is   expected that was not the
case.
Whether MHC class II and class I-mediated restriction are determined in the thymus or not cannot be deduced from the
human observations. In the mouse it seemed that this education can occur at a prethymic level or intra-thymically (1,
2,19). It remains that peculiar situation of HLA mismatched
BMT for patients with immunodeficiencies could help in a
better understanding of the mechanisms of self education.
In that respect mismatched BM transplantations for patients
with alymphocytosis but normal presence of monocytes could
distinct the respective roles of B lymphocytes and monocytes
as host Ia bearing cells and HLA mismatched BMT for patients
with defective expression of HLA antigens may represent another original model.

Table VII - Role of HLA class II expressing cells in self
tolerance and restriction education.

	Origin of HLA class II+ cells	
	a,b	a,b + b,c
T cell allorepertoire	c,d, ... x	d, ... ,x
Restriction of T cell Responses	a,b	a,b,c

Recipient HLA haplotypes = a,b , Donor HLA haplotypes = b,c,

1   ZINKERNAGEL R.M., CALLAHAN G. N., ALTHAGE A., COOPER S.,
    KLEIN P. A., KLEIN J. J Exp Med 147, 882-96 (1978)

2   ZINKERNAGEL R. M. Immunol Rev 42, 225-70 (1978)

3   FINK P. J. and BEVAN M. J J Exp Med 148, 766-75 (1978)

4   LONGO D. L. and SCHWARTZ R. H. Nature (Lond) 287, 44-46
    (1980)

5   LONGO D. L. and DAVIS M. J Immunol 130, 2525-7 (1983)

6   KENNY A.B. and HITZIG W. H. Eur J Paediatr 131, 155-77
    (1979)

7   FISCHER A., DURANDY A., DE VILLARTAY J. P., et al.
    Transpl Proc. in Press (1984)

8   REISNER Y., KAPOOR N., KIRKPATRICK D. et al. Blood 61,
    341-8 (1983)

9   REINHERZ E. L., GEHA R., RAPPEPORT J. M. et al. Proc
    Natl Acad Sci USA 79, 6047-51 (1982)

10 TUTSCHKA P.J., HESS A. D., BESCHORNER W. E. et al.
    Transplantation 32 , 32 - 5 (1981)

11 DEEG H. J., STORB R., WEIDEN P. L. et al Transplantation
    34, 30-4 (1982)

12 HESS A. D. and TUTSCHKA P. J. J Immunol 124, 2601-8
    (1980)

13 LAMB J. R. and FELDMANN M. Nature 300, 456-8 (1982)

14 FISCHER A., BEVERLEY P. C. L., FELDMAN M. Nature (Lond)
    294, 166-68 (1981)

15 FISCHER A., STERKERS G., CHARRON D., et al. Eur J Immunol
    in Press (1984)

16 CHU E., UMETSU D., ROSEN F. et al. J Clin Invest 72,
    1124-29 (1983)

17 BRADLEY S. M., KRUISBEEK A. M., SINGER A. J Exp Med
    156, 1650-64 (1982)

18 CHENEY R., SPRENT J. Abstract F-3 10th International
   Congress of Transplantation. Minneapolis 1984

19 BRADLEY S. M., MORRISSEY P. J., SHARROW S. O. et al
   J Exp Med 155, 1638-52 (1982)

HUMAN T-CELL LEUKEMIA VIRUSES, T-CELL LEUKEMIA AND AIDS

R. C. Gallo, M. G. Sarngadharan, J. Schupbach,
M. Popovic, P. Markham, S. Z. Salahuddin,
S. Arya, and M. S. Reitz, Jr.

Laboratory of Tumor Cell Biology, Developmental
Therapeutics Program, Division of Cancer
Treatment, National Cancer Institute,
Bethesda, Maryland 20205.

INTRODUCTION

HTLV is the name we gave the first retrovirus isolates.
Most of these are very closely related, and are called
human T-cell leukemia virus type I (HTLV-I). HTLV-I is
endemic, but at low rates, in southern Japan, the Caribbean,
South and Central America, the southeastern U.S., and
especially Africa. Viruses closely related to, but distinct
from, HTLV-I have been demonstrated in Old World monkeys.
This finding, as well as seroepidemiology, led us to propose that HTLV originated in Africa. HTLV-I has been shown
to be the direct cause of an aggressive form of adult T-
cell leukemia/lymphoma. The mechanisms which result in in
vitro immortalization and in vivo malignancy are not yet
known but apparently do not seem to involve visible consistent chromosomal changes, continuous expression of virus,
or any of the known onc genes. Whatever the mechanism for
growth induction in vitro by HTLV-I, its efficiency in
causing malignancy may be because of its dual major effects
on infected cells. These are: (1) immortalization of some
T cells, especially those which are OKT4+, and (2) abroga-
tion of function and/or cytopathic changes in others. We
have discovered a second class of human T-lymphotropic
retroviruses (HTLV-II), in collaboration with D. Golde and
colleagues. It shares many of the properties of HTLV-I
but has major difference in the genome. It has been
isolated only twice, once from a patient with hairy cell
leukemia, and recently from a patient with AIDS. HTLV-III
is the third member of the HTLV family. We have at present

obtained at least 96 isolates of HTLV-III. This retrovirus
shares limited antigenic cross-reactivity and genomic
homology with HTLV-I and II, and is also highly tropic
for OKT4+ T cells, but appears to have only cytopathic and
not immortalizing effects. All isolates of HTLV-III to
date have come from patients with AIDS or from people who
are in one of the high risk groups for AIDS. Sera from
the overwhelming majority of AIDS and pre-AIDS patients
have specific antibodies against this virus, while only 1%
of healthy heterosexuals are seropositive. These data, as
well as some prospective studies, indicate that HTLV-III
is the cause of AIDS.

HTLV-I AND ADULT T-CELL LEUKEMIA

The discovery of T-cell growth factor (TCGF), present
in the media of short-term cultures of lectin-stimulated
human peripheral blood cells (1,2), permitted the long-term
culture of cells from malignancies involving relatively
mature T cells. The availability of such cultures permitted
the identification and isolation of the first human retrovirus isolates, which we now refer to as HTLV-I. These
isolates were from black patients in the United States with
what appeared to be unusually aggressive variants of cutaneous T-cell lymphoma/leukemia (Sézary syndrome and mycosis
fungoides) (3-5). The morphology of HTLV-I is typical for
type C viruses (Fig. 1), and it contains a reverse transcriptase and high molecular weight polyadenylated RNA.
HTLV-I is not significantly related to other animal retroviruses by protein serology (6-8) and nucleic acid hybridization (5), and is completely exogenous to man (3). Transmission of the virus is by infection (perhaps including
congenital infections) and does not occur through the germ
line (9,10).

The availability of purified HTLV-I proteins and antibodies against those proteins made it feasible to test sera
for evidence of exposure to this virus. It was apparent
that the great majority of the population in the United
States was seronegative for HTLV-I. The sera tested
included those of persons with various leukemias and
lymphomas. HTLV-I was sporadically detected in persons
from the United States with cutaneous T-cell neoplasms
(11), most of whom were blacks in the southeastern United
States or of Caribbean origin (12). The great majority of
these sera, however, were also negative.

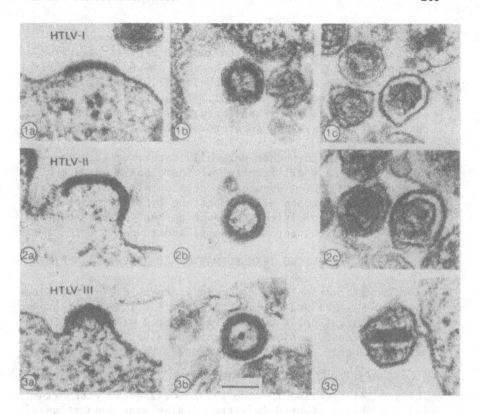

FIGURE 1. Electron microscopy of HTLV-I, II and III.
Shown are budding (panels a), immature (panels b) and
mature virions of the three types of HTLV. The bar in
panel 3b equals 100 nm.

     Two regions of the world were noted, however, in which
diseases clinically similar to those from which the first
two HTLV isolates originated were endemic. These were the
Caribbean region (13) and the southwestern part of Japan
(14). Both the disease in the Caribbean, then described as
lymphosarcoma cell leukemia, and that in Japan, which was
called adult T-cell leukemia, were highly associated with
the presence of serum antibodies to HTLV-I (15-17). Both
of these diseases are now known to be the same, and are
called adult T-cell leukemia/lymphoma, or ATLL.

These results have been confirmed by Japanese colleagues, who also were able to isolate retroviruses from
patients with ATLL (10,18). These Japanese isolates are
now known to be examples of HTLV-I (19). Sporadic cases of
both ATLL and infection with HTLV-I have also been identified in many other geographic areas (20), and certain
regions of Africa also appear to be endemic for HTLV-I (21).

As is true for other naturally occurring leukemia
viruses, only a small fraction of individuals who are
infected with HTLV-I eventually develop ATLL (22). There
are thus likely to be other important factors in determining the outcome of infection, such as host immune response,
age of first exposure, virus dose, and route of infection.

IN VITRO TRANSFORMATION BY HTLV-I

Transformation of T cells in vitro by HTLV-I was first
shown by Miyoshi and colleagues (23), but it was not proven
that the target cells were initially free of virus. Subsequently, transformation was reported using T cells which
were previously shown to be HTLV-negative (24,25).

HTLV-I is selectively infectious for T cells (particularly OKT4+ T cells) in vivo (7) as well as in vitro (24-
26). T cells infected in vitro display many properties of
transformed ATLL cells, including altered morphology,
increased growth rate, the tendency to grow in clumps,
reduced dependence on (or independence from) exogenous
T-cell growth factor (TCGF), and high level of cell surface
expression of the TCGF receptor and HLA-DR antigens (25-27).
Infection with HTLV-I also abrogates the crisis period
usually observed with uninfected T cells 4 to 5 weeks after
their initiation into culture. Transformation by HTLV-I in
vitro thus appears to be a much more rapid and effective
event than leukemogenesis in vivo.

Infection by HTLV-I of immunocompetent T cells causes
losses of some of their immune functions. In one example,
a T-cell line derived from a long-term survivor of ATLL was
found to be selectively cytotoxic for autologous HTLV-I-
infected tumor cells (28). The cytotoxic T cells were themselves able to be infected with HTLV-I, with a subsequent
loss of some immune functions. One clone (K7) infected
with HTLV-I no longer killed infected cells, but instead

stopped dividing and died when presented with the target
cells (29). Other changes in immune function following
infection with HTLV-I have also been noted (30,31).

HTLV-I also infects and transforms bone marrow cells
(32). The phenotype of these infected cells can be either
OKT4+T8-, OKT4-T8+, or OKT4-T8-.

HTLV-II

HTLV-II was originally isolated from one patient with
a hairy cell leukemia (33). Although it is related to
HTLV-I by antigenic determinants on the major gag protein,
p24, and the envelope proteins (33,34), it is readily distinguishable both by protein serology (35) and by nucleic
acid hybridization (36). It has many biochemical and biological properties in common with HTLV-I (see Table 1),
including the ability to transform T cells and to abrogate
certain immune functions (31). It has only been isolated
twice, and in spite of its ability to transform T cells,
as well as its origin from a leukemia, it has not at this
time been linked to any diseases.

COMPARISON OF THE HTLV-I AND HTLV-II GENOMES

The complete HTLV-I genome has been sequenced (37).
As with other retroviruses, HTLV-I proviral DNA contains
two large terminal repeat (LTR) sequences (containing
transcriptional promoters and termination signals) and the
usual gag, pol, and env genes. In addition, 3' to the env
gene is a large segment of DNA which contains four open
reading frames able to code for proteins of 10, 11, 12 and
27 kilodaltons. This region has been called the pX region,
and does not have a known role in viral replication.
Although its function is unknown, it is possible that it
may play a role in cell transformation. The pX region, as
is true of the rest of the HTLV-I genome, has no apparent
homology with uninfected human DNA. The structure of the
HTLV-I genome is shown in Figure 2.

The provirus of HTLV-II has also been shown to contain
a pX region, and has the same gene order as HTLV-I (38).
Using relaxed hybridization conditions, it is apparent that
HTLV-I and II are at least distantly related over their

Table 1.   Properties of HTLV-I, II and III

Property	Subgroup of HTLV		
	I	II	III
1. General infectivity	Lym	Lym	Lym
2. Particular tropism	T4	T4	T4
3. RT size	λ100K	λ100K	λ100K
4. RT divalent cation	Mg^{++}	Mg^{++}	Mg^{++}
5. Major core	p24	p24	p24
6. Common envelope epitope	+	+	+
7. Common p24 epitope	+	+	+
8. Nucleic acid homology to I (stringent)		$\pm$	−
9. Nucleic acid homology to I (moderate stringency)		++	+
10. Homology to other retroviruses	0	0	0
11. pX	+	+	+
12. Produces giant multinucleated cells	+	+	+
13. African origin	Likely	?	Likely

entire genomes.   The pX region appears to be the most
closely conserved genes of these two viruses.   The pX
region of HTLV-II has recently been sequenced (39).   There
is a large open reading frame in the 3' part of the HTLV-II
pX region which is capable of coding for a protein of at
least 38 kilodatons.   This region is closely related to and
analogous region of HTLV-I, suggesting that the resultant
protein is important for the biological activities of these
viruses.

The env gene of HTLV-II has also been sequenced (40).
The envelope genes of HTLV-I and II are significantly
related to each other (50% overall at the DNA sequence
level), except for the sequences at the extreme carboxy
and amino termini of the gene.

The LTRs of I and II differ substantially through most
of their length (41), but the sequences near the RNA cap
site, the primer binding site, and a 21 base pair sequence

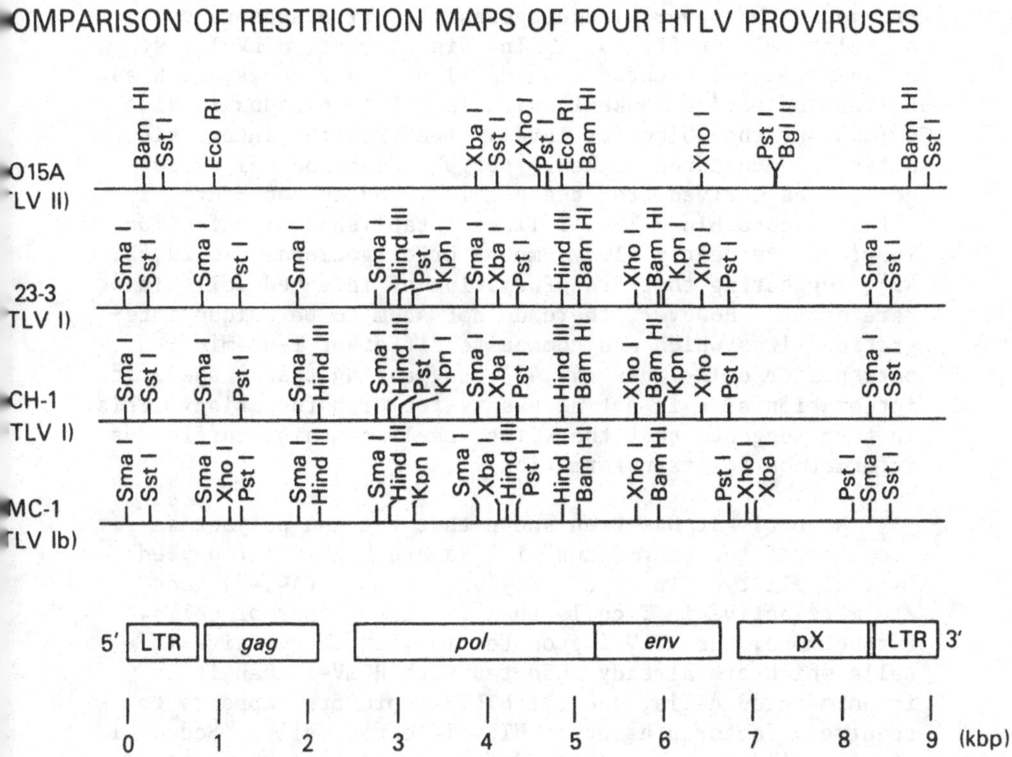

COMPARISON OF RESTRICTION MAPS OF FOUR HTLV PROVIRUSES

FIGURE 2. Genomes and restriction maps of HTLV-I and II. λMO15A is an example of HTLV-II, λ23-3 and λCH-1 are examples of HTLV-I, and λMC-1 is HTLV-Ib. Genomic regions corresponding to LTR, gag, pol, env, and pX are drawn to scale according to the published nucleotide sequence of an HTLV-I isolate. Two BglII sites in the 5' end of λMO15A are not shown.

which is repeated four times in the HTLV-II LTR and three times in that of HTLV-I are highly related. These 21 base pair repeats may represent RNA transcriptional enhancers.

POSSIBLE MECHANISMS OF TRANSFORMATION BY HTLV-I AND II

An unusual feature of the biology of HTLV-I (and II) is that although transformation of infected T cells appears to be rapid, the viral genome, unlike that of other rapidly transforming retroviruses, does not contain a cell-derived

onc gene. Moreover, leukemogenesis in vivo appears to
be relatively inefficient. In this respect, HTLV-I most
closely resembles chronic animal leukemia viruses, such as
feline and bovine leukemia viruses. This paradox is also
evident at the molecular level. The proviral integration
sites in uncultured leukemic peripheral blood cells, in
cell lines derived from these cells, and in long-term
infected cord blood T-cell lines established by infection
in vitro are nearly always mono- or oligoclonal (10,29,42,
43), suggesting that transformation of infected cells is a
rare event. However, there do not seem to be unique integration sites which are common to different leukemic
patients or cell lines (42,43), suggesting that a specific
integration site is not necessary for transformation. This
in turn suggests that the virus itself contains sufficient
information for transformation.

Recently it has been shown that the RNA polymerase
promoter of the HTLV-I and II LTRs are highly influenced
by the cell type in which they are present (44,45), and
are more active in T cells than in other types of cells.
Furthermore, the HTLV-I promoter is much more active in
cells which are already infected with HTLV-I than it is
in uninfected cells, and the HTLV-II promoter appears to
require a factor present in HTLV-infected cells. Sodroski
et al. (44) interpret these data as indicating that a
trans-acting factor (which could be encoded by the pX gene)
is present in HTLV cells which activates the HTLV promoter.
If this factor were indeed the pX product, and were also
able to affect the promoters of cellular genes critical
for T-cell function and proliferation, it could explain
rapid transformation of T cells without the requirement
for a specific integration site, as well as a cytopathic
or dysfunctional effect on infected T cells. This model
does not, however, explain the rapid proviral monoclonality
observed after infection and transformation of T cells.

HTLV-III AND AIDS

Acquired immunodeficiency syndrome (AIDS) is a recently
described, usually fatal disease involving a severe depletion of helper T cells and various opportunistic infections
of life-threatening proportions and/or malignancies. AIDS
is prevalent primarily in certain high-risk groups, including promiscuous homosexuals, hemophiliacs, Haitians,

intravenous drug abusers, and infants born to members of
high-risk groups. Epidemiologic data suggest the involvement of a transmissible agent. Because of this and because
of the involvement of OKT4+ T cells in the disease, it was
possible that an HTLV-like retrovirus could be involved.
In this respect, Essex and his colleagues hae shown an
antibody present in sera from a large percentage of AIDS
patients and high-risk populations which specifically
detect a protein present on the surface of HTLV-I-infected
cells (46,47).

  Recently, we developed a cell line for HTLV-III replication which allowed the reproducible detection of retrovirus from AIDS and pre-AIDS patients (48). Some of these
target cells support the production of high levels of
virus, and to date more than 90 isolates from this group
of patients have been obtained (49, P. Markham et al.,
submitted). By electron microphotographs, biochemical
properties of viral reverse transcriptase (48), antigenic
determinants of env and gag proteins (50), and distant but
significant nucleic acid homology, particularly in the gag-
pol region (51,52), summarized in Table 1, this new virus
is distantly related to both HTLV-I and II. Its OKT4+
T cell tropism, likely African origins, and seeming
presence of pX sequences also indicate that these viruses
belong to the same family. It has been designated HTLV-III.
This suggests that the antibody activity detected by Essex
and colleagues reflects a cross-reactivity of HTLV-I
proteins with antibody to HTLV-III. We have now isolated
HTLV-III from the majority of pre-AIDS patients and a large
fraction of actual AIDS patients (49), while isolation from
the normal population is rare. Moreover, the overwhelming
majority of patients with AIDS or pre-AIDS have antibodies
to HTLV-III (53). A typical Western blot using these antibodies is shown in Figure 3. The major reactivity is
against a 41 Kd protein, the presumed env protein of HTLV-
III. More recent data show that the incidence of antibodies
to HTLV-III in these patients is virtually 100% (54). This
striking association of antibodies to HTLV-III with AIDS
suggests that this virus is in fact the etiologic agent of
AIDS. The HTLV family of viruses can thus cause T-cell
depletion as well as the clonal T-cell proliferation seen
in ATLL. Recent evidence indicates that the virus called
LAV or IDAV detected previously by Sinoussi-Barre et al.
is also a member of the HTLV-III subgroup (55).

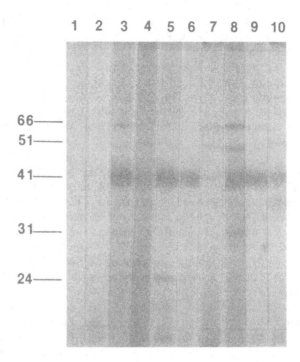

FIGURE 3. Identification of HTLV-III antigens recognized by
sera of AIDS patients. HTLV-III was lysed and fractionated
by electrophoresis on a 12% polyacrylamide slab gel in the
presence of SDS. The protein bands on the gel were electro-
phoretically transferred to a nitrocellulose sheet and
strip solid-phase radioimmunoassays were then performed.
The strips were washed, dried, mounted, and exposed to
x-ray film. Strip 1, adult T-cell leukemia; strip 2, normal
donor; strip 3, mother of a child with AIDS; strips 4 and 6
to 10, AIDS patients; and strip 5, patient with pre-AIDS.

DISCUSSION

We have used the term HTLV to designate what is at
present a family of three highly distinct but related virus
groups, HTLV-I, II, and III, all of which infect and have
major effects on OKT4+ cells. HTLV-I appears to be the
etiologic agent of adult T-cell leukemia/lymphoma (ATLL),

and its identification has helped to identify ATLL as a distinct worldwide clinicopathologic entity. Its biology in vitro resembles in many respects its activity in vivo, and may provide a model system for the disease. Infection in vitro results in cell transformation (22-24), the loss of immune functions (29-31), and in some instances selective T-cell death (29).

HTLV-II, although it has many of the same effects in vitro which are seen with T cells infected with HTLV-I, is at present not associated with any diseases and has only been isolated twice. Its geographic distribution and etiologic role in human disease require clarification.

HTLV-III is highly likely to be the cause of AIDS. Not only is it present in the overwhelming majority of AIDS and pre-AIDS patients, but its cytopathic effect in vitro against OKT4+ cells resembles the situation in vivo in AIDS.

These viruses are thus a group of related human retro-viruses with disparate effects on the same target cell, the OKT4+ T cell. It will be of interest to see if other members of this virus family exist. The identification of the presently recognized members of this group provides an opportunity to study T-cell biology, as well as the possibility for intervention in certain now fatal (and in the case of AIDS, increasingly prevalent) T-cell diseases.

REFERENCES

1. D. A. Morgan, F. W. Ruscetti, R. C. Gallo, Science 193, 1007 (1976).
2. F. W. Ruscetti, D. A. Morgan, R. C. Gallo, J. Immunol. 119, 131 (1977).
3. B. J. Poiesz et al, Proc. Natl. Acad. Sci. USA 77, 7415 (1980).
4. B. J. Poiesz, F. W. Ruscetti, M. S. Reitz, V. S. Kalyanaraman, R. C. Gallo, Nature 294, 268 (1981).
5. M. S. Reitz, B. J. Poiesz, F. W. Ruscetti, R. C. Gallo, Proc. Natl. Acad. Sci. USA 78, 1887 (1981).
6. V. S. Kalyanaraman, M. G. Sarngadharan, B. J. Poiesz, F. W. Ruscetti, R. C. Gallo, J. Virol. 38, 906 (1981).
7. M. Robert-Guroff, F. W. Ruscetti, L. E. Posner, B. J. Poiesz, R. C. Gallo, J. Exp. Med. 154, 1957 (1981).

8. H. M. Rho, B. J. Poiesz, F. W. Ruscetti, R. C. Gallo, Virology 112, 355 (1981).

9. R. C. Gallo et al., Proc. Natl. Acad. Sci. USA 79, 4680 (1982).

10. M. Yoshida, I. Miyoshi, Y. Hinuma, Proc. Natl. Acad. Sci. USA 79, 2031 (1982).

11. L. E. Posner et al., J. Exp. Med. 154, 333 (1981).

12. D. W. Blayney et al., JAMA 250, 1048 (1983).

13. D. Catovsky et al., Lancet i, 639, (1982).

14. K. Takatsuki, J. Uchiyama, K. Sagawa, J. Yodoi, in Topics in Hematology, S. Seno, F. Takaku, S. Irino, Eds. (Excerpta Medica, Amsterdam-Oxford, 1977), pp 73-77.

15. V. S. Kalyanaraman et al., Proc. Natl. Acad. Sci. USA 79, 1653 (1982).

16. M. Robert-Guroff et al., Science 215, 975 (1982).

17. W. A. Blattner, et al., Int. J. Cancer 30, 257 (1982).

18. I. Miyoshi et al., Nature 294, 770 (1981).

19. T. Watanabe, M. Seiki, M. Yoshida, Virology 133, 238 (1984).

20. R. C. Gallo et al., Cancer Res. 43, 3892 (1983).

21. W. C. Saxinger et al., Science (in press).

22. K. Tajima et al., Gann (in press).

23. T. Miyoshi et al., Gann 71, 155 (1981).

24. M. Popovic et al., Science 219, 856 (1983).

25. M. Popovic, G. Lange-Wantzin, P. S. Sarin, D. Mann, R. C. Gallo, Proc. Natl. Acad. Sci. USA 80, 5402 (1983).

26. D. L. Mann et al., J. Immunol. 131, 2021 (1983).

27. D. L. Mann et al., Nature 305, 58 (1983).

28. H. Mitsuya et al., J. Exp. Med. 158, 994 (1983).

29. H. Mitsuya et al., Science 223, 1293 (1984).

30. H. Mitsuya et al., Science (in press).

31. M. Popovic et al., Science (in press).

32. P. D. Markham, S. Z. Salahuddin, B. Macchi, M. Robert-Guroff, R. C. Gallo, Int. J. Cancer 33, 13 (1984).

33. V. S. Kalyanaraman et al., Science 218, 571 (1982).

34. T. H. Lee et al., Proc. Natl. Acad. Sci. USA (in press)

35. V. S. Kalyanaraman, M. Jarvis-Morar, M. G. Sarngadharan, R. C. Gallo, Virology 132, 61 (1984).

36. M. S. Reitz, Jr., M. Popovic, B. F. Haynes, S. C. Clark, R. C. Gallo, Virology 126, 688 (1983).

37. M. Seiki, S. Hattori, Y. Hirayama, M. Yoshida, Proc. Natl. Acad. Sci. USA 80, 3618 (1983).

38. G. M. Shaw et al., Proc. Natl. Acad. Sci. USA 81,
     4544 (1984).
39. W. A. Haseltine et al., Science 225, 419 (1984).
40. J. Sodroski et al., Science 225, 421 (1984).
41. J. Sodroski et al., Proc. Natl. Acad. Sci. USA (in
     press).
42. F. Wong-Staal et al., Nature 302, 626 (1983).
43. M. Yoshida, M. Seiki, K. Yamaguchi, K. Takatsuki,
     Proc. Natl. Acad. Sci. USA 81, 2534 (1984).
44. J. G. Sodroski, C. A. Rosen, W. A. Haseltine, Science
     225, 381 (1984).
45. I. S. Y. Chen, J. McLaughlin, D. W. Golde, Nature
     309, 276 (1980).
46. M. Essex et al., Science 220, 859 (1983).
47. M. Essex et al., Science 221, 1061 (1983).
48. M. Popovic, M. G. Sarngadharan, E. Read, R. C. Gallo,
     Science 224, 497, (1984).
49. R. C. Gallo et al., Science 224, 500 (1984).
50. J. Schupbach et al., Science 224, 503 (1984).
51. S. K. Arya et al., Science (in press).
52. B. H. Hahn et al., (submitted)
53. M. G. Sarngadharan, M. Popovic, L. Bruch, J.
     Schupbach, R. C. Gallo, Science 224, 506 (1984).
54. B. Safai et al., Lancet (June 30), 1438 (1984).
55. F. Barré-Sinoussi et al., Science 220, 868 (1983).

SESSION VI
Immuneregulation

Chairpersons: K. Smith and H. Wagner

The best characterized regulators of T cell functions are antigen and IL-2. Each interacts with defined receptors and sets in train a sequence of events culminating in proliferation and/or differentiation. A recent insight has been that antigen often functions via the intermediary action of IL-2 acting as a growth factor with the major role of antigenic recognition being the regulation of the expression of the receptors for IL-2. Thus this session examined current concepts of T cell growth induction and antigen induce growth inhibition in the phenomenon of tolerance.

Dr Smith reviewed the paradox that whereas antibodies to the IL-2 receptor (e.g. anti Tac) all recognize a single entity, not all anti Tac binding molecules represent active IL-2 receptors. IL-2, while inducing increased expression of Tac antigen, diminishes IL-2 binding sites (presumably by saturation).

Dr Waldmann reviewed the characterization of the Tac antigen, its identity with IL-2 receptors and aspects of its molecular cloning. Because adult T leukaemia, especially those involving HTLV-1 express Tac antigen at levels $\sim$ 10 times greater than normal, anti Tac by itself or coupled to a toxin has been used in vivo in attempts at immunotherapy. Preliminary results have been encouraging.

Drs Feldmann and Lamb reviewed their work on the antigen induced regulation of the function of antigen specific T cell clones, a phenomenon closely resembling (if not identical to) immunological tolerance. They reported work on the structural requirements for tolerance, and on the surface events: loss of the T3 and antigen receptor complex. The relevance of this form of tolerance to that occuring in vivo is substantiated by the fact that both are MHC restricted. One possible difference may be the greater sensitivity of unprimed or even immature T cells to tolerance induction in vivo. However tolerance of helper function rather than of proliferation was much more sensitive to antigen concentration suggesting that the difference may not be as pronounced as initially appeared. The capacity of T cells to be tolerized varies: after periods of rapid IL-2 driven growth, the resulting 'mutant' cells were not tolerizable. Whether this is a form of

277

regulation, or of genetic selection remains to be investigated.

Dr Pawalec discussed results with alloreactive T cell clones which aged perceptably in culture, changing their growth properties as well as their function. The significance of these changes is not known. One possibility is that this represents a class switching, as seen in much more rapid form in B cells during their driven maturation.

However other workers have not noted this aging at around ∿30 generations, nor change of function, suggesting that such changes are not an immutable part of the T cell developmental program, raising the possibility that adverse culture conditions are responsible. Further analysis is necessary to understand this process.

AUTOREGULATION OF T-CELL PROLIFERATION

Kendall A. Smith

Dartmouth Medical School

Hanover, New Hampshire

One of the unique characteristics of the immune system is the exquisite specificity of reactivity. The introduction of an antigen, either in vivo or in vitro, results in a clone-specific proliferative expansion and differentiation to effector function. Of course, this specificity of reactivity resides in the clonal distribution of antigen receptors on B cells and T cells; each cell reacts with high affinity only to one antigen epitope. As such, this phenomenon precludes the expression of interleukin 2 (IL-2) receptors by lymphocytes that have yet to encounter their specific antigen, since multiple clonal antigen specificities would react if non-antigen-specific cells were also capable of responding to IL-2. In practice, IL-2 receptors can not be detected on freshly isolated lymphocytes[1]. Moreover, immunoaffinity-purified, homogeneous IL-2 does not generate a proliferative response provided potential antigens are excluded from the culture system[2]. Accordingly, one of the unique aspects of the IL-2 hormone-receptor system is the **inducibility** of IL-2 receptors[3]: the immune system remains quiescent until environmental, foreign material is introduced, whereupon the IL-2 hormone-receptor system functions to transfer these environmental molecular signals to an internal, endocrine-like control mechanism. Consequently, the rapidity of induction, magnitude, and duration of T-cell proliferative responses are dictated by the rate and extent of IL-2 and IL-2 receptor gene expression[3,4].

An exceptional characteristic of the IL-2 hormone-receptor system relates to the "autocrine" nature of the response. Individual T-cells, primarily of the helper T-cell category, both produce and respond to IL-2[5,6]. Appropriate antigen stimulation of T-cell clones leads to the specific transcriptional activation of **both** the IL-2 gene and the IL-2 receptor gene. Given that a cell functions physiologically to make and respond to its own specific growth hormone, the question arises immediately as to what mechanisms, if any, regulate this process so that the cell does not proliferate continuously after antigen triggering. Certainly, antigen-triggered T cells do not proliferate indefinitely; rather, after several days in culture, the proliferative rate of the cell population gradually declines and eventually all of the cells reaccumulate in the resting (G_0/G_1) phase of the cell cycle[3]. As well, in vivo, antigen-initiated T-cell clonal expansion is a transient affair, culminating in long-term memory cells and cells that perform differentiated T-cell functions. Until very recently, the controlling influence on antigen-initiated, IL-2-dependent T-cell clonal expansion was thought to reside solely in the continued presence of antigen. The removal of antigen through clearance by the reticuloendothelial system necessarily results in a lack of sustained antigen-receptor interaction, thought to be essential for IL-2 and IL-2 receptor gene expression. This notion implies that the continued expression of both of these genes requires the constant generation of signals derived from the antigen receptor; the system is envisioned as driven only by positive signals. However, most biologic systems, especially endocrinologic, are known to have feedback regulatory controls that ensure homeostasis and prevent wide fluctuations in responses. A classic example is the feedback regulatory control inherent in the hypothalamic-pituitary-endocrine gland axis.

In a recent series of experiments, new information indicates that IL-2 responsiveness is under a reciprocal control mechanism mediated by antigen receptors and IL-2 receptors[7]. Antigen receptor triggering results in the appearance of high-affinity IL-2 binding sites. For normal human peripheral blood T cells, these sites exhibit an equilibrium dissociation constant (K_d) of 10 pM[1]. Consequently, the physiologic IL-2 concentration range responsible for binding to these sites varies between 1 X

10-12M and 1 X 10^{-10}M. However, we have discovered that saturation of high-affinity IL-2 binding sites results in a disappearance of as many as 50% of these receptors within 2 hr, at the very time the threshold of signals is generated that leads to DNA replication[7]. Simultaneously, different receptors appear, which have a 1000-fold lower affinity for IL-2 (K_d = 10 nM), and gradually accumulate on the cell membrane, ultimately exceeding by 10-fold the number of high-affinity sites (i.e., 100,000 vs. 10,000). Accordingly, IL-2 finely regulates the potential magnitude of its own biologic response by diminishing the cellular expression of high-affinity receptors, while promoting the expression of low-affinity receptors.

The concept of polypeptide hormone "down-regulation" of hormone receptors has evolved over the past 10 years and has been explained as a membrane event. Detailed morphologic and metabolic studies have revealed that hormone-occupied receptors migrate in the plane of the membrane to clathrin-coated pits, resulting in a more rapid internalization through invagination and the formation of endosomes or "receptosomes"[8]. Assuming an unaltered rate of new receptor synthesis, the consequence of hormone-receptor interaction is the establishment of a new, lower steady-state level of receptors. Turnover studies of the IL-2 receptor in the presence and absence of IL-2 indicate a more rapid disappearance of detectable high-affinity binding sites in the presence of IL-2 than in its absence (D.Cantrell and K. Smith, in prep.). Therefore, a ligand-mediated, accelerated disappearance of IL-2 receptors can account for diminished expression of high affinity binding sites. However, on a numerical basis alone, a 50% decrease in high-affinity IL-2 binding sites cannot possibly account for a simultaneous 10-fold increase in low-affinity IL-2 binding sites. Accordingly, it appears that IL-2 binding to antigen-induced high-affinity IL-2 receptors generates two signals; one results in DNA replication, the other results in a switch in the expression of molecules to those that now bind IL-2 with a 1000-fold lower affinity. The implications of such a system are that IL-2 regulates the potential responsiveness of T-cells by a unique process, which subtly influences the affinity of the receptor molecules expressed. Consequently, this unusual reciprocal regulation of expression of IL-2 receptors guarantees the eventual loss of IL-2 responsiveness and the return to a resting G_0 cell population, especially as antigen is cleared in vivo.

If one contemplates the ultimate consequences of the antigen-T-cell-IL-2 system, it is intuitive that the IL-2 autoregulation of IL-2 receptors serves as an efficient safeguard against IL-2-mediated autocrine growth. In situations where the positive influence in expression of high-affinity IL-2 binding sites (i.e., antigen stimulation) is not removed from the organism rapidly, the negative influence of IL-2 serves to restrain the expression of high-affinity sites, thereby dampening the ongoing T-cell proliferative response. Thus, chronic inflammatory or infectious diseases would be expected to maintain antigen-reactive T-cells in an IL-2-responsive state, owing to the continued presence of antigen. However, the IL-2 mediated down-regulation of high-affinity binding sites would prevent a gross overexpansion of antigen-specific T-cell clones. The selective advantage of such a system resides in the maintenance of a more homeostatic control over the extent of T-cell proliferation.

Another distinctive feature of the system favoring the selection of a mechanism of IL-2-mediated control of the extent of its own response can be inferred from the autocrine nature of helper T-cells. One might imagine that a distinct mechanism that dampens IL-2 responsiveness of IL-2 producing T-cells could have been selected for and conserved, thus preventing uncontrolled IL-2 autocrine-like neoplastic T-cell growth. A switch of 1000-fold in the affinity of the IL-2-receptor interaction would necessitate 1000-fold-higher concentrations of IL-2 to saturate the newly expressed receptor molecules. Such high concentrations of IL-2 (i.e., 100 nM) have yet to be encountered in vivo. Moreover, IL-2 concentrations supplied in vitro in excess of 1 μM fail to promote T-cell proliferation to a greater extent than those required to saturate high-affinity IL-2 binding sites (i.e., 100 pM). Thus, we have no evidence that low-affinity IL-2-binding sites function at all to promote or supress DNA replication and mitosis.

The mechanism responsible for the appearance of newly expressed low affinity IL-2 receptor molecules remains ill-defined and could be quite complex. The appearance of new, low-affinity binding sites only occurs at 37°C and requires 18-24 hr. Since IL-2 receptor turnover studies indicate that the membrane residence time for the low-affinity sites is much longer than for the high-affinity sites[7], it is conceivable that IL-2 promotes changes in the molecular conformation of high-affinity sites, resulting in low binding affinity. The "switched" molecules could then be imagined to accumulate on the membrane, owing to their slower turnover, or to participate in a recycling phenomenon, much as do receptors for transferrin, asialoglycoprotein, and low-density lipoprotein. An equally plausible hypothesis could be that IL-2-high affinity receptor interaction changes the molecular nature of the IL-2 receptor more centrally. Although restriction enzyme studies reveal that there is only one IL-2 receptor gene, there are at least two detectable mRNA transcripts[9,10]. Moreover, sequence analysis of cDNA clones reveals that a 216 bp region may be missing from the external coding domain of some of the transcripts, leading to 4 mRNA molecules. Of particular interest, there are RNA donor and acceptor splice sites adjacent to the missing region, suggesting that RNA splicing may be operative[9]. Since this change occurs in the external domain of the receptor translation product, it is tempting to speculate that the resulting molecule retains its Tac antibody and IL-2 binding regions but that the conformational change in the molecule results in a different IL-2-binding affinity. If so, then IL-2 may regulate its own biologic response by promoting a change of mRNA transcripts expressed.

Regardless of the precise mechanism responsible for the variable nature of the IL-2 receptor molecules expressed, it is hardly coincidental that many other polypeptide hormone receptors exist in both high affinity and low affinity forms; including insulin, platelet-derived growth factor, nerve growth factor and epidermal growth factor receptors. So far, only insulin is known to bind to two structurally similar but functionally different receptors; insulin binds with a 100-fold lower affinity to insulin-like growth factor I receptors[11]. The unusual aspect of the IL-2-receptor system, yet to be demonstrated for any other hormone-receptor system, relates to the induction of low affinity binding sites by IL-2 itself. This discovery leads to the inevitable prediction that such a phenomenon may be general, constituting a means by which hormones dictate the magnitude of the very responses they elicit.

1. Robb, R.J., Munck, A., & Smith, K.A. J. Exp. Med. **154**, 1455-1474 (1981).
2. Smith, K.A. Ann. Rev. Immunol. **2**, 319-333 (1984).
3. Cantrell, D.A., Smith, K.A. J. Exp. Med. **158**, 1895-1911 (1983).
4. Cantrell, D.A., Smith, K.A. Science **224**, 1312-1316 (1984).
5. Schreier, M.H., Isacove, N.N., Tees, R., Aarden, L, & von Boehmer, H. Immunol. Rev. **51**, 315-336 (1980).
6. Meuer, S.C., Hussey, R.E., Cantrell, D.A., Hodgdon, J.C., Schlossman, S.F., Smith, K.A. & Reinherz, E.L. Proc. Natl. Acad. Sci. U.S.A. **81**, 1509-1513 (1984).
7. Smith, K.A. & Cantrell, D.A. Proc. Natl. Acad. Sci. U.S.A. (in press).
8. Hanover, J. Willingham, M. & Pastan, I. Cell **39**, 283-288 (1984).
9. Leonard, W.J., Depper, J.M., Crabtree, G.R., Rudikoff, S. Pumphrey, J., Robb, R.J., Kronke, M., Svetlik, P.B., Peffer, N.J., Waldman, T.A. & Greene, W.C. Nature **311**, 626-631 (1984).
10. Nikaido, T., Shimizu, A., Ishida, N., Sabe, H., Teshigawara, K., Maeda, M., Uchiyama, T., Yodoi, J. & Honjo, T. Nature **311**, 631-635 (1984).
11. Massague', J. & Czech, M.P., J. Biol. Chem. **257**, 5038-5054 (1982).

INTERLEUKIN-2 RECEPTORS

Thomas A. Waldmann, Warren J. Leonard, Joel M.

Depper, Martin Kronke, Carolyn K. Goldman,

Kathleen Bongiovanni, and Warner C. Greene

Metabolism Branch, National Cancer Institute,

NIH, Bethesda, Maryland 20205

ABSTRACT

Interleukin-2 (IL-2) is a lymphokine synthesized by some
T-cells following activation. Resting T-cells do not express IL-2 receptors but receptors are rapidly expressed
on T-cells following the interaction of antigens, mitogens, or monoclonal antibodies with the antigen specific
T-cell receptor complex. Using anti-Tac a monoclonal
antibody that recognizes the IL-2 receptor, the receptor
has been purified. The receptor is a 33kd peptide that
is posttranslationally glycosylated to a 55kd mature
form. Mature receptors contain both N-linked and O-linked
sugars and are both sulfated and phosphorylated. Using
an oligonucleotide probe, based on the N-terminal amino
acid sequence, cDNAs encoding this receptor have been
cloned, sequenced and expressed. The addition of anti-Tac
to in vitro culture systems blocks the IL-2 induced DNA
synthesis of IL-2 dependent T-cell lines and inhibits
soluble auto- and alloantigen induced T-cell proliferation. Furthermore, it prevents the generation of cytotoxic and suppressor effector T cells. The anti-receptor
antibody also inhibits lectin stimulated immunoglobulin
synthesis and the sequential expression of late appearing
activation antigens on T-cells. Normal resting T-cells
and most leukemic T-cell populations do not express IL-
2 receptors however the leukemic cells of all patients
with human T-cell leukemia/lymphoma virus (HTLV-1) asso-

ciated, adult T-cell leukemia (ATL) examined expressed
the Tac antigen. In HTLV-I infected cells the 42kd LOR
protein encoded in part, by the pX region of HTLV-I may
act as a transacting transcriptional activator that induces transcription of the IL-2 receptor gene thus providing an explanation for the constant association of HTLV-I
infection of lymphoid cells and IL-2 receptor expression.
The constant display of large numbers of IL-2 receptors
which may be aberrant in the ATL cells may play a role in
the uncontrolled growth of these leukemic T-cells. Patients with the Tac positive adult T-cell leukemia are
being treated with the anti-Tac monoclonal antibody
directed towards this growth factor receptor.

INTRODUCTION

The induction of an immune response to a foreign antigen
requires the activation of T lymphocytes with receptors
for the specific antigen. The human antigen specific
T-cell receptor has been shown to be a polymorphic heterodimer of alpha and beta chains of approximately 49 and
43kd associated with three 20-28,000 dalton nonpolymorphic
peptide chains identified by the T-3 monoclonal antibody
(1-3). T-cell activation is initiated following the interaction of antigen, mitogens or antibodies with this
complex antigen specific T-cell receptor. Two principle
events occur at this point which are required for T-cell
proliferation and the development of functionally active
effector T-cells. First, following interaction with
antigen and the macrophage derived interleukin-1, T-cells
express the gene encoding the lymphokine T-cell growth
factor or Interleukin-2 (4,5). In order to exert its
biological effects IL-2 must interact with high affinity
specific membrane receptors (6). Resting T-cells do not
express IL-2 receptors but receptors are rapidly expressed
on T-cells following activation with antigen or mitogen.
Thus, both the growth factor Interleukin-2, and its receptor are absent in resting T-cells but following activation the genes for both proteins become expressed. Failure of the production of either the growth factor or its
receptor results in failure of the T-cell immune response.
Thus, both the production of interleukin-2 and the display
of the interleukin-2 receptors are pivotal events in the
full expression of the human immune response. While the

antigen confers specificity for a given immune response,
the interaction of IL-2 with IL-2 receptors determines
its magnitude and duration. Furthermore, IL-2 is required
for the development of the functional capacities of the T
lymphocyte.

The specific membrane receptor for IL-2 on human lymphocytes has been identified using a monoclonal antibody
(anti-Tac) directed towards this molecule (7-9). As
outlined in the review below, we have utilized the anti-
Tac monoclonal antibody to: characterize the human receptor for IL-2; Molecularly clone cDNAs for the human
IL-2 receptor; define the immunoregulatory affects of
this antibody on lymphocyte activation and function;
characterize the expression of the Tac antigen (IL-2 receptor) in leukemias of mature T lymphocytes and treat
patients with the Tac expressing adult T-cell leukemia.
<u>Demonstration that anti-Tac recognizes the human IL-2 re-
ceptor</u> The anti-Tac monoclonal antibody prepared by
Uchiyama, Broder and Waldmann (7) was selected on the
basis of its ability to bind to activated T-cells but
not to resting T-cells, B-cells or monocytes. This pattern of cellular reactivity was identical with the distribution of IL-2 receptors reported by Robb and coworkers (6).
We therefore, hypothesized that anti-Tac recognizes the
human receptor for IL-2 (8,9). Data in support of this
hypothesis are as follows: anti-Tac blocks the IL-2 induced
DNA synthesis of IL-2 dependent continuous T-cell lines but
does not inhibit DNA synthesis of IL-2 independent T-cell
lines; Anti-Tac blocks over 95% of the binding of ^{3}H-IL-2
to HUT 102-B2 cells and PHA activated lymphoblasts and IL-2
at high concentration blocks the binding of ^{3}H-anti-Tac to
PHA activated lymphoblasts. The requirement for high
concentrations of IL-2 is explained by the observation
that anti-Tac identifies two species of IL-2 receptors,
one with a high (10^{-12}M) and one with a lower affinity
of IL-2 binding. Furthermore, Robb and Greene (10)
demonstrated that an initial passage of radiolabeled
proteins from PHA lymphoblasts through either an IL-2
coupled affinity support or a column of anti-Tac coupled to
sepharose effectively removed molecules reactive with the
alternative support. Thus, under the conditions used all
anti-Tac reactive molecules appeared capable of binding
IL-2 and the ability to bind IL-2 was limited to the Tac
protein.

Chemical Characterization of the IL-2 Receptor

The anti-Tac monoclonal antibody was utilized to characterize the IL-2 receptor on PHA activated normal lymphocytes (8,9). Anti-Tac immunoprecipitations of ^{125}I-surface-
labeled PHA-activated normal lymphocytes were analyzed
on 8.75% SDS-polyacrylamide gels under reducing conditions.
A diffuse band of 55kd was readily identified as the
putative IL-2 receptor. This protein was also identified
in immunoprecipitations from cells precultured with
^{3}H-D-glucosamine thus demonstrating that it is a glycoprotein. Furthermore, when cells were biosynthetically
labeled with ^{35}-S-methionine and the immunoprecipitates
analyzed on 7.5% SDS-polyacrylamide gels a similar band
was identified. Furthermore, additional bands of 113kd
and approximately 180kd were also identified. None of
these bands was identified in immunoprecipitations using
control monoclonal antibodies. Since the 113 and 180kd
peptides were not labeled by either ^{125}I using lactoper-
oxidase labeling of intact cells or by ^{3}H-D-glucosamine
they do not appear to be surface membrane receptors and
the roles of these molecules is unknown. One or both may
be part of a theoretical receptor complex and therefore,
coimmunoprecipitated due to strong hydrophobic interactions with the 55kd peptide. It is also possible that
neither has any functional relationship to the IL-2 receptor but rather that they contain antigenic determinants
that result in their precipitation by anti-Tac. The post
translational processing of the 55kd glycoprotein was defined employing a combination of pulse-chase and tunicamycin experiments (9,11) PHA lymphoblasts were labeled with
^{35}S-methionine for 15 minutes and then chased with a
large excess of unlabeled methionine for 0,15,30,60,120,
or 240 minutes. A precursor doublet of 35 and 37kd was
identified early, and by 60 minutes of chase, the mature
form of the 55kd receptor was evident. When cells were
labeled in the presence of tunicamycin which prevents addition of N-linked sugars the sizes of both the precursor
and mature forms of the PHA activated lymphoblast IL-2
receptor decreased by 2-4kd. The 35/37kd doublet was
then seen as a 33kd band and the 55kd band was seen as
approximately 52kd band. In summary, on the basis of
these and additional studies the IL-2 receptor is a 55kd

sites. Furthermore there is a single hydrophobic transmembrane region and a very short (13 amino acid) cytoplasmic domain. The cytoplasmic domain of interleukin-2
receptor appears to be too small for enzymatic function.
Thus this receptor differs from other known growth factor
receptors that are tyrosine kinases. Potential phosphate
acceptor sites (serine and threonine, but not tyrosine)
are present within the intracytoplasmic domain.

Effects of Anti-Tac on Lymphocyte Activation
Utilizing the anti-Tac monoclonal antibody, we have defined those lymphocyte functions that require an interaction of IL-2 with its induceable receptor on activated
T-cells (13-15). The addition of anti-Tac to the cultures
of human periferal blood mononuclear cells inhibited a
variety of immune reactions. Anti-Tac blocked the proliferation of human T-cells stimulated with soluble, autologous and allogeneic antigens (14). In addition, anti-Tac
inhibited T-cell proliferation induced by mitogenic lectins. The degree of inhibition was inversely correlated
with the potency of the mitogeneic stimulus and its
ability to induce IL-2 production by the cultured T-cells.
Anti-Tac inhibition of antigen and mitogen induced T-cell
proliferation was reversed by the addition of purified
IL-2. Anti-Tac abrogated the generation of cytotoxic T
lymphocytes in allogeneic cell cultures but did not inhibit their action once generated. Furthermore, anti-Tac
inhibited the generation of suppressor T-cells activated
by lectins or by the sepharose bound T3 monoclonal antibody. Anti-Tac also inhibited the sequential development
of certain late appearing activation antigens on T-cells.
A series of activation antigens that in large measure
represent receptors for growth factors appear on T-cells
following the interaction of lectins or T3 antibody with
the antigen-specific T-cell receptor complex. The order
of receptor appearance is IL-2 receptor at 4-12 hours,
insulin, somatomedin-I and somatomedin-II receptors at 24
hours, transferrin receptors at 24-72 hours and Ia antigens at 5-7 days. It has been reported (16,17) that the
addition anti-Tac at the initiation of cultures inhibited
the appearance of the activation antigens examined, the
transferrin receptors and Ia antigens. Finally, anti-Tac
inhibited immunoglobulin production by B lymphocytes
activated by pokeweed mitogen, wheat-germ agglutanin,

glycoprotein composed of a 33kd peptide precursor. Mature receptors contain both N-linked and O-linked sugars
and are both sulfated and phosphorylated.

Molecular Cloning and Expression of cDNAs for the Human
Interleukin-2 Receptor

cDNAs encoding the human interleukin-2 receptor have been
molecularly cloned (12). For these studies the human
receptor for interleukin-2 was purified by immunoaffinity
chromatography using the anti-Tac monoclonal antibody.
The sequence of the 29 N-terminal amino acids was determined by gas phase microsequencing and a nucleotide probe
corresponding to the amino acids 3-8 was synthesized.
Using this probe, 11 candidate IL-2 receptor clones were
isolated from a HUT 102-B2 cDNA library prepared in lambda
gt 10 bacteriophage. Three of these clones were selected
for further study and were shown to correspond to the
IL-2 receptor based on selective hybridization of mRNA,
DNA sequencing, and expression in COS-1 cells. Southern
blot analysis of human geneomic DNA suggested that a
single gene encodes the IL-2 receptor. In contrast mRNAs
of two different sizes approximately 1500 and 3500 bases
long, were identified. These two classes of mRNA differ
because of the utilization of different polyadenylation
signals. Sequence analysis of the cloned cDNAs also
suggested an alternative pathway of mRNA processing
whereby a 216 base pair segment flanked by classical mRNA
splice signals within the protein coding region may be
removed. Using expression studies of cDNAs in COS-1
cells Leonard and coworkers (12) demonstrated that the
unspliced but not the spliced form of the mRNA was translated into the IL-2 receptor. These data raised the
possibility that the IL-2 receptor expression may be
regulated not only through initiation of transcription
but through post-transcriptional splicing as well.
However, alternative possibilities for the deletion of
this internal segment exist.

The deduced amino acid sequence of the IL-2 receptor
indicates that this peptide is composed of 272 amino
acids including a 21 amino acid signal peptide. The
receptor contains two potential N-linked glycosylation
sites as well as multiple possible O-linked carboydrate

sites. Furthermore there is a single hydrophobic transmembrane region and a very short (13 amino acid) cytoplasmic domain. The cytoplasmic domain of interleukin-2
receptor appears to be too small for enzymatic function.
Thus this receptor differs from other known growth factor
receptors that are tyrosine kinases. Potential phosphate
acceptor sites (serine and threonine, but not tyrosine)
are present within the intracytoplasmic domain.

Effects of Anti-Tac on Lymphocyte Activation
Utilizing the anti-Tac monoclonal antibody, we have defined those lymphocyte functions that require an interaction of IL-2 with its induceable receptor on activated
T-cells (13-15). The addition of anti-Tac to the cultures
of human periferal blood mononuclear cells inhibited a
variety of immune reactions. Anti-Tac blocked the proliferation of human T-cells stimulated with soluble, autologous and allogeneic antigens (14). In addition, anti-Tac
inhibited T-cell proliferation induced by mitogenic lectins. The degree of inhibition was inversly correlated
with the potency of the mitogeneic stimulus and its
ability to induce IL-2 production by the cultured T-cells.
Anti-Tac inhibition of antigen and mitogen induced T-cell
proliferation was reversed by the addition of purified
IL-2. Anti-Tac abrogated the generation of cytotoxic T
lymphocytes in allogeneic cell cultures but did not inhibit their action once generated. Furthermore, anti-Tac
inhibited the generation of suppressor T-cells activated
by lectins or by the sepharose bound T3 monoclonal antibody. Anti-Tac also inhibited the sequential development
of certain late appearing activation antigens on T-cells.
A series of activation antigens that in large measure
represent receptors for growth factors appear on T-cells
following the interaction of lectins or T3 antibody with
the antigen-specific T-cell receptor complex. The order
of receptor appearance is IL-2 receptor at 4-12 hours,
insulin, somatomedin-I and somatomedin-II receptors at 24
hours, transferrin receptors at 24-72 hours and Ia antigens at 5-7 days. It has been reported (16,17) that the
addition anti-Tac at the initiation of cultures inhibited
the appearance of the activation antigens examined, the
transferrin receptors and Ia antigens. Finally, anti-Tac
inhibited immunoglobulin production by B lymphocytes
activated by pokeweed mitogen, wheat-germ agglutanin,

streptolysin O or Nocardia water soluble mitogen (15).
The inhibition of immunoglobulin synthesis by B-cells
could theoretically reflect either an inhibition of the
secretion of B-cell growth and differentiation factors by
helper T-cells or a direct action on the B-cells themselves. The prevailing view has been that B-cells do not
display receptors for IL-2 (18). However utilizing the
anti-Tac monoclonal antibody we explored the possibility
that certain activated B cells display receptors for IL-2
(15). Normal resting B-cells and most unselected B cell
lines established from normal individuals with the Epstein-
Barr virus were Tac antigen negative. In contrast, cell
surface Tac antigen expression was demonstrable on six of
ten B-cell lines derived from patients with Burkitt's
lymphoma, on 14 of 15 leukemic cell populations from
patients with the B-cell form of Hairy Cell Leukemia (19)
and on all B-cell lines infected with HTLV-1 obtained
from patients with adult T-cell leukemia (20). Finally,
the Tac antigen was demonstrable on a proportion of
normal B-cells activated with either pokeweed mitogen or
Staphlococcus Aureus Cowan strain I organisms (SAC).
Furthermore, cloned EBV transformed B-cell lines derived
from such Tac positive pokeweed mitogen activated normal
B-cells continued to express the Tac antigen in long-term
culture and manifested high affinity IL-2 receptors
identified utilizing radiolabeled IL-2. One B-cell line
derived from a normal individual developed in this study
could be induced by the addition of the ligand, purified
or recombinant IL-2 to increase the number of Tac receptors
expressed from 500 to 4500 per cell. This up-regulation
of the number of IL-2 receptors expressed required protein
synthesis and RNA transcription but not cell division or
DNA replication. These studies suggest that de novo
receptor synthesis was occurring rather than the unmasking
of cryptic receptors. The size of the IL-2 receptors on
the Tac positive cloned normal B cells was similar (53 to
57kd) to that of receptors on PHA stimulated T lymphoblasts. Futhermore, Tac positive B-cells were shown to
transcribe mRNA for the IL-2 receptor. Thus, certain
malignant as well as activated normal B cells display the
Tac antigen and manifest high affinity receptors for IL-2.

In functional studies, peripheral blood B-cells from normal individuals activated with SAC could be induced to
proliferate and to synthesize immunoglobulin molecules by
the addition of recombinant IL-2. These responses were
abrogated if anti-Tac was added to the cultures. These
data suggest that IL-2 may play a role in the proliferation of activated B-cells as well as their differentiation
into immunoglobulin synthesizing and secreting cells.

IL-2 Receptor Expression in Adult T-cell Leukemia

We have analyzed the IL-2 receptor expression on three
forms of T-cell leukemia, acute T-cell leukemia, the
Sèzary leukemia and adult T-cell leukemia (ATL) (20).
Acute T-cell leukemia is a malignant proliferation of
immature T-cells that frequently do not express surface
antigens such as the T3 antigen that are associated with
mature T-cells. Both the adult T-cell leukemia and the
Sèzary leukemia are malignant proliferations of mature
T-cells with a propensity to infiltrate the skin. They
share similar cell morphology and clinical features.
However, certain features aid in distinguishing these
leukemias. Cases of adult T-cell leukemia in contrast
to those with the Sèzary leukemia are clustered within
families and geographically occurring in the southwest of
Japan, the Carribean basin and certain areas of the southeastern united states. Furthermore, adult T-cell leukemia
has been shown to be caused by the human T-cell leukemia/
lymphoma virus (HTLV-I) a human type c retrovirus whereas
patients with the Sèzary syndrome do not have circulating
antibodies to this virus (21,22). The acute T-cell leukemic populations and lines derived from such cells we
examined did not express the IL-2 receptor. Furthermore,
nine of the ten populations of Sèzary leukemic T-cells
not associated with HTLV-I examined were Tac antigen negative (20). In contrast, all of populations of leukemic
cells from patients with the adult T-cell leukemia, associated with HTLV-I expressed the Tac antigen. Thus, the
demonstration of IL-2 receptors on leukemic T-cells may
aid in differentiating leukemias caused by HTLV-I which
are Tac antigen positive from other forms of T-cell leukemia which are, in general, Tac antigen negative.
The IL-2 receptor expression on adult T-cell leukemic
cells differs from that on normal T-cells. Firstly,
unlike normal T-cells ATL cells do not require prior
activation to express the IL-2 receptors. Furthermore,

using the ^{3}H-anti-Tac receptor assay, HTLV-I infected
leukemic T-cell lines characteristically expressed five
to ten fold more receptors per cell (270,000-640,000)
then did maximally PHA stimulated T lymphoblasts (30,000-
60,000) (23). Since the cell volume of these leukemic
cells was only 13% greater than that of PHA lymphoblasts
the density of IL-2 receptors on these leukemic cells was
correspondingly increased. In addition, whereas normal
human T lymphocytes maintained in long-term culture with
IL-2 demonstrate a rapid decline in receptor number ATL
lines do not show a similar decline. Furthermore, we
have noted that some but not all HTLV-I infected cell
lines display aberently sized IL-2 receptors (11,24).
For example, the receptor on HTLV-I infected HUT 102-B2
cells is approximately 5,000 daltons smaller than that on
PHA lymphoblasts. Using pulse-chase, tunicamycin, endo-
glycosidase and neurominindase analyses the difference in
receptor size was shown to be due to differences in post
translational modification of the 33kd protein backbone
(11, 24). Furthermore, the receptors on the HUT 102 B2
cells manifested less sulfation than did normal receptors.
Finally in studies by Uchiyama and coworkers (25), IL-2
receptors on ATL cells unlike normal activated T-cells
were not modulated (down regulated) by anti-Tac and IL-2
receptors on ATL cell lines were spontaneously (IL-2 independently) phosphorylated whereas the phosphorylation
of receptors on PHA stimulated T-cells required the
addition of IL-2. It is conceivable that the constant
presence of high numbers of IL-2 receptors on the adult
T-cell leukemic cells and/or the aberancy of these receptors may play a major role in the pathogenesis of uncontrolled growth of these malignant T-cells. As noted
above the T-cell leukemias caused by HTLV-I as well as
all T-cell and B-cell lines infected with HTLV-1 universally express large numbers of IL-2 receptors. A recent
report by Haseltine and colleagues (26) suggests a potential mechanism for this association between HTLV-1 and
IL-2 receptor expression. The complete sequence of
HTLV-1 has been determined by Seiki and colleagues (27).
In addition to the GAG, POL, ENV, and LTR (long terminal
repeats) sequences common to other groups of retro-viruses,

HTLV-1 contains an additional genomic region between env
and the LTR referred to as pX. Haseltine and colleagues
(26) demonstrated that this pX region encodes a Mr 38-42
kd protein termed LOR (long open reading frame) protein
that may act as a transacting regulator of transcription.
They demonstrated that the LOR protein acts on the LTRs
(promoter and regulatory sequences) of HTLV-I, II and III
stimulating transcription. The LOR protein could theoretically also play a central role in increasing the
transcription of host genes such as the IL-2 receptor
gene involved in T-cell activation and HTLV-I mediated
leukemogenesis. With the cloning of the gene encoding
the IL-2 receptor, this hypothesis that the LOR protein
acts as a transacting regulator of transcription of the
IL-2 receptor gene can now be readily tested.

Treatment of Patients with Adult T-Cell Leukemia with the Anti-Tac Monoclonal Antibody

We have initiated a clinical trial to evaluate the efficacy of intravenously administered anti-Tac monoclonal
antibody in the treatment of patients with the adult
T-cell leukemia. The scientific basis for these studies
is the observation that adult T-cell leukemia cells
express the Tac antigen whereas normal resting T-cells
and their precursors do not (20). Two patients with
adult T-cell leukemia have been treated with intravenously administered anti-Tac. Neither patient suffered any
ontoward reactions nor did they produce antibodies reactive with mouse immunoglobulin or the idiotype of the
anti-Tac monoclonal. One patient with a very rapidly
developing form of adult T-cell leukemia had a very
transient response. However, therapy of the other patient was followed by a six month remission as assessed
by routine hematological tests, by immunofluorescense
analysis of circulating T-cells and by molecular genetic
analysis of the arrangement of T-cell beta receptor
genes. Prior to anti-Tac therapy the patient had 2200
circulating malignant T-cells/mm^3 as assessed by immunofluorescence analysis using the anti-Tac monoclonal
antibody. Furthermore, some (1200/mm^3) but not all of
these circulating leukemic lymphocytes reacted with an
antibody to the transferrin receptor, a receptor expressed
on malignant T-cells but not on normal circulating cells.
Following anti-Tac therapy there was a decline in the

number of circulating T-cells bearing the Tac antigen from 2,200 to less than $100/mm^3$ and in transferrin receptor expressing T cells from 1,200 to less than $100/mm^3$. During the four week period following the anti-Tac infusions there were no cells with free IL-2 receptors that is with receptors unblocked by the infused anti-Tac monoclonal. Cells with blocked IL-2 receptors were identified as cells that were not reactive with FITC-conjugated anti-Tac but were reactive with FITC conjugated anti-mouse IgG and with the 7G7 monoclonal antibody, an antibody that identifies an epitope of the IL-2 receptor peptide other than that identified by anti-Tac. The remission of the T-cell leukemia in this patient was confirmed utilizing molecular genetic analysis of the arrangement of the gene encoding the beta chain of the antigen specific T-cell receptor. Prior to therapy Southern analysis of the arrangement of the T-cell beta receptor gene utilizing a radiolabeled probe to the constant region of the T beta chain (28), revealed a new band not present with germ line tissues, the hallmark of a clonal expansion of T-lymphocytes. This band reflecting the clonally rearranged T-cell receptor gene was not demonstrable on specimens obtained following anti-Tac therapy when the patient was in remission. Approximately six months following the initial remission, the leukemia recurred with a reappearance of circulating leukemic cells identified by immunofluorescence and molecular genetic analysis. The patient also developed large (5x7x1 cm) malignant skin lesions. A new course of intravenous infusions of anti-Tac was followed by the virtual dissappearance of the skin lesions and an over 90% reduction in the number of circulating leukemic cells. Three months subsequently leukemic cells were again demonstrable in the circulation. At this time the leukemia was no longer responsive to infusions of anti-Tac and the patient required chemotherapy. These therapeutic studies have been extended in vitro by examining the efficacy of toxins coupled to anti-Tac in selectively inhibiting protein synthesis and viability of Tac positive adult T-cell leukemic cell lines. The addition of anti-Tac antibody coupled to the A chain of the toxin ricin effectively inhibited protein synthesis by the HTLV-I

associated, Tac positive adult T cell leukemia line HUT
102-B2. In contrast conjugates of ricin A with a control
monoclonal of the same isotype did not inhibit protein
synthesis when used in the same concentration (29). The
inhibitory action of anti-Tac conjugated with ricin A
could be abolished by the addition of excess unlabeled
anti-Tac or IL-2. In parallel studies performed in
collaboration with David Fitzgerald, Mark Willingham and
Ira Pastan (30) pseudomonas exotoxin conjugates of anti-
Tac inhibited the protein synthesis by HUT 102-B2 cells
but not that of the Tac negative acute T cell line Molt-4
that does not express the Tac antigen. Again, the toxicity of the anti-Tac toxin conjugates could be inhibited
by adding excess unlabeled anti-Tac. Thus, the development of toxin conjugates of the monoclonal anti-Tac that
is directed toward the IL-2 receptor expressed on adult
T-cell leukemic cells may permit the development of a
rational approach for the treatment of this almost uni-
formly fatal form of leukemia.

REFERENCES

1. Allison, J.P., McIntyre, B.W. and Bloch, D.
   J. Immunol. 129:2293, 1982.
2. Haskins, K., Kubo, R., White, J., Pigeon, M., Kappler,
   J., Marrack, P. J. Exp. Med. 157:1149, 1983.
3. Meuer, S.C., Fitzgerald, K.A., Hussey, R.E., Hodgdon,
   J.C., Schlossman, S.F. and Reinherz, E.L. J. Exp.
   Med. 157:705, 1983.
4. Morgan, D.A., Roscetti, F.W., and Gallo, R.C. Science
   (Wash. DC) 193:1007, 1983.
5. Smith, K.A. Immunol. Rev. 51:337, 1980.
6. Robb, R.J., Munck, A., Smith, K.A. J. Exp. Med.
   154:1455, 1981.
7. Uchiyama, T., Broder, S., and Waldmann, T.A. J.
   Immunol. 126:1393, 1981.
8. Leonard, W.J., Depper, J.M., Uchiyama, T., Smith, K.A.,
   Waldmann, T.A. and Greene, W.C. Nature (Lond.).
   300:267, 1982.
9. Leonard, W.J., Depper, J.M., Robb, R.J., Waldmann,
   T.A., and Greene, W.C. Proc. Natl. Acad. Sci. USA
   80:6957, 1983.
10. Robb, R.J., and Greene, W.C. J. Exp. Med. 158:1332,
    1983.

11. Leonard, W.J., Deper, J.M., Waldmann, T.A. and Greene,
    W.C. (Receptors and Recognition. Series B. Volume
    17) (M.F. Greaves ed. pp. 45-46. Chapman and Hall
    publishers London.

12. Leonard, W.J., Depper, J.M., Crabtree, G.R., Rudikoff,
    S., Pumphrey, J., Robb, R.J., Kronke, M., Svetlik,
    P.B., Peffer, N.J., Waldmann, T.A., and Greene, W.C.
    Nature. 311:626, 1984.

13. Uchiyama, T., Nelson, D.L., Fleisher, T.A., and
    Waldmann, T.A. J. Immunol. 126:1398, 1981.

14. Depper, J.M., Leonard, W.J., Waldmann, T.A., and
    Greene, W.C. J. Immunol. 131:690, 1983.

15. Waldmann, T.A., Goldman, C.K., Robb, R.J., Depper,
    J.M., Leonard, W.J., Sharrow, S.O., Bongiovanni,
    K.F., Korsmeyer, S.J. and Greene, W.C. J.
    Exp. Med. 160:1450, 1984.

16. Neckers, L.M., and Cossman, J. Proc. Natl. Acad.
    Sci. USA 80:3494, 1983.

17. Tsudo, M., Uchiyama, T., Takatsuki, K., Uchino, H.,
    and Yodoi, J. J. Immunol. 129:592, 1982.

18. Howard, M. and Paul, W.E. Ann. Rev. Immunol. 1:307,
    1983.

19. Korsmeyer, S.J., Greene, W.C., Cossman, J., Hsu, S.M.,
    Jensen, J.P., Neckers, .LM., Marshall, S.L., Bakhshi,
    A., Leonard, W.J., Jaffe, E.S., and Waldmann, T.A.
    Proc. Natl. Acad. Sci. USA. 80:4522, 1983.

20. Waldmann, T.A., Greene, W.C., Sarin, P.S., Saxinger,
    C., Blayney, W., Blattner, W.A., Goldman, C.K.,
    Bongiovanni, K., Sharrow, S., Depper, J.M., Leonard,
    W., Uchiyama, T., and Gallo, R.C. J. Clin. Invest.
    73:1711, 1984.

21. Poiesz, B.J., Ruscetti, F.W., Gazdar, A.F., Bunn, P.A.,
    Minna, J.D., and Gallo, R.C. Proc. Natl. Acad.
    Sci. USA. 77:7415, 1980.

22. Gallo, R.C., and Wong-Staal, F. Blood. 60:545, 1982.

23. Depper, J.M., Leonard, W.J., Kronke, M., Waldmann, T.A.
    and Greene, W.C. J. Immunol. 133:1691, 1984.

24. Leonard, W.J., Depper, J.M., Roth, J.S., Rudikoff, S.,
    Waldmann, T.A. and Greene, W.C. Clin. Res. 31:348A,
    1983.

25. Uchiyama, T., Wano, Y., Tsudo, M., Umadome, H., Hori,
    T., Tamori, S., Yodoi, J. and Maeda, M.
    Miwa, M. (ed.) Japan Sci. Soc. Press. in press.

26. Haseltine, W.A., Sodroski, J.G., Patarca, R., Briggs,
    D., Perkins, D. and Wong-Staal, F. Science. 225:
    419, 1984.

27. Seiki, M., Hattori, S., Hirayama, Y., and Yoshida, M.
       Proc. Natl. Acad. Sci. USA. 80:3618, 1983.
28. Hedrick, S.M., Cohen, D.I., Nielsen, E.A., and Davis,
       M.M. Nature 308:149, 1984.
29. Kronke, M., Depper, J.M., Leonard, W.J., Vitetta, E.S.,
       Waldmann, T.A. and Greene, W.C. Blood. in press.
30. Fitzgerald, D.J.P., Waldmann, T.A., Willingham, M.C.,
       and Pastan, I. J. Clin. Invest. 74: 966, 1984.

RESPONSE OF T CELLS TO SYNTHETIC PEPTIDE ANTIGENS: SPECIFIC

UNRESPONSIVENESS ANALOGOUS TO TOLERANCE

Marc Feldmann, E.D. Zanders, P.C.L. Beverley[+] and J.R. Lamb

Imperial Cancer Research Fund, Tumour Immunology Unit, Department of Zoology, University College London, Gower Street, London WC1E 6BT.

[+] Human Tumour Immunology Group, School of Medicine, University College Hospital, University Street, London WC1E 6JJ

INTRODUCTION

Regulated immune responses require that the magnitude of responses be under strict control. They also necessitate an accurate discrimination of self from non self antigens. The regulatory mechanisms involved in these processes are undoubtedly complex, but certain components have been identified, namely suppressor cells, and immunological tolerance (1,2). The latter process, a state of antigen induced, antigen specific unresponsiveness has been relatively ignored in recent years, due partly to the interest in the analysis of suppressor T cells, and also to the lack of suitable models for the analysis of T cell tolerance (unlike B cell tolerance) in vitro. It had even been proposed that tolerance was due to the action of suppressor T cells. The availability of homogeneous populations of cloned T cells (3) provided us with a opportunity to determine whether antigen could directly inhibit T cell function, in the absence of suppressor cells, and if so, to investigate its mechansism.

MATERIALS AND METHODS

The isolation and characterisation of T lymphocyte clones reactive with peptides of the haemagglutinin

301

molecule of Influenza virus have been described in detail elsewhere, as have methods for the induction and assay of tolerance in vitro (3,4).

RESULTS AND DISCUSSION

Typically, immune responses of complex cell populations in vitro or in vivo show bell shaped dose response kinetics. An optimum is gradually reached, with excess antigen this is reduced. Various human clones reactive with synthetic peptides of the HA-1 molecule of Influenza A/Texas were tested in this way, and it was found that clear optima were detected, as in mice or tissue culture using complex populations responding to more complex antigens (6,7).

There is evidence that both tolerance and T cell suppression are induced preferentially in the absence of

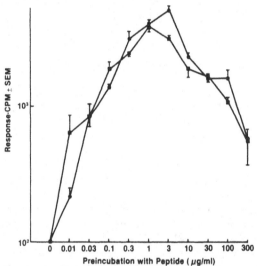

Fig. 1. Inactivation of antigen-induced proliferation of TLC with high concentration of specific antigen. TLC cells (HA1.7 [●], HA2.61 [■]; 5 × 10³) were cultured with irradiated autologous E⁻ cells (5 × 10³) in the presence of differing concentrations of antigen (0.01–300 μg/ml of peptides 20 and 11, respectively, for HA1.7 and HA2.61). Proliferation as correlated with [³H]TdR incorporation was determined for 72-h cultures. The results are expressed as the mean counts per minute (cpm) ± SEM of triplicate cultures. Background responses of HA1.7 and HA2.61 in the absence of irradiated E⁻ cells for any of the antigen concentrations used was <50 cpm as was that of E⁻ cells alone cultured with antigen. The response of HA1.7 and HA2.61 cultured with E⁻ cells in the absence of antigen were 29 ± 4 and 21 ± 6 cpm, respectively.

Reprinted with permission from J. Exp. Med. (1983) 157: 1434.

accessory cells (8,9) and so the preincubation experiments, necessary to determine whether the unresponsiveness lasts once the high antigen concentration is removed, were performed in the absence of any antigen presenting cells.

It was found that the degree of antigen induced inhibition by preincubation overnight with p20 was much greater in the absence of antigen presenting cells (APC) than in the presence of antigen presenting cells (APC), even with high p20 concentrations left in culture for 3 days (see Figs. 1 and 2).

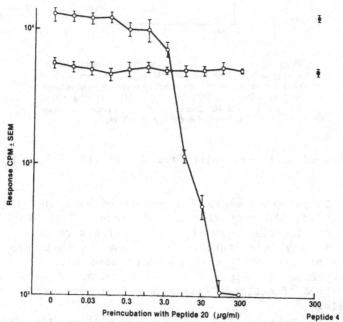

FIG. 2. Dose dependency of tolerance induced by preincubating T cells with specific antigen. Clone HA1.7 (10^6 cells/ml) was incubated in the presence or absence of varying concentrations of specific peptide (peptide 20; 0.01–300 μg/ml). The pretreatment was performed in round-bottomed 96-well microtiter plates for 16 h at 37°C. The plates were washed twice and 5×10^3 viable TLC cells were added to 5×10^3 irradiated antigen-pulsed E⁻ cells. Cells from each group were assayed for their ability to proliferate in the absence of TCGF alone. Proliferation was determined by [³H]TdR incorporation as described in legend to Fig. 1. O, HA1.7 preincubated with specific antigen (HA peptide 20) and then tested for the response to peptide 20 in the presence of accessory cells. □, HA1.7 preincubated with specific antigen (HA peptide 20) and then tested for the response to TCGF in the absence of accessory cells. ●, HA1.7 preincubated with non–cross-reactive antigen (HA peptide 4; 300 μg/ml) and then tested for the response to peptide 20 in the presence of accessory cells. ■, HA1.7 preincubated with non–cross-reactive antigen (HA peptide 4; 300 μg/ml) and then tested for the response to TCGF in the absence of accessory cells.

Reprinted with permission from J. Exp. Med. (1983) 157: 1434.

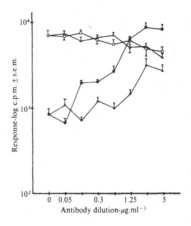

Fig. 3 Dose–response curve of the inhibition of tolerance induction by anti-HLA-DC and anti-HLA-DR antibodies. Cells of HA1.7 were pretreated with various concentrations of antibody (anti-HLA-DC, SG 465[27] ●, ○; anti-HLA-DR, DA2[23] ▲, △) and the antigen specific (●, ▲) and TCGF (○, △) responses assayed as described in the legend to Table 1.

Reprinted with permission from Nature (1984) 308: No. 5954, p72

These experiments (4) permitted certain conclusions concerning the mechanism of tolerance. The first is that tolerant T cells do exist, at least for a certain period of time (7 day in culture). The second is that suppressor T cells are not obligatory for high dose antigen regulation as a clone of helper T cells is tolerized, and this has permitted functional analysis of tolerance at several levels.

The role of the APC in diminishing the degree of tolerance is not understood. But one possibility was that MHC Class II antigen recognition on an antigen presenting cell was involved in immunity, but not in tolerance. This concept led to a series of experiments to determine whether tolerance, induced in vitro, was 'MHC restricted', i.e. whether MHC Class II antigens were recognised during tolerance induction. The simplest approach was to use monoclonal antibodies to MHC Class II, and to determine whether those antibodies blocking antigen induced stimulation also inhibited antigen induced tolerance. This was indeed the case, indicating that tolerance induced in vitro involved recognition of MHC, (see Fig. 3), and leaving unresolved the mechanism by which APC tend to inhibit tolerance. We are currently testing the effects of macrophage supernatants, IL-1 etc.

One possible mechanism for tolerance is receptor blockade. In B cell systems, Schrader and Nossal (10), and subsequently others demonstrated that antibody forming cells, even at the secreting stage could be inhibited, transiently and reversibly by high concentrations of polymeric antigens. The mechanism of tolerance induced by p20 is different: it is long lasting (> 7 days), and induced by very small antigen (a synthetic peptide), and thus this form of tolerance does not resemble effector cell blockade. It is of interest that in earlier studies (11) T cell tolerance induced, in whole spleen populations, in vitro was somewhat more efficient with polymeric rather than monomeric flagellin, and so it will be of interest to examine whether receptor cross linking is necessary for tolerance induction. Effects of p20 on the cell surface were investigated. It was found that the expression of the T3 complex (as detected by the monoclonal antibody UCHT1) was markedly reduced, in proportion to the antigen concentration used, but never as effectively as using an anti T3 antibody. Other cell surface changes were noted: some reduction of T1, none of T4 antigen or E rosette receptor, but enhancement of Tac antigen (IL-2 receptor). These results emphasise that active "signalling" occurs during tolerance induction, in the absence of APC but do not as yet discriminate between events occurring during activation and those occuring in tolerance.

Attempts were made to analyse biochemically the events occurring during tolerance and immunity. Total RNA and protein synthesis were unaffected, but total RNA synthesis was augmented both by low and high concentrations of antigen. Synthesis of certain proteins, of unknown function, of MW 24, 29, 44, 47, 60, 70 and 135 Kd was enhanced, while those of 42 and 92 Kd was diminished by high antigen exposure (12).

Lymphocyte function involves both cell proliferation, to increase the size of the antigen sensitive cell pool, and differentiation, which permits the cells to mediate their respective functions. It was thus of interest to determine whether inhibition of helper function was induced just as readily as inhibition of proliferation, by high concentrations of peptide antigen. Overnight preincubation experiments were performed, using a range of p20 concentrations, prior to washing the cells and restimulating them

TABLE 1

DIFFERENTIAL EFFECT OF ANTIGEN INCUBATION ON HELP AND
PROLIFERATION

Antigen Preincubation (µg/ml)	Help	Proliferation
–	+	+
0.1	+	+
0.3	±	+
1	–	+
3	–	+
10	–	–
30	–	–
100	–	–

Clone HA1.7 was incubated with various concentrations of synthetic antigen p20 for 16 hours at 37°C, prior to washing the cells and stimulation with 0.1 µg/ml p20 and E⁻ cells as a source of antigen presenting cells for 3 days (proliferation assay) or Influenza A/Texas and E⁻ cells for 6 days prior to assay of supernatant antibody.

with APC and an immunogenic concentration of p20. The results obtained, represented in Table 1 indicate that tolerance of helper function the differentiated function of these cells was induced much more readily than of cell proliferation. This observation implies that the tolerance phenomenon we have been analysing is probably of much wider significance than we had hitherto envisaged. As tolerance of proliferation occurred at 10-100 µg/ml of p20, corresponding to a molarity of $10^{-5-6}M$, very few antigens would be potential tolerogens (13), e.g. high concentration serum proteins, albumin, Ig, C3. But with a threshold 2 $\log_{10}$ lower, at $10^{-7-8}M$, many more antigens may be potential tolerogens in vivo, including tumour surface antigens, as the tumour grows.

Recently there have been reports that in certain conditions, T cells lacking the T3 antigen can be found in the blood. This has been noted in the elderly (14), and also in certain autoimmune diseases (L. Terry, R.N. Maini and M. Feldmann, unpublished data). These may conceivably be circulating tolerant T cells, inhibited by excess exposure to antigen.

CONCLUSION

Despite extensive analysis, we still do not know how lymphocytes decide whether to be activated by antigen, or inactivated. We are optimistic that further investigation especially using gene probes for T cell receptors, IL-2, IL-2 receptor will reveal the mechanism, which will be of importance in rationalization of immunization protocols and vaccine development.

REFERENCES

1. Nossal, G.J.V. Ann. Rev. Immunol. 1, 33-62 (1983).
2. Feldmann, M., Doniach, D., Bottazzo, G.F. In: "Immunology of Rheumatic Diseases" (Eds N. Talal and S. Gupta) Plenum Press Inc (in press).
3. Lamb, J.R., Eckels, D.D., Lake, P., Woody, J.N. and Green, N. Nature. 300, 66-69 (1982).
4. Lamb, J.R., Skidmore, B.J., Green, N., Chiller, J.M. and Feldmann, M. J. Exp. Med. 157, 1434-1447 (1983).
5. Zanders, E.D., Lamb, J.R., Feldmann, M., Green, N. and Beverley, P.C.L. Nature. 303, 625-627 (1983).
6. Chiller, J.M., Habicht, G.S., Weigle, W.O. Proc. Natl. Acad. Sci. USA. 65, 551-556 (1970).
7. Feldmann, M. J. Exp. Med. 135, 735-753 (1972).
8. Feldmann, M. and Kontiainen, S. Eur. J. Immunol. 6, 302-305.
9. Katz, D.H. and Benacerraf, B. (eds) Immunological Tolerance: Mechanism and Potential Therapeutic Applications. Academic Press, N.Y. (1974).
10. Schrader, J.W. and Nossal, G.J.V. J. Exp. Med. 139, 1582-1598 (1974).
11. Feldmann, M. and Nossal, G.J.V. Transplant. Rev. 13, 3-34 (1972).
12. Zanders, E.D., Feldmann, M., Green, N. and Lamb, J.R. Eur. J. Immunol. (in press).
13. Mitchison, N.A. In: "Cell Interactions and Receptor Antibodies in Immune Responses" (eds O. Makela, A. Cross, T.U. Kosuren. Academic Press, N.Y. pp 249-260 (1971).
14. Hallgren, H.M., Tackola, D.R. and O'Leary, J.J. J. Immunol. 131, 191-194 (1983).

ANTIGEN-T LYMPHOCYTE INTERACTIONS IN THE INDUCTION

OF FUNCTIONAL UNRESPONSIVENESS

J.R. Lamb, P.C.L. Beverley*, Marc Feldmann and E.D. Zanders

Imperial Cancer Research Fund, Tumour Immunology Unit, Department of Zoology, University College London, Gower Street, London WC1E 6BT.

* Imperial Cancer Research Fund, Human Tumour Immunology Group, University College London, Faculty of Clinical Sciences, University Street, London WC1E 6JJ

INTRODUCTION

In the initiation of an immune response helper/inducer T lymphocytes are activated by antigen presented in association with Class II major histocompatibility complex (MHC) gene products[1,2]. Even though there is now extensive information on the structure of both MHC Class II determinants[3,4] and the T cell receptor[5,6] their physical interaction with antigen in the induction of an activation signal is unclear. As a preliminary step in the analysis of receptor antigen interactions it is necessary to demonstrate specific binding of that ligand to the appropriate receptor. Recently employing T lymphocyte clones reactive with defined antigens the specific binding to T cells of antigen in the presence of antigen presenting cells[7] or in isolation[8,9] has been reported. We have isolated human T lymphocyte clones reactive with a 24 amino acid peptide (p20) located at the carboxyl terminus (306-329) of the HA-1 molecule of influenza virus haemagglutinin (HA)[10], that after incubation with a supraimmunogenic concentration of p20 in the absence of presenting cells fail to respond to an immunogenic challenge[11]. With these reagents we have begun to investigate antigen-T lymphocyte interactions in the induction of functional unresponsiveness.

MATERIALS AND METHODS

The isolation and characterisation of T lymphocyte clones reactive with peptides of the HA molecule of influenza virus have been described in detail elsewhere[10], as have the methods for the in vitro induction and assay of T cell unresponsiveness[11].

RESULTS AND DISCUSSION
Antigen dependency in the induction of unresponsiveness

Cloned helper T cells (HA1.7), in isolation from other lymphoid cells were cultured with increasing concentration of specific peptide (p20, 0.3-100 µg/ml), and the challenged with an immunogenic dose of p20 in the presence of presenting cells (irradiated histocompatible E⁻ cells). Preincubation with p20 at concentrations < 3 µg/ml rendered the T cells unresponsive to stimulation with antigen at an immunogenic dose (Table 1). This induction of unresponsiveness was not the result of cell death since the T cells were still able to proliferate in response to IL-2 (Table 1).

Table 1
Antigen dose dependency of T cell tolerance induction

Concentration[a] of p20 (µg/ml)	Response E⁻ + p20	IL-2
0	+	+
0.3	+	+
1.0	+	+
3.0	+	+
10	−	+
30	−	+
100	−	+

[a] T cells of clone HA1.7 (p20 specific) were pretreated with antigen and assayed for their ability to respond to an immunogenic challenge of p20 or IL-2[11].

Since HA1.7 is a cloned helper T cell it would appear that T cell unresponsiveness induced by supraoptimal concentrations of antigen can occur in the absence of suppressor T cells, suggesting a direct interaction between antigen and T cells.

The binding of activated and tolerized T cell clones to antigen pulsed accessory cell monolayers

It has recently been reported that murine T cell hybridomas can bind to antigen in association with MHC Class II molecules on accessory cells[7]. Therefore experiments were designed to determine whether or not radiolabelled helper T cells reactive with p20 (HA1.7) could bind to accessory cells pulsed with specific antigen. The results of these experiments are shown in Table 2. Cells of HA1.7 bound to E⁻ cells (source of B cells and macrophages) pulsed with p20, but not the unrelated peptide, p11 (residues 105-140). Furthermore, the binding of the tritiated T cells could be inhibited by the addition of an excess of p20 (100 µg/ml) or anti-MHC Class II antibody of the appropriate specificity (Table 2).

Table 2
Specific binding of cloned T cells to antigen pulsed accessory cells

Cloned[a] T cells	Tolerance induction	Accessory Cells	Inhibitory Peptide	Inhibitory Antibody	Counts Bound
TH p2-	-	-	-	-	-
+	-	p20	-	-	+
+	-	p11	-	-	-
+	-	p20	p20	-	-
+	-	p20	p11	-	+
+	-	p20	-	Anti-DR	+/-
+	-	p20	-	Anti-DQ	-
+	p20	p20	-	-	-
+	p11	p20	-	-	+

a   T cells of clone HA1.7 were labelled with ³H-TdR and assayed for their ability to bind to accessory cells pulsed with antigen[12].

If cloned T cells are pretreated with a supraimmunogenic dose of p20, they fail to bind to the p20 accessory cell monolayer. No inhibition was observed after pretreatment with p11 (Table 2). Thus human IL-2 dependent helper T cells are able to bind specific antigen in association with accessory cell Class II determinants. However, following pretreatment with a high concentration of p20 the T cells failed to bind to specific antigen in the presence of accessory cells which indirectly suggests that the antigen recognition structures have been lost from the surface of the T cells during the induction of unresponsiveness[13].

Binding of peptide to cloned T lymphocytes

Since the induction of unresponsiveness (Table 1)[11] implied that antigen was binding directly to the peptide specific T cells, binding experiments were performed using tritiated p20. The binding of ^{3}H-p20 to p20 reactive T cells (HA1.7) was temperature dependent, with the amount of peptide bound (21 fmol) at 37°C being three fold that observd at 4°C (Table 3).

The addition of unlabelled p20, but not p11, in excess was able to inhibit the binding of ^{3}H-p20 (Table 3) confirming the antigen specificity of the reaction. From these results it would appear that the helper T cells are able to bind specific antigen in the absence of accessory cells. However, since the T cells themselves express MHC

Table 3
Specific binding of ^{3}H-p20 to cloned T lymphocytes[a]

Cold peptide (10 µg/ml)	Temperature (°C)	Antigen bound (fmol)
0	4	6
p20	4	0
0	37	21
p20	37	0
p11	37	22

[a] T cells were incubated for 1 hr with 0.005 µg/ml of ^{3}H-p20. Data summarized from reference 12.

Class II determinants and the induction of T cell unresponsiveness in the absence of accessory cells can be inhibited by the appropriate anti-MHC Class II antibody[14], the binding of antigen to the T cell may involve T cell MHC Class II.

Functional analysis of normal and variant populations of T cell clone HA1.7

The results in the previous tables are suggestive that the T cells of clone HA1.7 are able to bind p20 in isolation or in association with accessory cell MHC Class II determinants. In addition, exposure of the T cells to a supraimmunogenic concentration of p20 resulted in a reduction in the surface expression of the T3/Ti complex[14,15] and a loss of function[11]. After prolonged in vitro culture it was observed that a variant(s) of HA1.7 had evolved, since a population of cells were not present that could neither be rendered functionally unresponsive nor showed a loss of T3 after exposure to a tolerizing dose of p20 (Table 4).

Following incubation with 20 µg/ml of p20 the variant population of T cells expressing T3 (TV; Table 4) were sorted under sterile conditions on the FACS. The TV

Table 4
Functional analysis of normal (TN) and variant (TV) populations of HA1.7

Cloned T cells	Tolerance induction	Response pll	p20	IL-2
TN	-	-	+	+
+	p20	-	-	+
+	pll	-	+	+
TV	-	-	+	+
+	p20	-	+	+
+	pll	-	+	+
TM	-	-	+	+
+	p20	-	+/-	+
+	pll	-	+	+

TM is mixed population of TN and TV

population was passaged over filler cells, antigen and IL-2 and then compared with normal HAl.7 (TN) for the ability to respond to or be inactivated by specific antigen. These results are summarized in Table 4. Both TN and TV were activated by immunogenic doses of p20, but not pll, in the presence of histocompatible accessory cells. In contrast p20 (at 20 μg/ml) induced unresponsiveness in only TN and not TV when challenged with p20 at an immunogenic dose. These findings imply that the variant population has lost its ability to bind antigen in isolation, the molecule(s) in the antigen recognition structures where the lesion has occurred is not clear. However, since TV can be activated by p20 in association with MHC Class II it seems likely that the mutation is not in the T cell receptor (Ti) but may involve the T cell MHC Class II determinants. A comparative analysis of the structure and function of mutant and normal populations of cloned T cells may be of value in determining requirements of T cell activation and tolerance induction.

CONCLUSIONS

The results reported here demonstrate that cloned human helper T cells reactive with a defined peptide antigen, can bind that antigen in isolation or in association with accessory cell MHC Class II determinants. The specificity of the antigen binding was confirmed by inhibition with the appropriate unlabelled peptide. These findings are in agreement with those on murine T cell clones[9] and hybridomas[7,8]. The pretreatment of cloned T cells with supraimmunogenic concentrations of peptide in isolation resulted in functional unresponsiveness[11] and a failure to bind to antigen pulsed accessory cells, substantiating our earlier findings that the Ti/T3 complex is downregulated during the induction of unresponsive-ness[13]. Since the induction of T cell unresponsiveness can be inhibited by the relevant anti-MHC Class II antibody[14], Class II determinants on the T cells themselves may be involved in antigen binding. From a long term culture of HAl.7 was have isolated a variant that although it could be activated by peptide in the presence of accessory cells, high concentrations of antigen failed to tolerize it in contrast to the parent cells. This suggests that the mutation is likely to have occurred in a molecule of the antigen recognition structures other than the specific receptor.

REFERENCES

1.   Klein, J. and Nagy, Z.A.   Adv. Cancer. Res. 37,
     233-317 (1982).
2.   Bodmer, W.F.   In: Mammalian Genetics and Cancer (ed.
     Russel, E.) 213-240 (Alan Liss, New York, 1981).
3.   Kaufman, J.F., Auffray, C., Korman, A.J., Shackelford,
     D.A. and Strominger, J.   Cell. 36, 1-13 (1984).
4.   Travers, P., Blundell, T.L., Sternberg, M.J.E. and
     Bodmer, W.F. Nature 310, 235-238 (1984).
5.   Hedrick, S.M., Nielsen, E.A., Kavaler, J., Cohen,
     D.I. and Davis, M.M. Nature. 308, 153-158 (1984).
6.   Saito, H. et al. Nature. 309, 757-762 (1984).
7.   Marrack, P., Skidmore, B. and Kappler, J.W.   J.
     Immunol. 130, 2088-2092 (1983).
8.   Carel, S., Bron, C. and Corradin, G.   Proc. Natl.
     Acad. Sci. USA. 80, 4832-4836 (1983).
9.   Rao, A., Ko, W.W-P., Faas, S.J. and Cantor, H.   Cell.
     36, 879-888 (1984).
10. Lamb, J.R., Eckels, D.D., Lake, P., Woody, J.N. and
     Green, N. Nature 300, 66-69 (1982).
11. Lamb, J.R., Skidmore, B.J., Green, N., Chiller, J.M.
     and Feldmann, M.   J. Exp. Med.   157,   1434-1447
     (1983).
12. Zanders, E.D., Feldmann, M., Green, N. and Lamb, J.R.
     Eur. J. Immunol. (in press).
13. Zanders, E.D., Lamb, J.R., Green, N., Feldmann, M. and
     Beverley, P.C.L. Nature 303, 625-627 (1983).
14. Lamb, J.R. and Feldmann, M. Nature 308, 72-74 (1984).
15. Meuer, S.C. et al. J. Exp. Med. 157, 705-719 (1983).

PATHWAYS AND MECHANISMS OF HUMAN T CELL ACTIVATION

Stefan C. Meuer

I.Med.Klinik u.Poliklinik d.Universität Mainz

Langenbeckstrasse 1, D-6500 Mainz, FRG

Introduction

The antigen receptor of T lymphocytes was recently identified
as a complex consisting of a 90 KD disulfide linked heterodimer, termed Ti which is functionally and structurally associated with three additional molecular components, termed
T3 (1). Whereas the former contains clonally unique epitopes
and displays peptide variability among T cell clones of distinct specificities, no variability could be detected within any of the known three subunits of T3 (2,3). Monoclonal
antibodies to T3 and Ti, respectively, in soluble form were
capable of blocking antigen specific clonal T cell responses
(4,5). Perhaps more importantly, when coupled to the surface
of a solid support these antibodies produced functional effects that were undistinguishable from those produced by
the natural ligand of this molecular complex, namely antigen itself (6,7).
Most recently, a T cell receptor independent "alternative"
pathway of activation was identified: monoclonal antibodies,
directed at the T3-Ti unrelated, yet T lineage restricted
50 KD T11 glycoprotein were demonstrated to induce T cell
activation in the absence of accessory cells and antigen
(8).
In the present report we employed monoclonal antibodies to
T3 in order to analyse precisely the mechanisms underlying
T cell activation in primary immune responses and compared
this mode of T cell triggering with activation via the T11
glycoprotein.

317

Results

The mitogenic activity of monoclonal antibodies directed at epitopes contained within the T3-Ti antigen receptor complex was previously shown to require their presentation in multimeric form to the T lymphocyte surface. This could be achieved by either immobilizing antibodies on a solid support, e.g. Sepharose-beads (6), or, alternatively, employing monocytes which most likely bind anti-T3/anti-Ti via membrane Fc-receptors. That monocyte Fc-receptor activity is indeed involved in producing T cell activation by antibodies reactive with the antigen receptor is demonstrated in Table 1.

Table 1

T cell triggering involves crosslinking of antigen receptors

	medium	anti-T3 (soluble)	anti-T3- Sepharose	anti-T11- Sepharose
A)	450*	4.265	8.974	383
B)	549	1.106	10.408	475

* cpm ^{3}HTdR uptake (SD $\leqslant$ 15%)

A) represents T cell proliferation to various monoclonal antibodies in medium containing 10% FCS.
B) represents T cell proliferation in medium containing 20% HS and pool of unrelated monoclonal antibodies (ascites, 1:100 final concentration).

Thus, blocking of Fc-receptors utilizing high serum concentrations (20% human serum) and a pool of unrelated monoclonal antibodies abolishes the mitogenic activity of soluble anti-T3. In contrast, this treatment did not alter PHA responses (not shown) and, perhaps more importantly, did not reduce the capacity of Sepharose-bound anti-T3 to induce T cell proliferation. In addition, this experiment excludes the possibility that the mitogenic effects of Sepharose-anti-T3 were due to antibody leaking from the bead surface. Thus, these data provide further support for the view that multimeric ligation and crosslinking of antigen receptors represent a critical signal in efficient antigen recognition by T cells. Note that a monoclonal anti-T11 antibody, even in surface linked form, did not induce T cell proliferation under these experimental circumstances. The next set of experiments was aimed at investigating the contributions of accessory cells in the activation of rest-

ing T lymphocytes, i.e. primary immune responses. The possibility to replace one of the potential accessory cell activities, namely, presentation of antigens in multimeric
form to the responding T lymphocyte by a monoclonal antibody
now affords the opportunity to dissect sterical from metabolic effects involved in this process. To this end, a preparation of purified resting T lymphocytes (T_R) was obtained by removing monocytes via adherence, E-rosetting and
complement lysis employing monoclonal antibodies directed
at human monocytes (anti-Mo1) and Ia antigens (anti-I2).
The latter antibody was utilized to allow a more vigorous
depletion of monocytes and, in addition, to eliminate Ia
positive "preactivated" T lymphocytes. This measure was necessary since previous studies had indicated that activated
T lymphocytes can be triggered to proliferate by mere crosslinking of antigen receptors and in the absence of accessory
cells (6). Table 2 (subsequent page) demonstrates that in
the course of the purification procedure monocytes are efficiently removed as judged by the loss of responsiveness
by peripheral blood lymphocytes (PBL) to PHA. Perhaps more
importantly, there was also a loss of proliferative responses to anti-T3-Sepharose which could be restored by addition of 5% autologous adherent cells. Note that anti-T11
covalently linked to Sepharose had no effect on either monocyte depleted or reconstituted T_R. Thus, in striking contrast to activated T lymphocytes (T_A) (Table 2) antigen receptor crosslinking (signal 1) is in itself not sufficient
to trigger proliferation of T_R. Additional signals, most
likely provided by accessory cells, appear to be required
(signal 2).
Given the well-established fact that monocyte-Ia-antigens
play a critical role in antigen presentation (10), it was
necessary to investigate whether class II gene products of
the major histocompatibility complex were involved in providing this second signal for T cell activation. To test
this possibility, allogeneic monocytes were utilized to replace autologous adherent cells in the experimental system.
As demonstrated in Table 3, the former functioned equally
well as the latter provided resting T cells had been triggered by anti-T3-Sepharose. Moreover, Table 4 indicates
that blocking concentrations of a monoclonal antibody (9-49)
directed at a monomorphic portion of human Ia antigens and
known to strongly inhibit class II dependent immune responses (11) had no blocking effect on accessory cell activity in promoting anti-T3 triggered T cell proliferation.
These findings indicate that whereas Ia-antigens may func-

tion in signal 1 of MØ-T cell interaction, i.e. antigen recognition, they are apparently unrelated to signal 2.

Table 2

Activation of <u>resting</u> T lymphocytes by monoclonal antibodies
via T3 requires an accessory cell dependent signal

responder population	stimulus			
	medium	T3-Sepharose	T11-Sepharose	PHA
PBL	483*	16.311	389	27.845
E^+	686	2.688	572	24.381
$E^+(Ab+C) = T_R$	892	686	486	1.054
$E^+(Ab+C) + MØ$	752	23.835	601	24.935
blasts $= T_A$	513	8.816	321	1.973

* cpm ^{3}HTdR; SD $\leq$ 15%

Table 3

Signal 2 is unrelated to autologous MHC-gene products

responder population		stimulus		
		medium	T3-Sepharose	T11-Sepharose
T_R		307	1.252	331
T_R+autologous MØ	5%	112*	12.648	511
	10%	997	13.843	766
	20%	1.112	12.229	1.216
T_R+allogeneic MØ	5%	1.447	7.871	1.188
	10%	2.058	11.783	1.706
	20%	2.260	14.128	2.196

* cpm ^{3}HTdR uptake; SD $\leq$ 15%

Table 4

Signal 2 does not involve Ia-antigens of accessory cells

responder population	stimulus		
	medium	T3-Sepharose	T11-Sepharose
T_R	100*	194	176
T_R + MØ 5%	718	5.993	824
T_R + MØ 5% (anti-Ia treated)	526	5.485	545

* cpm ^{3}HTdR uptake; SD $\leq$ 15%

A number of previous studies had suggested that Interleukin-1, a soluble monocyte product, may play a role in primary T cell activation (12,13). Therefore, a source of affinity purified human Interleukin-1 was utilized to investigate the question whether this lymphokine instead of adherent cells would be capable to serve as signal 2 in the response of resting T lymphocytes to Sepharose-anti-T3. As shown in Table 5 this is indeed the case. Thus, triggering of monocyte depleted T_R via their antigen receptor by anti-T3-Sepharose induces receptiveness to Interleukin-1 as indicated by a dose dependent proliferative in vitro response.

Table 5

Antigen receptor crosslinking leads to expression of IL-1 receptors

responder population	stimulus		
	medium	T3-Sepharose	T11-Sepharose
T_R	439*	491	539
T_R + IL-1 (2 U/ml)	378	5.661	353
T_R + IL-1 (0.4 U/ml)	182	3.224	180

* ^{3}HTdR; SD $\leq$ 15%

Since previous studies firmly established the concept that T cell proliferation is mediated through a hormonal system based on the activity of Interleukin-2 and the presence of Interleukin-2 receptors (14,15) it was necessary to in-

vestigate the effects of the above defined signals 1 and 2
on the activation of the IL-2 hormonal system. We reasoned
that if antigen receptor crosslinking (signal 1) which in
itself did not lead to T cell proliferation (Table 2) was
at all related to this system, then signal 1 could only induce its partial activation, i.e. IL-2 receptor expression
without IL-2 secretion or vice versa. If the former were
the case then incubation of T_R with Sepharose-anti-T3
should establish responsiveness to a source of recombinant
Interleukin-2 indicative of IL-2-receptor induction. As
shown in Table 6, T_R do not respond to Interleukin-2. However, following incubation with immobilized anti-T cell receptor antibody a dose dependent proliferative response to
IL-2 was observed. Although not shown, no IL-2 activity was
present in supernatants collected from anti-T3-Sepharose
treated T_R at various points of time (up to 72h following
initiation of culture). Moreover, the presence of IL-2 receptors could be detected by means of indirect immune fluorescence employing a monoclonal antibody known to react
with this structure (not shown).
Thus, we conclude that signal 1 serves to induce expression
of receptors for Interleukin-1 and Interleukin-2 whereas
signal 2 is required to trigger IL-2 production and secretion.

Table 6

Antigen receptor crosslinking leads to expression of IL-2
receptors

responder population	stimulus			
	medium	T3-Sepharose	T11-Sepharose	$\alpha T11_2 + \alpha T11_3$
T_R	430*	539	491	18.647
T_R + IL-2 (20 ng/ml)	457	12.803	600	n.t.
T_R + IL-2 (4 ng/ml)	553	6.982	565	n.t.

* ^{3}HTdR; SD $\leq$ 15%

Table 6 also demonstrates the proliferative T cell response
to a combination of monoclonal antibodies that react with
two out of three individual epitopes known to exist on the

T cell receptor unrelated 50 KD T11 glycoprotein (8). In
contrast to the antigen receptor mediated pathway of T cell
activation, triggering via T11 occurs independent of accessory cells. However, as reported previously, both modes of
T cell activation are dependent on the IL-2/IL-2 receptor
system. Thus, in vitro proliferation to either stimulus is
strongly inhibitable by monoclonal antibodies to the IL-2
receptor and to the lymphokine IL-2 itself (not shown).

Discussion

The antigen receptor of T lymphocytes has recently been identified as complex consisting of a 90 KD disulfide linked heterodimer, termed Ti, which is structurally and functionally
associated with three additional components, termed T3 (1).
Whereas the former contains clonally unique epitopes and
displays peptide variability among individual clonal T lymphocyte populations, no variability could be detected within the known three subunits of T3 (2,3). Thus, Ti most likely represents the antigen-binding portion of the antigen
receptor complex, although this remains to be formally demonstrated. In contrast, as yet very little is known about
the function of T3. Moreover, the precise association of
the T3 subcomponents with each other and with the Ti heterodimer as well as their expression during T cell ontogeny
remains elusive. Nevertheless, the functional activities of
monoclonal antibodies directed at clonotypic Ti determinants
and anti-T3 reagents were found to be identical. Whereas
anti-Ti or anti-T3, respectively, in soluble form inhibited
antigen specific clonal activities (4,5), they were capable
of activating responder populations in a fashion analogous
to the natural ligand of the Ti-T3 molecular complex, namely antigen itself, provided they were linked to the surface
of a solid support (e.g. Sepharose beads) (6,7).
From these studies it seems justified to assume that employing anti-T3 monoclonal antibodies indeed produces an antigen-
like effect on T cells, i.e. mimics antigen-recognition similar to the interaction of antigen-presenting cells and T
cells. At the level of activated T lymphocytes such as T cell
clones it was shown that this multimeric surface attachment
of antigen receptors appeared to be sufficient for re-stimu-
lation, hence leading to IL-2 receptor expression, IL-2 secretion and induction of the cells' immunoregulatory activities (7,15).
In contrast, the present experiments demonstrate that primary T cell activation requires an additional sign provid-

ed by accessory cells. Thus, the process of MØ-T cell interaction appears to occur as a series of precisely orchestrat-
ed events in which antigen-receptor crosslinking leads to
receptiveness for a second signal, i.e. Interleukin-1, the
latter serving to enable IL-2 production. However, antigen
recognition alone partially activates the IL-2 hormonal
system since IL-2 receptor expression occurs in the absence
of additional monocyte activities, i.e. IL-2. Supernatants
obtained from resting monocytes did not contain detectable
IL-1 activity. Therefore, the present data can only be explained by the existence of an additional signal which,
following multimeric antigen receptor ligation, is directed
from the responding T cell towards the accessory cell in
order to enable IL-1 production. The nature of this activity
is currently under investigation. Whereas Ia antigens may
be critical to enable efficient antigen recognition by T
lymphocytes (signal 1) they are not involved in providing
the second signal. Thus, allogeneic monocytes or anti-Ia
treated autologous monocytes were equally effective to support T cell activation once the T cell receptor was suf-
ficiently triggered (Tables 3 and 4).

The function of Interleukin-1 in the process of primary T
cell activation appears to mediate a differentiation step
that engages the mechanism of IL-2 production and/or secretion. However, once a T cell has received this signal it becomes more independent of Interleukin-1 in that antigen -
receptor triggering alone is now sufficient for restimulation. The finding that activated T lymphocytes did not respond to Interleukin-1 (not shown) provides further support
for this notion.

In line with recent data, a combination of two monoclonal
antibodies (anti-T11$_2$ + anti-T11$_3$) directed at distinct
epitopes of the T lineage restricted T11 glycoprotein was
found to produce a strong stimulus which apparently bypasses
the accessory cell/IL-1 requirement in inducing T cell proliferation (8). Since T11 is clearly unrelated to the T3-Ti
antigen receptor complex, this mode of T cell triggering
has to be considered as a previously unknown "alternative
pathway" of T cell activation.

As yet, a natural ligand which could engage this alternative
pathway remains to be identified. Nevertheless, both pathways eventually induce T cell proliferation via the IL-2/
IL-2-receptor system. In addition, it was recently demonstrated that activation of human T lymphocytes via T3-Ti
prevents further activation through T11 triggering (8).
This finding may indicate that intracellular control mechan-

isms exist which induce a temporary state of unresponsiveness following activation and thus secure well regulated T
cell activity in the immune response.
Taken together, the possibility to replace natural signals
involved in T cell activation by monoclonal antibodies now
affords the opportunity to analyse in detail the mechanisms
and signals necessary for generation of functional immunoregulatory and effector T cells such as helper, suppressor
and cytotoxic lymphocytes. In addition, the present experimental system should allow to more precisely analyse failures
underlying certain stages of primary and acquired immunodeficiency.

Acknowledgement

The author wants to thank Ms. M. Hauer and Ms. G. Rasch for
their excellent technical assistance and Prof. Meyer zum
Büschenfelde for support and encouragement in this project.
(Supported by grant DFG Me 693/3-1).

References

1. Meuer, S.C. et al. Nature 303, 808-810 (1983).
2. Acuto, O. et al. J.Exp.Med. 158, 1368-1373 (1983).
3. Borst, J. et al. J.Biol.Chem. 8, 5135-5141 (1983).
4. Reinherz, E.L. et al. Cell 30, 735-743 (1982).
5. Meuer, S.C. et al. J.Exp.Med. 157, 705-719 (1983).
6. Meuer, S.C. et al. J.Exp.Med. 158, 988-993 (1983).
7. Meuer, S.C. et al. Science 222, 1239-1242 (1983).
8. Meuer, S.C. et al. Cell 36, 897-906 (1984).
9. Kaneoka, H. J.Immunol. 131, 158-164 (1983).
10. Bergholtz, B.O. & Thorsby, E. Scand.J.Immunol. 8, 63-67
    (1978).
11. Todd III, R.F. Human Immunol. 10, 23-40 (1984).
12. Lachman, L.B. Federation Proc. 42, 2639-2645 (1983).
13. Conlon, P.J., Henney, C.S. & Gillis, S. J.Immunol. 128,
    797-801 (1982).
14. Cantrell, D.A. & Smith, K.A. J.Exp.Med. 158, 1895-1911
    (1983).
15. Meuer, S.C. et al. Proc.Natl.Acad.Sci. 81, 1509-1513
    (1984).

LOSS OF ALLOREACTIVITY ASSOCIATED WITH ACQUIRED SUPPRESSIVE AND NATURAL KILLER-LIKE ACTIVITIES OF AGED T CELL CLONES.

G. Pawelec and P. Wernet,

Immunology Laboratory,
Medizinische Klinik,
D-7400 Tübingen, FRG.

INTRODUCTION

The production of human T cell clones is now an established procedure in a number of laboratories. The relative ease with which antigen-specific or alloreactive lymphoblasts can be cloned and propagated in interleukin 2 (IL 2) makes this technique attractive for analysing the molecular and genetic bases of lymphocyte activation, regulation and effector functions of isolated populations. A widespread expectation amongst investigators in this area was that such cloned lines could be established as functionally stable, immortal sources of homogeneous reagents. However, few reports in the literature system- atically address the question of the long-term functional stability, longevity, or percentage of immortal clones obtained in each particular experiment, and whether the generation of "permanent" lines is the exception rather than the rule. In several cases, the continuous culture of cloned human T cells with various reactivities for periods of many months or even years has been reported (1-11). Nonetheless, this is not necessarily a universal finding, particularly for T cell clones which respond proliferative- ly against alloantigens and which are thus of value as primed lymphocyte typing (PLT) reagents (12-19). In this chapter we review results obtained with, and present new data on, a panel of more than 50 PLT clones which suggest that lymphocytes classifiable as "helper" T cells on the basis of their antigen-specific proliferative responses,

IL 2-secretory capacity, T4+ T8- Leu8- surface phenotypes,
and lack of suppressive activity on lymphoproliferative
(LP) responses (20-22), undergo a switch of function after
a culture period corresponding to the time required for 30
population doublings (PD). At this time they lose alloreactivity (22,23) and acquire strong non-specific MHC
unrestricted constitutive suppressive activity on LP
responses (22,24). In addition they may acquire a
previously absent lytic activity predominantly for target
cells susceptible to destruction by natural killer (NK)
effectors.

CONSISTENCY OF THE "SWITCH" FROM HELPER TO SUPPRESSOR
STATUS IN ALLOREACTIVE PLT CLONES.

     To date, 53 PLT clones have been followed up with
regard to their loss of alloproliferative capacity and
acquisition of suppressive activity. The clones were
derived from limiting dilution (LD) cloning of lymphocytes
from nine different donors activated in mixed lymphocyte
cultures (MLC), cloned in the presence of autologous,
stimulator-specific, or third-party filler cells, and
expanded in unpurified PHA-conditioned medium, partially
purified IL 2 or recombinant IL 2. The cloned cells were
propagated by weekly readdition of filler cells and twice
weekly readdition of IL 2, by readdition of both filler
cells and IL 2 every 3 - 5 days, or by readdition of filler
cells every 3 days and IL 2 weekly. All the various
permutations of the above which have been tested thus far
have failed to influence the loss of alloproliferative
capacity, as measured either by thymidine incorporation or
by secretion of IL 2, observed in these clones after
approximately 30 PD. At this time, the cloned cells
continued to divide without noticeable impact on their
growth curves and with retention of their dependency on
IL 2 and filler cells. Their predominantly T4+ T8- Leu8-
phenotypes remained unchanged, and quantitative FACS
analysis demonstrated an identical, or even increased,
amount of T3 molecules at the cell surface. 14 out of 15
clones examined still possessed apparently normal
karyotypes. There was no obvious de novo contamination by
mycoplasma occurring only at this time (varying between 30
and 85 days to achieve 30 PD) as assessed by staining with
Hoechst 33258, 4 week agar colony formation, depressed
viability or growth rates of the clones, or ability of

their unfiltered culture supernatants to incorporate
tritiated thymidine (3H-TdR), or infect other cell lines.
The cloned cells themselves could still incorporate 3H-TdR,
and apparent loss of alloreactivity was not caused by
altered kinetics of the response or the requirement for
different concentrations of stimulating antigen. "Starving"
the clones for short periods in the absence of IL 2, or for
longer periods with concentrations of IL 2 suboptimal for
the growth of the cells, failed to reconstitute alloreactivity. The addition of other lymphokines (IL 1, IL 3,
or gamma interferon) to the growth and/or test medium also
had no effect. Thus, to all intents and purposes, the
cloned cells were "arrested" in a tolerised state, that is,
one refractory to antigen-specific stimulation. Such clones
were designated "ex-PLT" clones.

ACQUISITION OF SUPPRESSIVE ACTIVITY BY EX-PLT CLONES.

Prior to their attaining 30 PD, the majority of
irradiated PLT clones specific for stimulatory determinants
associated with HLA-DR, Dw, DQ, or DP specificities failed
to suppress primary or secondary MLC when added at the
initiation of culture. However, the same clones in their
ex-PLT phase strongly suppressed LP responses in MLC.
Suppression was constitutive in that the test MLC were
inhibited equally well whether or not the stimulating cells
carried alloantigens to which the ex-PLT clones had been
able to respond, and was not MHC restricted since
HLA-mismatched responding cells were as well suppressed as
autologous or HLA-matched donors. Suppression was not
caused by absorption of IL 2, or by altering the kinetics
of the test MLC.

The acquisition of suppressive activity by ex-PLT
clones was paralleled by their ability to stimulate LP
responses in, and to induce suppressor effectors in, normal
peripheral blood mononuclear cells (PBMC), both being
properties which PLT-active clones lacked. An example of
these activities for a representative ex-PLT clone is shown
in Fig. 1, in which the suppressive capacity of the cloned
cells titrated directly into MLC is compared with the
suppressive activity of PBMC co-cultured for 3 days with
the same ex-PLT clone.

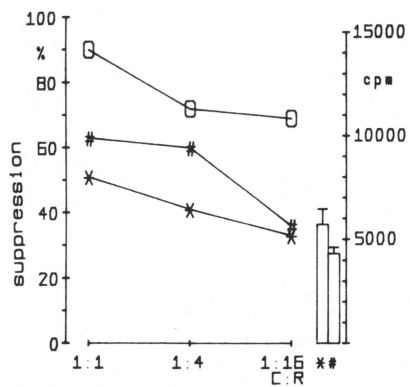

Fig. 1. Suppressor-inducing, and direct suppressive
activities of ex-PLT clone 124-6 with two different donors
✕ and #. Percent suppression of test MLC caused by
irradiated cloned cells (○——○), and caused by PBMC
previously incubated with cloned cells (✕——✕ and
#——#). C:R = ratio of added cells to responding cells
in test MLC. LP responses stimulated by the ex-PLT clones
in these two donors are shown in the histograms on the
right (cpm + SEM).

      The degree of inhibition caused by the latter is lower
than by the cloned cells themselves, but still very marked.
Suppression was not caused by carry over of the cloned
cells themselves into the test cultures, since irradiated
clones cultured alone for 3 days failed to inhibit on
transfer to test MLC. On the right hand side of the Fig.,
the LP responses of the two donors stimulated by the ex-PLT
clone are also shown. The same clone tested in the PLT-

Table 1.   Reduction of suppressor-inducing activity of
            ex-PLT clones by moAb to class II molecules.

	Ratio of transferred:responding cells		
Cells transferred	1:1	1:4	1:16
Normal PBMC	4	3	6
PBMC + TÜ34	2	0	5
PBMC + TÜ39	7	8	3
PBMC + clone	67	61	42
PBMC + clone + TÜ34	59	52	37
PBMC + clone + TÜ39	13	10	9

After 3 days culture in the combinations shown, cells were
thoroughly washed, 20 Gy irradiated, and transferred into
test MLC. The clone used to stimulate normal PBMC in this
experiment was ex-PLT clone 124-6 (see Fig. 1). MoAb TÜ34
binds HLA-DR molecules only, whereas TÜ39 binds both DR and
DP molecules. Results are given as percent suppression of
the test MLC in the absence of added cells.

active phase failed to induce suppressor effector cells or
to stimulate LP responses (data not shown). LP responses
stimulated by ex-PLT clones, as measured by 3H-TdR
incorporation, peaked much earlier (72 h) than those
stimulated by allogeneic PBMC (144 h). Stimulation was
observed whether or not the responding cells were
autologous with the clone, or HLA-D mismatched allogeneic,
but was inhibited by certain monoclonal antibodies (moAb)
specific for class II MHC molecules in a manner reminiscent
of DP-directed stimulation inhibition (25). Such stimulated
PBMC, when irradiated and titrated into a second MLC, were
themselves capable of strong non-specific suppression of LP
responses (as exemplified in Fig. 1), suggesting that the
lymphocytes stimulated to proliferate by ex-PLT clones were
suppressive cells. Consistent with this idea was the
finding that the inclusion in the suppressor-induction
cultures of moAb which inhibited the early LP responses
stimulated by ex-PLT clones resulted in a marked reduction
of the suppressive activity of such cells on transfer to a
second MLC (Table 1).

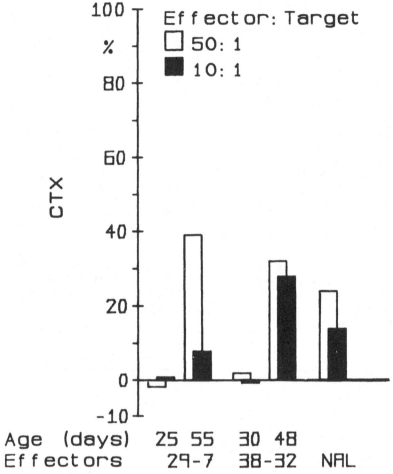

Fig. 2. Ex-PLT clones may acquire NK-like CTX. Clones 29-7
and 38-32 were tested on NK-susceptible HSB2 target cells
during their PLT phase (25 and 30 days old respectively)
and their ex-PLT phase (55 and 48 days old).

ACQUISITION OF NK-LIKE ACTIVITY BY EX-PLT CLONES.

The stimulation of early LP responses and the induction of suppressor cells by ex-PLT clones is phenomeno-
logically identical to the activities of MLC-derived T cell
clones with NK-like cytotoxicity (CTX), which concomitantly
exert suppressive effects (21,26). Because of these
remarkable similarities, ex-PLT clones were retested for

Table 2.
Cold target competition suggests different target
determinants on NK-susceptible and normal target cells

	Ratio of labelled : unlabelled targets				
Effector	1:100	1:10	1:1	1:0	Competing cells
38-32, 41 PD	3.3	18.5	29.7	42.6	K562
(50:1)	39.7	43.3	41.8		B-LCL
29-7, 37 PD	-1.2	3.6	39.5	68.2	K562
(37:1)	63.4	61.8	65.7		B-LCL
29-15, 35 PD	2.6	7.3	28.3	25.4	K562
(25:1)	27.3	29.4	26.1		B-LCL
38-27, 51 PD	0.4	17.6	55.1	59.8	K562
(50:1)	47.5	58.6	54.2		B-LCL
38-27*	42.6	47.5	54.5		K562
(50:1)	12.1	40.4	48.7	49.6	B-LCL

Unlabelled K562 or B-LCL cells were added in different
numbers to 2×10^3 51 Cr-labelled K562 target cells (or, in
the case of 38-27* only, B-LCL target cells). The effector
cells were ex-PLT clones 38-32 and 29-7, NK-like clone
29-15, or dually allospecific and NK-active clone 38-27.
Age is given in PD, and in parentheses the effector:target
ratio used in the CTX assay. Results given as percent
specific 51 Cr-release.

their NK-like CTX. Fig. 2 shows an example of the acquired
NK-like CTX of ex-PLT clones on HSB2 target cells. The
level of killing of these NK-susceptible target cells was
as high as that mediated by freshly isolated effectors
(non-adherent lymphocytes, NAL). To summarise, of 24 ex-PLT
clones tested, 18 were found to have acquired a previously
absent ability to lyse the classical NK-susceptible target
cell K562, and two acquired a lytic activity on the
original allogeneic priming cells. These CTX activities
generally appeared at 35 - 40 PD and remained for the
finite lifespans of the clones (maximally about 85 PD). The

specificity of the NK-like CTX mediated by ex-PLT clones
was investigated in cold target cross-competition experiments using K562 cells and B-lymphoid cell lines from the
donor of the original MLC stimulating cells. Table 2 shows
that whereas unlabelled K562 competed very well for lysis
of 51 Cr-labelled K562 target cells by ex-PLT clones, as
well as by NK-like effectors, B cell lines carrying
specific alloantigen were unable to inhibit lysis of
labelled K562 targets. In the case of a class I-directed
CTX clone which simultaneously lysed K562 cells, again the
two target cells did not cross-compete, suggesting that
different determinants were being recognised on NK-
susceptible and normal target cells.

Another remarkable similarity between the CTX
activities of NK-like clones, ex-PLT clones, and freshly
isolated NAL was observed in experiments where CTX was
blocked by moAb 13.1. This moAb, which binds an epitope of
T200 molecules, was suggested to be directed against a
structure intimately associated with the NK "receptor"
(27). It specifically inhibits lysis, at the effector cell
level, of erythro/myeloid leukaemic, but not T leukaemic,
target cells by fresh NAL (28) and by NK-like T cell clones
(29). Exactly this specific pattern of lytic blockade was
mediated by 13.1 also on NK-active ex-PLT clones (illustrated in Table 3). Thus, lysis of K562 was strongly
inhibited, but lysis of HSB2 or B-LCL target cells was
practically unaffected in the presence of saturating
concentrations (10 µg/ml) of 13.1. This suggests that
ex-PLT clones employ the same receptor structures as fresh
NK cells to recognise NK-susceptible target cells, and
further implies that such receptors are different from the
T3-linked 49/43 kD heterodimeric T cell receptor complex.

CONCLUSION

The switch of function from putative help to strong
suppression occurring in aged human PLT clones has emerged
as a very reproducible phenomenon in the 53 lines thus far
examined in this laboratory, regardless of the culture
duration required for 30 PD (which ranged from 30 - 85
days). Several considerations argue against a trivial
explanation, such as mycoplasma contamination being
responsible for these results. The fact that the switch of
function takes place at almost exactly 30 PD in clones

Table 3   NK-like CTX against K562 target cells by ex-PLT
           clones specifically blocked by moAb 13.1

| | | Target cells | | | | | |
| | | minus 13.1 | | | plus 13.1 | | |
Effector	E:T	K562	HSB2	B-LCL	K562	HSB2	B-LCL
NAL	50:1	82.5	23.9	6.2	11.5	26.1	14.2
(fresh)	10:1	36.3	14.2	-1.6	-3.6	13.8	15.4
12-2	50:1	18.5	nt	nt	0.5	nt	nt
(65 PD)	10:1	7.3	nt	nt	0.8	nt	nt
29-15	50:1	39.4	37.5	0.4	6.8	29.5	-1.1
(43 PD)	10:1	15.1	4.2	0.9	-1.9	21.7	0.5
29-7	50:1	28.6	38.9	3.9	3.9	36.3	7.9
(51 PD)	10:1	21.9	8.4	9.1	5.9	7.0	5.2
38-27	50:1	93.1	40.3	75.0	13.0	44.2	65.0
(52 PD)	10:1	84.8	14.1	57.7	12.7	28.7	27.6
38-32	50:1	89.1	32.1	17.7	1.2	15.5	22.0
(49 PD)	10:1	39.7	27.8	8.4	1.1	7.0	3.0

Results are presented as percent specific 51 Cr-release
from target cells in the presence or absence of 10 μg/ml of
moAb 13.1. E:T = effector : target ratio. Age of clones
given in PD. Functions of clones as follows: 12-2, 29-7,
and 38-32 = ex-PLT, 29-15 = NK-like, and 38-27 = allo-
specific and NK-like. nt = not tested.

derived from a number of different donors, propagated using
various permutations of different media, filler cells,
stimulating antigen, or sources and concentrations of IL 2
& serum supplements already argues against a de novo
mycoplasma contamination, and requires that an initial
contamination needs such a long "incubation" period before
manifesting this sort of effect. In addition, clones
showing signs of mycoplasma prior to 30 PD still exhibit
the functional switch to suppression and suppressor-
induction at this time point, and not before. Conversely,

clones apparently free of any mycoplasma are not spared
this occurrence. The reproducibility of the phenomenon
argues more for a preprogrammed switch of regulatory
activity within the clone than for contamination or
selection of mutants in the lines. The reason that such a
switch is not universally observed amongst PLT clones in
some other laboratories is not clear. Whereas several
investigators have noted in passing a loss of alloproliferative capacity in such clones (12-16), this was
apparently not investigated further, and has not always
been reported (1,2,8). It may be less common in CTX
effector clones (3-7), or amongst antigen-specific clones
which could have been exposed in vivo to the relevant
antigens (6,10,11). It seems unlikely that small variations
in culture technique could account for these differences.
It may be the case that a small fraction of antigen-
reactive cells, previously primed in vivo, could be just
those which retain stable function during culture more
readily than after an entirely in vitro sensitisation.
Alternatively, a proportion of the clones which retain
functional integrity for extended periods may represent
"transformed" or abnormal cells, despite their continued
dependence on IL 2 for their growth. Little information
exists concerning the karyotypic state of these cells to
provide any indication of normality or abnormality (30,31).

The attainment of as many as 30 PD for a single
lymphocyte clone would probably be a rare occurrence in
vivo, and it may therefore not be surprising if at least
the majority of clones are unable to perpetuate specific
functional capacity beyond this point. Whether the
acquisition of suppressive activity and NK-like CTX could
be regarded as having potential biological advantage in
vivo, should this phenomenon occur at all in intact
organisms, is a moot point. One might speculate that T
lymphocytes in fact differentiate through a "window" of
immunological specificity, and would be able to mediate
quite different functions after, and perhaps also before,
this period. Thus, one possible source of NK cells in the
periphery could be such aged T cells. Indeed, these clones
do have many important characteristics of large granular
lymphocytes (LGL), thought to be the main components of the
NK system in vivo, although they continue to express rather
more T cell markers than most freshly isolated LGL (32).
Nonetheless, at least a large proportion of LGL might be
considered to be "poised" T cells, since after a very brief

period of culture with IL 2, to which they apparently react directly without further stimulation, they lose non-T markers, and gain a characteristic T cell phenotype (33).

The change of function from help to suppression may be viewed as a further example of unexpected flexibility within the immune network, in which the function of each interacting T cell clone is not necessarily immutably fixed (34). Several recent reports are beginning to hint at the inappropriateness and perhaps artificiality of consigning T cells to particular separate functional subsets, be they helper, suppressor, suppressor-inducer, cytotoxic or whatever. Thus, co-existence of helper and CTX activities (2,14,16,35-39), suppressor, suppressor-inducer and CTX activities, helper and suppressor activities (40-42), as well as the induction by experimental manipulation (43-45), or extended culture (46-50) of permanent or temporary changes of functional status in T cell clones are now becoming increasingly frequent. In the face of these results, it may be necessary to modify compartmentalised models of immune systems to take into account a functional flexibility not necessarily to be dismissed as merely inexplicable in vitro artefact.

REFERENCES

1. Eckels, D.D. & Hartzman, R.J. Immunogenetics 16, 117-133, (1982).
2. Friedman, S., Thompson, G.S. & Principato, M.A. J. Immun. 129, 2451-2457 (1982).
3. Malissen, B., Kristensen, T., Goridis, C., Madsen, M. & Mawas, C. Scand. J. Immun. 14, 213-224 (1981).
4. Meuer, S.C., Schlossman, S.F. & Reinherz, E.L. Proc. natn. Acad. Sci. U.S.A. 79, 4590-4595 (1982).
5. Kornbluth, J., Flomenberg, N. & Dupont, B. J. Immun. 129, 2831-2837 (1982).
6. DeVries, J. & Spits, H. J. Immun. 132, 510-519 (1984).
7. Hercend, T., Meuer, S., Reinherz, E.L., Schlossman, S.F. & Ritz, J. J. Immun. 129, 1299-1305 (1982).
8. Ramarli, D., Parodi, B., Fabbi, M., Corte, G. & Lanzavecchia, A. J. exp. Med. 159, 318-323 (1984).
9. Santoli, D., DeFreitas, E.L., Sandberg-Wolheim, M., Francis, M.K. & Koprowski, H. J. Immun. 132, 2386-2392 (1984).

10. Schmitt, C., Ballet, J.-J., Agrapart, M. & Bizzini, B.
    Eur. J. Immun. 12, 849-854 (1982).
11. Lamb, J.R., Eckels, D.D., Lake, P., Johnson, A.H.,
    Hartzman, R.J. & Woody, J.N. J. Immun. 128, 233-238
    (1982).
12. Malissen, B., Charmot, D. & Mawas, C. Hum. Immun. 2,
    1-13 (1981).
13. Duquesnoy, R.J. & Zeevi, A. Hum. Immun. 8, 17-23
    (1983).
14. Flomenberg, N., Russo, C., Ferrone, S. & Dupont, B.
    Immunogenetics 19, 39-54 (1984).
15. Fradelizi, D., Chouaib, S. & Wollman, E.
    Transplantation Clin. Immun. 13, 69-78 (1981).
16. Reinsmoen, N.L., Anichini, A. & Bach, F.H. Hum. Immun.
    8, 195-205 (1983).
17. Allavena, P. & Ortaldo, J.R. J. Immun. 132, 2363-2369
    (1984).
18. Sheehy, M.J., Quintieri, F.B., Leung, D.Y.M., Geha,
    R.S., Dubey, D.P., Limmer, C.E. & Yunis, E.J.
    J. Immun. 130, 524-526 (1983).
19. Sterkers, G., Hannoun, C. & Levy, J.-P. Immunogenetics
    17, 271-281 (1983).
20. Pawelec, G. & Wernet, P. Immunogenetics 11, 507-519
    (1980).
21. Pawelec, G., Kahle, P. & Wernet, P. Eur. J. Immun. 12,
    607-615 (1982).
22. Pawelec, G. in T Cell Clones (eds. von Boehmer, H.
    & Haas, W.) Elsevier, Amsterdam, in the press.
23. Pawelec, G., Schneider, E.M., Rehbein, A., Schaa, I.
    & Wernet, P. Scand. J. Immun. 17, 147-153 (1983).
24. Pawelec, G., Wernet, P., Rehbein, A., Balko, I. &
    Schneider, E.M. Hum. Immun. 10, 135-142 (1984).
25. Pawelec, G., Shaw, S., Ziegler, A., Müller, C. &
    Wernet, P. J. Immun. 129, 1070-1075 (1982).
26. Pawelec, G., Schneider, E.M. & Wernet, P. Eur.
    J. Immun. 14, 335-340 (1984).
27. Newman, W., Targan, S.R. & Fast, L.D. Molec.
    Immun., in the press.
28. Newman, W. Proc. natn. Acad. Sci. U.S.A. 79,
    3858-3862 (1982).
29. Pawelec, G., Newman, W., Schwulera, U. & Wernet, P.
    Cell. Immun., in the press.

30. Johnson, J.P., Cianfriglia, M., Glasebrook, A.L. & Nabholz, M. in Isolation, Characterisation and Utilisation of T Lymphocyte Clones (eds. Fathman, C.G. & Fitch, F.W.) 183-191 (Academic Press, New York, 1982).
31. Zagury, D., Morgan, D., Lenoir, G., Fouchard, M. & Feldman, M. Int. J. Cancer 31, 427-432 (1983).
32. Schneider, E.M., Pawelec, G., Shi, L. & Wernet, P. J. Immun. 133, 173-179 (1984).
33. Timonen, T., Ortaldo, J.R., Stadler, B.M., Bonnard, G.D., Sharrow, S.O. & Herberman, R.B. Cell. Immun. 72, 178-185 (1982).
34. Pawelec, G., Schneider, E.M. & Wernet, P. Immun. Today 4, 275-278 (1983).
35. Von Boehmer, H. & Turton, K. Eur. J. Immun. 13, 176-179 (1983).
36. Widmer, M.B. & Bach, F.H. Nature 294, 750-752 (1981).
37. Wee, S.-L., Chen, L.-K., Strassman, G. & Bach, F.H. J. exp. Med. 156, 1854-1859 (1982).
38. Dennert, G., Weiss, S. & Warner, N.L. Proc. natn. Acad. Sci. U.S.A. 78, 4540-4543 (1981).
39. Fischer-Lindahl, K., Nordin, A.A. & Schreier, M. Curr. Topics Microbiol. Immun. 100, 1-10 (1982).
40. Kurnick, J.T., Hayward, A.R. & Altevogt, P. J. Immun. 126, 1307-1311 (1981).
41. Clayberger, C., DeKruyff, R.H. & Cantor, H. J. Immun. 132, 2237-2243 (1984).
42. Zeevi, A., Chiu, K.M. & Duquesnoy, R.J. Hum. Immun. 5, 107-122 (1982).
43. Lamb, J.R., Skidmore, B.J., Green, N., Chiller, J.M. & Feldmann, M. J. exp. Med. 157, 1434-1447 (1983).
44. Spits, H., Yssel, H., Leeuwenberg, S. & DeVries, J.E. Eur. J. Immun., in the press.
45. Freeman, G.J., Clayberger, C., DeKruyff, R.H., Rosenblum, D.S. & Cantor, H. Proc. natn. Acad. Sci. U.S.A. 80, 4094-4098 (1983).
46. Brooks, C.G. Nature 305, 155-158 (1983).
47. Acha-Orbea, H., Groscurth, P., Lang, R., Stitz, L. & Hengartner, H. J. Immun. 130, 2952-2959 (1983).
48. Simon, M.M., Weltzien, H.U., Bühring, H.-J. & Eichmann, K. Nature 308, 367-370 (1984).
49. Fleischer, B. Nature 308, 365-367 (1984).
50. Shortman, K., Wilson, A. & Scollay, R. J.Immun. 132, 584-593 (1984).

PHORBOL ESTER INDUCED MODULATION OF LYMPHOCYTE

PHENOTYPE AND FUNCTION

I. Ando, P.C.L. Beverley, D.H. Crawford,
G. Hariri, M.A. Kissonerghis, M.J. Owen,
D. Wallace

ICRF, Human Tumour Immunology Unit,

Department of Haematology, Department of Zoology
University College London, London WC1E 6JJ

Phorbol esters are a family of compounds which act as tumour promoters in experimental animals and induce a variety of phenotypic changes as detected in cultured cells(1.2.). Studies of the cellular action of phorbol esters revealed that they act synergistically with many growth factors (platelet derived growth factor, epidermal growth factor) to induce DNA synthesis but fail to synergise with others (vasopressin, bombesin) (3.4.). These results suggest that the metabolic pathways for mitogenic effect utilised by phorbol esters and hormones are closely related.

The proliferation and differentiation of T and B lymphocytes is regulated via clonally distributed receptors for antigen and non-clonally distributed receptors for growth factors.

In this paper we summarize the results of an analysis (5.6.7.) of phorbol ester induced phenotypic changes in the pattern of the cell surface structures known to be involved in responses to specific antigen or the lymphocyte growth factor interleukin 2 (IL-2). Furthermore we examine the functional changes which parallel these alterations.

Since antigen recognition in T cells occurs via the T3 molecular complex and in B cells via surface Ig we studied first the modulation of the

density of these structures after phorbol ester
treatment. (5.6.).   A variety of T cells of
different origin, (T3 positive tumour cell lines,
E$^+$ cells of peripheral blood, a T-T cell hybridoma,
thymic cells and IL-2 dependent cloned cell lines)
were incubated with the most potent member of the
phorbol ester family, 12-0-tetradecanoylphorbol
13-acetate (TPA) (0.1-100ng/ml) and tested for
expression of the cell surface molecules defined
by UCHT1 and WT31 (8.9.) monoclonal antibodies.
It was found that in all cell types the density
of the cell surface molecules associated with the
T3 complex was reduced.   In peripheral B cells
and in Epstein-Barr virus transformed lymphoblastoid
Bcell lines (EBV lines) TPA reduced markedly the
density of surface Ig.

   Next we studied the expression of a non-
clonally distributed growth factor receptor - the
receptor for IL-2 (Tac) after stimulating T and B
cells with TPA.   In all the T cell lines and T
cell clones the IL-2 receptor detected by an
antibody (anti Tac)(10) to the IL-2 receptor was
induced.   Surprisingly when normal B cells and
EBV lines were stimulated with TPA (0.1-100ng/ml)
bright staining with anti Tac antibody was seen in
these cells also.   The intensity of the staining
in EBV cells is comparable to that of T cells
showing that IL-2 receptor is not exclusively
expressed on T cells and can be induced by phorbol
esters in B cells too.

   The functional consequences of the observed
phenotypic modulation in T cells have been studied
in an IL-2 dependent cloned helper type T cell
line specific to the haemagglutinin molecule of
the influenza virus, and in a cloned IL-2 dependent
cytotoxic T-cell line specific to EBV transformed
B cells.   It was found that the loss of the T3
receptor complex from the cell surface is paralleled
by unresponsiveness to antigen in the helper type
cell clone and a diminished cytotoxic activity in
the CTL line(7).The cloned IL-2 dependent T cell
lines showed an increased sensitivity to IL-2
which can be accounted for by the increased number
of IL-2 receptors on the cell surface.

The function of the IL-2 receptor on B cells was studied first by showing that recombinant IL-2 could be absorbed equally well by Tac[+] EBV lines as by a Tac[+] T-T hybridoma. Secondly, B cells were cultured in TPA or TPA + IL-2 containing tissue culture medium and the cultures assayed for cell proliferation. B cells cultured in the presence of TPA alone show increased DNA synthesis which added IL-2 induces a further elevation of ^{3}H-TdR uptake. This increased DNA synthesis is blocked by the addition of anti Tac antibody, showing that the B cell IL-2 receptor is able to transmit an effective signal.

The identity of the TPA induced IL-2 receptor in T and B cells was confirmed by SDS-PAGE. T and B cells were stimulated with TPA surface iodinated lysed and immunoprecipitated with anti Tac. Autoradiography revealed a broad band of molecular weight 55000 in both T and B cells. Further evidence for the identity of the 55000 molecular weight band in T and B cells was obtained by endo-B-N-acetylglucosamimidase F digestion experiments. Removal of the N-linked glycan units from the 55000 molecular weight band immunoprecipitation from either T or B cells resulted in the appearance of identical bands of 49000 molecular weight. These observations suggest that TPA treatment of T and B cells results in the expressio of functional IL-2 receptor with very similar biochemical properties.

It is well established that the intracellular level of hormone receptors is regulated by specific ligands(4.). In some cases phorbol esters mimic this hormone induced effect, by downregulating the expression of receptors to certain hormones. (4.). In lymphocytes TPA seems to mimic antigen induced changes in the pattern of cell surface molecules and in function that is, the downregulation of the T3 complex, temporary unresponsiveness to antigen and increased expression of IL-2 receptors and increased sensitivity for IL-2. There are therefore strong

parallels between the regulation of antigen
specific receptors in lymphocytes and receptors
for hormones in lymphocytes and other cells.

Acknowledgements.   Istvan Ando is the holder of
a long-term EMBO fellowship on leave from the
Institute of Genetics, Biological Research Centre
of Hungarian Academy of Sciences.

References

1. Cassel, L.D., Hoxie, J.A. and Cooper, R.A.,
Cancer Res. 43, 4582-4586 (1983)

2. Delia, D., Greaves, M.F., Newman, R.A.,
Sutherland, D.R., Minowada, J., Kung, P. and
Goldstein, G., Int. J. Cancer 29, 123-131 (1982)

3. Decker, P. and Rozengurt, E., Nature
287, 607-612 (1980)

4. Rozengurt, E. and Collins, M., Pathology
141, 309-331 (1983)

5. Ando, I., Hariri, G., Wallace, D.,
Beverley, P.C.L., Eur.J.Immunol. (in press)

6. Ando, I., Crawford, D.H., Kissonerghis, M.A.,
Owen, M.J., Beverley, P.C.L., Eur.J.Immunol
(in press)

7. Ando, I., Crawford, D.H., Beverley, P.C.L.,
in proceedings of the second international
workshop on Leucocyte differentiation antigens
(in press)

8. Beverley, P.C.L., and Callard, R.E.,
Eur. J. Immunol, 11, 329-334 (1981)

9. Tax, W.J.M., Willems, H.W., Reekers, P.P.M.,
Capel, P.J.A. and Koene, R.A.P., Nature
304, 445-447 (1983)

10. Uchiyama, T., Nelson, D.C., Fleisher, T.A. and
Waldman, T.A., J. Immunol. 126, 1398-1403 (1981)

11. Catt, K.J., Harwood, J.P., Aguilera, G.,
Dufau, M.L,. Nature 280, 109-116 (1979)

Regulatory Factors Produced by T Cell Clones

Chairpersons: B.A. Askonas and J.N. Woody

While molecular cloning has recently begun to resolve the issues of T cell receptor structure and function its impact on lymphokines research has been equally dramatic with the isolation and function expression of genes encoding for γ-interferon, interleukin 1 and interleukin 2 and its receptor.   However complete understanding of the biological role of these and other as yet uncloned lymhokines in immunoregulation requires the investigation of structure and function in parallel.   Since the biology of IL-2 and its receptor has been discussed in detail already (Session VI), in this session the current position of a number of other lymphokines as regards their functional role is discussed.

The first presentation by Dr Kishimoto described the growth regulation and differentiation of B cells.   From the supernatant of a human T cell line transformed with the T cell retrovirus HTLV-1, B cell differentiation factor (BCDF) was purified to homogeneity.   In analysis of the properties of BCDF of particular interest was the increased level of mRNA for secretory type heavy chains associated with the conversion of activated B cells to Ig secreting cells.   It was also demonstrated that the interaction of recombinant IL-2 with IL-2 receptors (Tac antigen) on B cells induced both proliferation and differentiation. Finally, Dr Kishimoto reported that transfection with a cloned c-myc gene sensitized resting B cells to respond to BCGF.

The regulatory affects of antigen specific T cell derived mediators on B cell function was reviewed by Drs Woody and Kilburn.   Dr Woody reported that cloned IL-2 dependent helper T cells, upon specific activation by antigen and antigen presenting cells released antigen specific factors that on serological analysis comprised of constant and variable regions complexed with MHC Class II determinants as reported previously with uncloned cells. The helper factor of Dr Kilburn although derived from human T cell hybrids displayed similar properties.   The molecular characterisation of these factors is now required to provide essential information of their physiological roles in the mechanisms of B cell activation.

In analysing the interaction between influenza virus immune murine T cells and γ-IFN, Dr Askonas observed that treatment with recombinant γ-IFN had no effect on the induction, proliferation and cytolytic function of cytotoxic T cells. In addition the secretion of γ-IFN by cloned T cells was H-2 restricted and dependent on contact with infected targets. The rate of secretion of γ-IFN and cytotoxic T cell proliferation were inversely related.

This session ended with a paper by Dr Lake on the role of interleukin-1 (IL-1) in human T cell activation. He observed that IL-1 enhanced the expression of the OKT11 antigen and of the IL-2 receptor. The response of T cells to phorbol ester could be restored by IL-1 alone, whereas Con A and PHA responses of highly purified T cells still required the presence of accessory cells.

So while molecular genetics continues to answer the questions of lymphokine structure it is clear from this session that the complete functional repertoire of these molecules still awaits resolution.

Regulation of growth and differentiation of human B cells

T. Kishimoto, T. Hirano, H. Kikutani, A. Muraguchi, K. Shimizu, H. Kishi, S. Kashiwamura, T. Taga, S. Inui, R. Kimura, N. Nakano, K. Ishibashi, and T. Tagawa

Institute for Molecular and Cellular Biology, Osaka University, 1-3. Yamada-Oka, Suita City, Osaka

Introduction

Activation process of B lymphocytes into immuno-globulin (Ig)-secreting cells can be dissected into three steps, i.e., activation, proliferation and differentiation (1-3). It has been demonstrated by several investigators that B cell specific growth and differentiation factors are involved in the process of proliferation and differentiation of activated B cells (4-10). The presence of two different kinds of B cell growth factors, BCGF-I or BSF-pI and BCGF-II, was reported in human (11) as well as in murine systems (12). BCGF-I induces proliferation of anti-IgM-stimulated human or murine B cells as well as SAC (Staphylococcus aureus Cowan I)-stimulated human B cells. Activated but not resting B cells are able to adsorb the activity of BCGF-I, suggesting the induction of the expression of receptors for BCGF-I on activated B cells. However, a recent study showed an increased expression of Ia antigen on resting B cells by stimulation with BCGF-I, suggesting the presence of BCGF-I receptors even on resting B cells, although BCGF-I induces proliferation only in activated B cells (13).

BCGF-II shows a reciprocal pattern of activity compared to BCGF-I. Human BCGF-II does not induce proliferation of anti-μ or SAC-stimulated B cells, but induces proliferation of Dextran-Sulfate (DXS)-stimulated murine B cells and a murine leukemic B cell line, BCL_1

Table 1
Biochemical and immunological properties
of BCGF-I and BCGF-II

	BCGF-I (or BSF-pI)	BCGF-II
M.W.	20 K	50K
P.I.	6.5	5.0-5.5
Function	Growth activity	Growth and differentiation activity
Induction of proliferation		
a) in anti-μ B	++	- or ±
b) in SAC B	++	- or ±
c) in B-blast	+	++
d) in DXS-B	-	++
e) in BCL$_1$ cells	-	++

(14). BCGF-I shows only the growth activity, while BCGF-II induces both proliferation and Ig-secretion in DXS-stimulated B cells as well as in BCL$_1$ cells (14). Several factors, such as BGDF by Pike et al. (5) and T151 TRF by Takatsu et al. (15), were shown to have both growth and differentiation activities. Therefore, those factors may belong to the category of BCGF-II. Physicochemical and immunological properties of BCGF-I and BCGF-II are summarized in Table 1. After the maximum proliferation of activated B cells in the presence of BCGF-I and BCGF-II, B cell specific differentiation factor (BCDF) induces the final maturation of B cells into high-rate Ig-secreting cells.

Activation process of B cells and the signals involved in this process have been delineated. Therefore, the study to be undertaken will be the isolation and the determination of the chemical structure of those B cell stimulatory factors and their receptors.

Isolation of BCDF
As is well known, the amount of B cell stimulatory factors released from activated T cells is so minute that

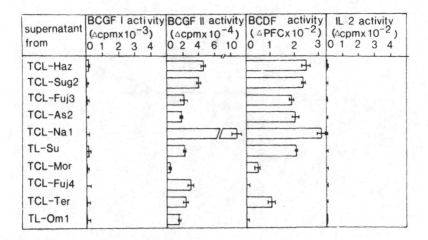

Fig.1   Immunoregulatory factors secreted from HTLV-transformed T cell lines.

it is essential to establish T cell lines which continuously secrete a relatively large amount of those
factors. In order to establish such T cell lines, human
T cell leukemia virus (HTLV) was employed for the
establishment of transformed human T cell lines. Culture
supernatants from many HTLV-transformed T cell lines were
tested for the activity of B cell stimulatory factors.
As shown in Fig.1, several interesting findings were
obtained, i.e. i) many cell lines secreted a relatively
large amount of BCDF and BCGF-II, ii) none of the cell
lines tested secreted any BCGF-I, iii) none of the cell
lines tested secreted any IL-2 and mRNA for IL-2 was not
detected. BCDF secreted from one of the T cell lines
(TcL-Na1) was approximately 1,000 fold as much as that of
PHA-stimulated T cells. Thus, the culture supernatant
from this cell line was employed for the isolation of
BCDF.
        As a simple, sensitive and quantitative assay system
for BCDF activity, a BCDF-responsive human B cell line
(CESS) was employed.   As reported (16), CESS cells
expressed BCDF-receptors and BCDF induced IgG secretion

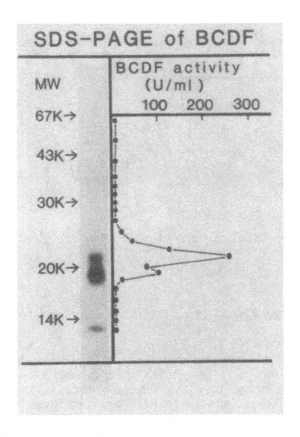

Fig.2   SDS-PAGE   analysis   of ^{125}I-labelled   BCDF
preparation purified from culture supernatant from a
HTLV-transformed T cell line.

in these cells without any effect on cell growth. Thus,
1×10^3 CESS   cells   were   incubated   with   varing
concentrations of BCDF for 48 hr and the concentration of
IgG in culture supernatants was measured by ELISA. CESS
cells were also incubated with test samples with several
dilutions and the activity to induce 50% of the maximum
response was designated as 1 unit.
      Culture supernatant from a HTLV-transformed T cells
was fractionated by gel filtration on AcA 34 column and
the active fraction with the m.w. of 30 K was applied to

Table 2

Physicochemical and immunological properties of human BCDF

---

1. M.W.: 21K on SDS-PAGE

2. P.I.: 5.5 on IEF

3. The minimum protein concentration for the activity: 0.1-0.01 ng/ml

4. Induce an increase in mRNA for secretory type heavy chains in activated B cells

5. Induce both IgM and IgG secretion (no isotype specificity)

6. No growth activity

---

preparative isoelectric focusing. BCDF activity was focused at pI 5.5 and this fraction was applied to Mono P column on FPLC. Then, the active fraction was further purified on a reverse column on HPLC. A small protein peak with BCDF activity was isolated. In order to examine the purity of this fraction, the active fraction was iodinated by Bolton-Hunter method and applied to SDS-PAGE analysis. As shown in Fig.2, two radioactive, bands, 18 and 21 K were observed and BCDF activity was detected in the 21 K fraction when each eluted sample was tested. These results strongly suggest that human BCDF has been purified to an apparent homogeneity. Thus, the determination of the partial amino acid sequence for gene cloning will be possible. By employing highly purified BCDF preparation, some physicochemical and immunological properties were studied, and the result was summarized in Table 2.

Effect of IL-2 on B cells

Several recent studies including ourselves (17-20) have suggested that IL-2 is able to act directly on B cells and to induce proliferation or Ig-secretion in B cells. However, as those studies employed highly purified normal B cells, the possibility that IL-2 stimulated a small number of contaminated T cells to secrete B cell stimulatory factors could not be excluded. Thus, in this study a B cell clone responsive to IL-2 was established. As shown in Fig.3 incubation of a human B cell clone (SGB3) either with purified BCDF or with

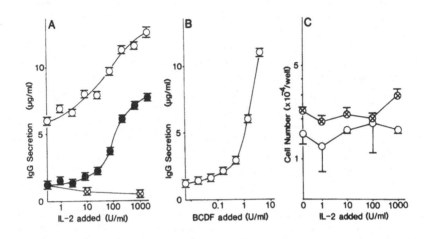

Fig.3   IgG induction in a human B cell line with recombinant IL-2 or BCDF.

A)   ●-● with varing concentrations of IL-2
       ○-○ with 1 unit/ml BCDF + varing concentrations of IL-2.
B)   ○-○ with varing concentrations of BCDF.
C)   Effect of varing concentrations of IL-2 on cell growth.
       ○-○ after 2 days
       ⊗-⊗ after 4 days

recombinant IL-2 could induce IgG secretion in a dose-dependent manner.   Growth of SGB3 cells was not affected at all by the incubation with any concentration of IL-2. More than 1,000 units/ml of IL-2 were required for the maximum IgG secretion in SGB3 cells, whereas only 0.5 unit/ml of IL-2 could induce the maximum proliferation of activated T cells.   Anti-Tac antibody could completely inhibited IL-2-induced IgG secretion, but showed no inhibitory effect on BCDF-induced IgG secretion in the same cells.   The concentration of anti-Tac antibody for the complete inhibition of SGB3 cells was only 100 ng/ml, while 10 µg/ml anti-Tac antibody was required for the inhibition of IL-2-induced proliferation of T cells. All of these results obtained with an IL-2 responsive human B cell clone provide several informations, i.e. i) IL-2 can act directly on B cells, ii) B cells can express IL-2 receptor (Tac antigen), iii) interaction of IL-2 and IL-2 receptors can generate the signal responsible for Ig-secretion but not for proliferation in a certain differentiation stage of B cells, iv) affinity of IL-2 receptors on B cells may be much lower than that on T cells.

B cell activation and c-myc gene expression

As described, anti-Ig-stimulation of resting B cells does not induce any proliferation or Ig-secretion, but it renders B cells responsive to BCGF-I. Therefore, the process of B cell proliferation can be dissected into two steps, i.e., anti-Ig-induced activation and BCGF-induced proliferation. Several recent studies (21,22) demonstrated that c-myc oncogene expression may be responsible for the early stage of cell activation from G_0 to G_1, i.e., platelet-derived growth factor (PDGF) activates 3T3 cells and induces an increase in c-myc expression, while EGF, which induces proliferation of activated 3T3 cells, does not induce any increase in c-myc expression. In order to study whether this principle obtained with a cell line can be applied to the activation of resting B cells and whether c-myc expression is essential for the activation of B cells to the responsive stage to BCGF-I, the change of c-myc expression in B cells stimulated with anti-Ig or BCGF and the effect of transfection of c-myc gene into resting B cells were studied.

Small resting human B cells were stimulated with 5 µg/ml anti-µ antibody, total RNA was extracted every 2 hr after anti-Ig stimulation and c-myc mRNA was measured by dot hybridization with Cla-EcoRI fragment of exon III of human c-myc genomic DNA as a probe. A significant increase in c-myc expression was observed 2 hr after anti-µ stimulation and this increased expression was quickly returned to the original level within 24 hr. BCGF-stimulation of anti-µ activated B cells at 24 hr did not affect the level of c-myc expression. This result suggests that an increase in c-myc expression my be responsible for the early activation stage of resting B cells from G_0 to G_1.

In order to study whether an increase in c-myc

Table 3
Intorduction of cloned c-myc DNA can
substitute for anti-μ stimulation

Treatment of B cells	^{3}H-Thymidine uptake
	cpm
-	2,387 ± 65
anti-μ	3,165 ± 160
BCGF	3,722 ± 856
anti-μ + BCGF	8,887 ± 25
DEAE-Dextran	864 ± 122
DEAE-Dextran + BCGF	1,000 ± 590
pSV2. gpt	1,080 ± 519
pSV2. gpt + BCGF	1,257 ± 387
pSV2.26	1,192 ± 700
pSV2.26 + BCGF	5,935 ± 217

expression is essential for B cell activation, attempt
was made to introduce cloned c-myc gene into resting B
cells and examine whether transient expression of c-myc
gene in B cells could substitute for anti-μ-stimulation.
The translocated c-myc gene of a non-Hodgkin's lymphoma
was employed, since the cryptic promoter of this c-myc
gene was activated by adjacent Ig-enhancer element,
resulting in high level of c-myc expression. The
plasmid, pSV2.26, that was kindly provided by Dr. S.
Tonegawa (MIT, Mass.), was prepared by cloning the EcoRI
fragment containing IInd and IIIrd exons of c-myc and
enhancer element into pSV2 gpt. DEAE-dextran method was
employed for the transient expression of c-myc gene in
resting B cells.

The result depicted in Table 3 showed that the
transient expression of c-myc gene in resting B cells
activated them to the responsive stage to BCGF. In each
experiment, 3 to 4 fold increase in ^{3}H-thymidine uptake
was observed in B cells treated with pSV2.26 when they
were cultured with BCGF. The proliferation induced with
c-myc and BCGF was comparable to that observed in anti-μ-

stimulated B cells. No increase in proliferation was observed in B cells treated with pSV2 gpt or only with DEAE-dextran, even when they were cultured with BCGF. These results strongly suggest that c-myc expression can substitute for anti-μ stimulation and may have an essential role in the early activation process of resting B cells. Recent study done by Armelin et al. (22) also showed that the expression of the c-myc gene in 3T3 cells sensitized them to the growth promoting action of EGF. The present study together with their work illustrates the common role of c-myc gene products as intracellular mediators of the growth response to widely divergent mitogens.

Conclusion
     A HTLV-transformed human T cell line, which secreted a relatively large amount of BCDF, was established and a human BCDF was highly purified to an apparent homogeneity by employing a large volume of the culture supernatant from this cell line. BCDF induced a final maturation of activated B cells to high-rate Ig-secreting cells by inducing an increase in mRNA specific for secretory type heavy chains.
     Recombinant IL-2 could also induce Ig-secretion in a B cell line at a certain differentiation stage. An affinity of IL-2 receptors (Tac antigen) on this B cell line was much lower than that on T cells. However, IL-2 and IL-2 receptor interaction could generate the same signals as those provided by BCDF in this particular cell line. The result indicated that IL-2 could provide signals not only for proliferation but also for differentiation through IL-2 receptors.
     Anti-μ-stimulation, but not BCGF-stimulation of human B cells caused a transient spike of c-myc gene expression and transfection with a cloned c-myc gene sensitized resting B cells to respond to BCGF. The result suggests that c-myc gene expression plays a common role as an intracellular mediator of the growth response to widely divergent mitogens.
     Isolation and chemical characterization of B cell stimulatory factors, their receptors and intracellular mediators will provide essential informations for the elucidation of the mechanism of B cell differentiation at the molecular level.

358   Kishimoto et al.

References

1. Yoshizaki, K., Nakagawa, T., Kaieda, T., Muraguchi, A., Yamamura, Y., and Kishimoto, T.   J. Immunol. 128, 1296 (1982)
2. Nakanishi, K., Howard, M., Muraguchi, A., Farrar, J., Takatsu, K., Hamaoka, T., and Paul, W.E.   J. Immunol. 130, 2219 (1983)
3. Kishimoto, T., Yoshizaki, K., Kimoto, M., Okada, M., Kuritani, T., Kikutani, H., Shimizu, K., Nakagawa, T., Nakagawa, N., Miki, Y., Kishi, H., Fukunaga, K., Yoshikubo, T., and Taga, T. Immunological Rev. 78, 97 (1984)
4. Howard, M., Farrar, J., Hilfiker, M., Johnson, B., Takatsu, K., Hamaoka, T., and Paul, W.E.   J. Exp. Med. 155, 914 (1982)
5. Pike, B.L., Vaux, D.L., Clark-Lewis, I., Shrader, J.W., and Nossal, G.J.V.   Proc. Natl. Acad. Sci., USA 79, 6350 (1982)
6. Okada, M., Sakaguchi, N., Yoshimura, N., Hara, H., Shimizu, K., Yoshida, N., Yoshizaki, K., Kishimoto, S., Yamamura, Y., and Kishimoto, T.   J. Exp. Med. 157, 583 (1983)
7. Maizel, A., Sahasrabuddhe, C., Mehta, S., Morgan, J., Lachman, L., and Ford, R.   Proc. Natl. Acad. Sci., USA 79, 5998 (1982)
8. Lernhardt, W., Corbel, C., Wall, R., and Melchers, F. Nature 300, 355 (1982)
9. Leanderson, T., Lundgren, E., Ruuth, E., Borg, H., Persson, H., and Countinho, A.   Proc. Natl. Acad. Sci., USA 79, 7455 (1982)
10. Butler, J.L., Muraguchi, A., Clifford, H., and Fauci, A.S. J. Exp. Med. 157, 60 (1983)
11. Yoshizaki, K., Nakagawa, T., Fukunaga, K., Kaieda, T., Maruyama, S., Kishimoto, S., Yamamura, Y., and Kishimoto, T. J. Immunol. 130, 1241 (1983)
12. Swain, S.L., Howard, M., Kappler, J., Marrack, P., Watson, J., Booth, R., Wetzel, G.D., and Dutton, R.W. J. Exp. Med. 158, 822 (1983)
13. Noelle, R., Krammer, P.H., Ohara, J., Uhr, J.W., and Vitetta, E.S. proc. Natl. Acad. Sci., USA 81, 6149 (1984)
14. Shimizu, K., Hirano, T., Ishibashi, K., Nakano, N., Taga, T., Sugamura, K., Yamamura, Y., and Kishimoto, T. J. Immunol. in press.
15. Takatsu, K., Tanaka, K., Tominaga, A., Kumaharam Y.,

and Hamaoka, T. J. Immunol. 125, 2646 (1980)

16. Muraguchi, A., Kishimoto, T., Miki, Y., Kuritani, T., Kaieda, T., Yoshizaki, K., Yamamura, Y. J. Immunol. 127, 412 (1981)

17. Nakagawa, T., Hirano, T., Nakagawa, N., Yoshizaki, K., and Kishimoto, T. J. Immunol. in press

18. Tsuda, M., Uchiyama, T., and Uchino, H. J. Exp. Med. 160, 612 (1984)

19. Muraguchi, A., Kehrl, J.H., Longo, D.L., Volkman, D.J., Smith, K.A., and Fauci, A. J. Exp. Med. in press

20. Nakanishi, K., Malek, T.R., Smith, K.A., Hamaoka, T., Shevach, E.M., and Paul, W.E. J. Exp. Med. in press

21. Kelly, K., Cochran, B.H., Stiles, C.D., and Leder, P. Cell 35, 603 (1983)

22. Armelin, H.A., Armelin, M.C.S., Kelly, K., Stewart, T., Leder, P., Cochran, B.H., and Stiles, C.D. Nature 310, 655 (1984)

ANTIGEN-SPECIFIC T CELL HELPER FACTORS

James N. Woody,[1] Jonathan R. Lamb,[2] Edward D. Zanders,[2] and Marc Feldman[2]

[1]Transplantation Research Program Center, Naval Medical Research Institute, Bethesda, Maryland 20814-5055.

[2]Imperial Cancer Research Fund, Tumor Immunology Unit, University College, London.

ABSTRACT. The mechanism by which antigen-specific T helper cells convey information to their B cell counterparts has received much attention in the immunologic literature. Recent studies with cloned T helper cells indicate that antigen-specific T helper factors (^{T}HF), capable of inducing specific antibody responses, are actively secreted in response to antigenic restimulation. Serologic analysis of such factors suggest the presence of constant and variable regions, as well as products of class II histocompatibility genes. Current models suggest that ^{T}HF represents the secreted variant form of the T cell receptor.

INTRODUCTION

The methods by which antigen-specific T cells communicate detailed information to their B cell counterparts, resulting in specific antibody production, has received considerable attention in the immunologic literature over the past two decades (reviewed in 1 and 2). With the development of methods to clone and propogate T cells, using IL-2 (3), and the demonstration that some of these clones are classical "helper cells" (4), the technology became available to analyze this issue in greater detail, using more definitive functional assays.

361

The past two years has seen meteoric progress on the
biochemistry and molecular biology of the elusive T cell
receptor. Initial evidence, suggesting that the T cell
receptor is an 85-90 Kd disulfide-linked heterodimer, was
provided for human (5) and murine (6) T cells, using monoclonal anti-"clonotypic" antibodies. The use of these reagents with antigen-specific T cells argues, convincingly,
that the T cell receptor for antigen has been identified,
and consists of an alpha chain and beta chain of approximately 46-49K and 40-43K, respectively, in human T cells.

In the past year, two independent groups have cloned
and sequenced the beta chain genes for human (7) and murine
(8) T cell receptors, with derived protein sequences being
in general agreement with the biochemical molecular weight
analysis. Similar studies for the alpha chain genes (9)
have now been reported, although confirmation by independent investigators has not been published. While most
workers (1,10,11) assume that [T]HF represents the secreted
form of the receptor, in analogy with immunoglobulin representing the secreted form of the B cell receptor; serologic
analysis provides clues that the [T]HF molecules may be more
complex.

RESULTS AND DISCUSSION

The Release of Immunoregulatory Factors from
T Helper Cell Lines and Clones

Over a decade ago, Feldmann and Basten (12) reported
that [T]HF passed through a nucleopore membrane and provided
classical antigen-specific B cell help. While this work
was performed with mixed cell populations, similar studies
have recently been reproduced with human antigen-specific
T cell lines by Fischer, et al. (4) and with T cell clones
by Lamb and colleagues (13), as well as by other groups of
workers, as summarized in ref. 14. TABLE 1 illustrates
some of the results we have obtained with influenza-
specific lines and clones.

TABLE 1

Summary Analysis of Functional Helper Activity
of Human T Cell Lines and Clones[*]

Helper Cells	No. of Cells	MPH/B Cells (E⁻)	Antibody Production (% Control)
$-$		$+$	1-5
E^+		$+$	100
Helper Lines	1×10^2	$+$	40
" "	5×10^2	$+$	90
" "	1×10^3	$+$	80
" "	1×10^4	$+$	85
" "	1×10^5	$+$	25
Helper Clones	1×10^1	$+$	10
" "	1×10^2	$+$	95
" "	5×10^2	$+$	80
" "	1×10^3	$+$	70
" "	5×10^3	$+$	30

[*] Various numbers of influenza A-specific helper cells were added to a mixture of 1×10^5 B cells and macrophages (double E rosetted). Antibody production was measured using influenza A or B adhered to polystyrene plates, in an ELISA assay. Except in the PBL T cell control (E^+), no antibody was induced to influenza B, indicating the appropriate antigen specificity of the helper cell lines and clones.

The study of supernatants from such antigen-specific helper cells provides information concerning the secretion of molecules capable of mediating help and inducing antigen-specific responses in B cells. A summary of the results is shown in TABLE 2, demonstrating the capacity of helper cells to produce such molecules.

Similar types of studies in murine systems by Lifshitz and colleagues (15) with T-G-A--L, and De Kruyff et al. (16), using hapten-specific clones, support the view that antigen-specific helper factors are produced and secreted by specific clones. Both Fischer et al. (12), and Lamb and colleagues (13), clearly demonstrated that the output of functionally active helper factor increased with stimulation of

TABLE 2

Summary Analysis of Functional Helper Activity
of Supernatants of (SN) of T Helper
Cell Lines and Clones[*]

Helper Factor	Final Concentration (%)	MPH/B Cells (E^-)	Antibody Production (% Control)
-		+	1-5
E^+ Cells		+	100
Helper Line SN	1×10^{-3}	+	25
" "	1×10^{-2}	+	60
" "	1×10^{-1}	+	100
" "	1×10^{0}	+	80
" "	5×10^{0}	+	85
" "	1×10^{1}	+	70
" "	2.5×10^{1}	+	20
Helper Clone SN	1×10^{-3}	+	40
" "	1×10^{-2}	+	95
" "	1×10^{-1}	+	90
" "	1×10^{0}	+	70
" "	5×10^{0}	+	30
" "	5×10^{1}	+	20

[*]Same format as for TABLE 1. Supernatant concentrations
from influenza A-specific helper cells represent "final
volume" percentages. Antibody responses to influenza B
were all under 5%, except for the E^+ control, indicating
antigen specificity for the SN's.

the clones by antigen and antigen-presenting cells (APC's),
suggesting that the helper factor was derived from viable
cells, and production could be modulated as with the release of lymphokines. Studies with metabolic inhibitors
have confirmed this view (reviewed 14).

Serologic Analysis of Helper Factors from
T Helper Cell Lines and Clones
_____

The serologic analysis of helper factors, using both
polyclonal and monoclonal antisera, has been fraught with
difficulties. Several reasons exist to explain these problems (14), the major one being that even minute amounts of
other antibodies present as contaminants, or perhaps a minor
crossreaction, may be sufficient to bind factors present at
very low levels. A summary of serologic work on helper
factors from T cell lines or clones, is presented in
TABLE 3.

TABLE 3

Summary of Analysis of Human Helper Factors
from T Helper Cell Lines or Clones[*]

Immunoadsorbent Column	Response of E- Cells to	
	Filtrate	Eluate
Antigen	-	+
Anti-human Ig	+	-
Protein A	-	+
Anti-beta-2 microglobulin	-	+
Anti-Ia (framework)	+	+

[*] Factors were eluted from columns to which the various
antibodies (or antigens) had been adhered. Filtrates or
eluates were tested for activity as described in the
legend for TABLE 2.

In order to accommodate the serologic findings, with
data on the biochemistry and molecular biology of the T
cell receptor (7-9), which demonstrates an 85-90 Kd heterodimer, one must offer the following hypothesis:

(a) Helper factors, which are the secretory form of the
     T cell membrane receptor for antigen, share common
     determinants with other molecules in this class of
     immunoregulatory proteins, which includes immunoglobu-
     lin, beta-2 microglobulin, Ia (class II) antigens, and
     possibly class I antigens, indicating a common
     ancestry.

(b)   These shared conformational regions (folds, etc.)
       account for the serologic reactivity observed. Initial
       analysis of the alpha and beta chains for the T cell
       receptor does not suggest a high degree (over 50%) of
       homology with beta-2 microglobulin or Ia antigens,
       although these are likely to share folding regions.
       Homology with immunoglublin of 40-60% has been
       reported (7).

(c)   The Ia antigenic determinants could derive from Ia
       molecules bound to the factor, as the T cell receptor
       has an Ia binding portion, and Ia molecules from APC's
       are always present in the ^{T}HF S/N due to the method
       of restimulation of the T helper cell clones. Binding
       of Ia antigens has been observed on alloreactive T
       cells (17).

Molecular weight analysis with ^{T}HF from one of antigen-
specific clones suggested a size of 65 Kd. The smaller
apparent size of the factor versus membrane receptor (85 Kd)
may be accounted for by the loss of cytoplasmic and transmembrane portions, in the secreted form, as seen with the
membrane and secreted forms of immunoglobulin. For B cells,
the membrane and secreted forms are represented by two
distinct mRNA's (18). In those T cell lines examined
(Jurkat) by TAk Mak (personal communication), two forms
of mRNA were found: a 1300 and 1000-base variety. Closer
examination of the smaller RNA showed a D-J recombination
rather than loss of the transmembrane and cytoplasmic portions. Analysis of classical "helper cell" clones, after
antigenic stimulation, for the two types of RNA may reveal
the secretory form of the receptor in RNA, lacking the
transmembrane portions, as is observed in B cells, as well
as the "membrane bound receptor" message, which would include the transmembrane portions (17).

CONCLUSIONS

The available information suggests that T cell clones
secrete an antigen-specific helper factor capable of inducing specific B cell responses. Current thought suggests
that ^{T}HF is the secreted form of the membrane T cell receptor for antigen. It shares homology with immunoglobulin
and has ancestral relationships with Ia and beta-2 microglobulin. Whether the factor has Ia as a structural component, or binds Ia via a portion of its receptor, is not

known. The presence of other non-specific molecules, such
as IL-2, IL-3, BCGF, BCDF, gamma interferon, and perhaps
prostaglandins and leukotrienes in most T_{HF} supernatants
makes analysis in functional assays difficult, but the
possibility of newer molecular forms of analysis may soon
resolve these issues. T_{HF} protein sequence will shortly
resolve this issue.

REFERENCES

1. Feldmann, M., Fischer, A., James, R., et al. In:
    Fabris, N., Garcia, E., Hadden, J. and Mitchison, N.A.
    (eds.). "Proceedings of the International Workshop on
    Immunoregulation, p. 93 (1981).

2. Melchers, F., and Andersson, J. Cell 37, 715 (1984).

3. Smith, K.A. Immunologic Rev. 51, 337 (1980).

4. Fischer, A., Beverley, P.C.L., Feldmann, M. Nature
    294, 166 (1981).

5. Meuer, S.C., Acuto, O., Hussey, R.E., Hodgdon, J.C.,
    Fitzgerald, K.A., Schlossman, S.F. and Reinherz, E.L.
    Nature 303, 808 (1983).

6. Allison, J.P., McIntyre, B.W. and Bloch, D. J of
    Immunol. 129, 2293 (1982).

7. Yanagi, Y., Yoshikai, Y., Leggett, K., Clark, S.P.,
    Aleksander, I. and Mak, T.W. Nature 308, 145 (1984).

8. Hedrick, S.M., Cohen, D.I., Nielsen, E.A., and Davis,
    M.M. Nature 308, 149 (1984).

9. Saito, H., Kranz, D.M., Takagaki, Y., Hayday, A.C.,
    Eisen, H. and Jonegawa, S. Nature 309, 757 (1984).

10. Tada, T., Okamura, K. Adv. Immunol. 28, 1 (1981).

11. Feldmann, M., Kontainen, S. Lymphokines 2, 87 (1981).

12. Feldmann, M., and Basten, A. J. Exp. Med. 136, 49
    (1972).

13. Lamb, J.R., Woody, J.N., Hartzman, R.J., and Eckels,
     D.D. J. Immunol. 129, 1465 (1982).

14. Feldmann, M., Zanders, E.D., Culbert, E.J., and Lamb,
     J.R. In: Regulation of the Immune System: UCLA
     Symposium on Molecular and Cellular Biology, Vol. 18,
     1984 (in press).

15. Lifshitz, R., Apte, R., and Mozes, E. PNAS 80, 5689
     (1983).

16. Dekruyff, R.H., Clayberger, C. and Cantor, H. J Exp.
     Med. 158, 1881 (1983).

17. Elliot, B.D., and Palfree, R.G. J. Immunol. Meth.
     72, 11 (1984).

18. Rogers, J. and Wall, R. Adv. in Immunol. 35, 39 (1984).

HUMAN T-CELL HYBRIDS PRODUCING ANTIGEN

SPECIFIC HELPER FACTORS

Muzaffer Altin, Douglas G. Kilburn and Robert C. Miller, Jr.

Department of Microbiology, University of British Columbia,

Vancouver, B.C., Canada V6T 1W5

The regulation of the immune system involves a complex series of interactions between different cell types and their soluble products. Regulatory T cells occupy a central position in this process and act to amplify or suppress the responses of both T and B cells.

Regulatory T cells produce antigen-specific factors which, at least in part, mediate the effector function of these cells (1-4). The structure and mode of action of these factors is not yet clear, primarily because the factors are produced in minute quantities and hence are extremely difficult to isolate. In order to study their chemical and biological characteristics and, ultimately to evaluate their potential for modulating immune responses in man, it is necessary to have a potent source of factors. With this objective in mind, we have sought to establish human T-cell hybridomas producing helper factors specific for tuberculin (PPD[1]). Tuberculin was chosen because

---

[1]. Abbreviations: PPD, tuberculin, purified protein derivative of Mycobacterium tuberculosis; PHS, pooled human serum; IL-2, interleukin 2; PHA, phytohemagglutinin; HAT, hypoxanthine, aminopterin, thymidine, selective medium; PEG, polyethylene glycol; DMSO, dimethylsulphoxide; ThF, antigen-specific T-cell derived helper factor, BSA, bovine serum albumin.

the response to this antigen is strongly biased towards T
cells and, in addition, a large population of sensitized
donors is available. Our approach involved the
development of a rapid screening assay, the establishment
of IL-2 dependent cell lines enriched in PPD reactive
cells and the generation from these cells of T-cell
hybrids producing PPD specific helper factors (ThF).

METHODS

1.   PPD Specific IL-2 lines (5,6,7)
     Fifty mls of blood from PPD positive donors were
diluted 1:1 with RPMI 1640 supplemented with 2.5% pooled
Human Serum (PHS), Penicillin-Streptomycin, 5×10^{-5} M
2-mercaptoethanol, 10 mM Hepes and 25 units of heparin
per ml (Medium A). Medium with 10% PHS will be referred
to as Medium B. The blood solution was layered onto
Ficoll-Hypaque (d=1.130 g/ml) and centrifuged for 20
minutes at 400xg. The cells at the interface were
collected and washed with Medium A. The PBL were
stimulated with PPD (100 µg/ml) at a cell density of
2.5×10^6/ml for 4 days at 37°C under 5% CO_2 in
microculture plates in 200 ul of Medium B. The cells
were harvested and washed twice with Medium A and
returned to culture at a cell density of 4×10^5/ml
without PPD in Medium A supplemented with human
Interleukin 2 (25%) in 1 ml per well of Costar 24-well
tissue culture plates. The cell density was maintained
at 4×10^5/ml by subculturing with fresh human IL 2
every 3-4 days. The supernatants of these cells were
used as the source of ThF-PPD.

     The supernatants of human tonsillar lymphocytes (2.5
$\times 10^6$/ml) stimulated with PHA (2.5 µg/ml) for 48
hours at 37°C under 5% CO_2 were used as the source of
human IL-2.

2.   Fusion of PPD-stimulated, IL 2-maintained long term
cells with a human T cell leukemia line (HTL-1).

     After three-four weeks in culture, ThF-PPD
producing, IL 2-maintained cells (shown to be >70% OKT
4+,   helper/inducer by FACS analysis) were mixed
with a HAT-sensitive human T cell leukemia line, HTL-1,
at 10:1. The cell mixture was centrifuged for 10 minutes

at 400xg, and the cell pellet was gently resuspended in a
solution of 41.6% PEG (Serva 1550) and 15% DMSO. The
fusion mixture was then diluted to 25 ml with warm Medium
C (supplemented with 10% FCS) and dispensed into 24-well
Costar plates in 0.5 ml. HTL-1 cells were added as
filler cells. After 24 hours at 37°C, the medium was
replaced with HAT medium. Fresh HAT medium was added
every 7 days for 4 - 5 weeks. The supernatants of
growing cells were tested in the antibody blocking assay
and positive wells were cloned immediately by limiting
dilution. The positive clones were maintained in Medium
C. The supernatants of these cells harvested at a cell
density of 1 x 10^6/ml were used as the source of
ThF-PPD.

3.   Purification of ThF-PPD
      The crude ThF-PPD from long term cell lines or T-T
cell hybridomas was applied to a PPD-Sepharose column
(1.5 x 10 cm). The column was washed exhaustively with
PBS and then eluted with either 2 M NaCl or 0.2 M
NH$_4$OH. The eluate was dialysed against PBS. ThF-PPD
was stored at 4°C until further use.

4.   RIA Inhibition Assay (8)
      Soft plastic plates were coated with 500 ng/ml PPD
or 250 ng/ml CGG (Chicken Gamma Globulin) or KLH (Keyhole
Limpet Hemocyanin) in carbonate/bicarbonate buffer
overnight at 4°C. Mouse anti PPD antibody (1/4,000) or
anti CGG antibody or anti KLH antibody (1/10,000) in PBS
containing 1% BSA was incubated overnight at 4°C either
alone or with antigen or ThF at various dilutions. The
next day, the plates were washed with PBS-Tween. The
antibody mixture was then added to the plate in
triplicates and incubated at room temperature for an
hour. After washing the plate with PBS-Tween, 10^5 cpm
per well of ^{125}I-goat anti mouse F(ab)$_2$ in 0.1 ml of
PBS+1% BSA was added and incubated at room temperature
for an hour. Finally, the plates were washed with tap
water, individual wells were cut out and radioactivity
was measured in a gamma counter.

5.   Immuno absorption of ThF-PPD by anti HLA-DR
      antibodies
      To verify that human ThF-PPD bears markers coded by
the I region of the MHC (I-A like determinants), we

absorbed ThF with anti HLA-DR monoclonal antibodies (MAS
053 Rat IgG against HLA-DR, Cedarlane, Hornby, Ontario)
bound to goat anti mouse Ig linked to Sepharose.
Briefly, ThF-PPD (400 µl) was incubated with 10, 20 and
60 µg of antibody for 30 minutes at 37°C in Eppendorf
plastic tubes. The goat anti-mouse Ig-Sepharose was
added to the above mixture (200 µl of 0.5 g/ml beads)
and incubated for an hour at room temperature. The tubes
were spun in an Eppendorf centrifuge for 3 minutes and
the supernatants were assayed in the RIA inhibition assay.

6.   Biological Assay of ThF-PPD
      The biological activity of human ThF-PPD was
measured by its enhancement of the _in vitro_ generation of
CTL by murine thymocytes stimulated with allogenic cells
(9). Briefly, normal DBA/2 spleen cells (10^7/ml) were
adhered to plastic tissue culture plates overnight at
37°C. The next day, non-adherent cells were removed by
washing three times with medium without serum. The
adherent cells were incubated with PPD (1 µg/ml). The
control plates (without PPD) were incubated with sterile
PBS. After one hour at 37°C, the plates were washed
three times with medium without serum and pulsed with
ThF-PPD or appropriate controls at various dilutions for
an hour at room temperature. Again, the plates were
washed with Medium C three times. Antigen and factor
pulsed as well as control plates were irradiated (2,000
rads) using a Cobalt source before C57/B6 thymocytes (3 x
10^6/ml) were added. After five days of incubation, the
effector cells were harvested from six identical wells
and pooled, washed once with Medium C. These cells were
assayed against ^{51}Cr labeled P815 tumor cells in a 4
hour Cr-release assay at varying E/T ratios. The percent
specific lysis was calculated as

$$\% \text{ Specific Lysis} = \frac{\text{Experimental cpm} - \text{Spontaneous cpm}}{\text{Maximum cpm} - \text{Spontaneous cpm}} \times 100.$$

RESULTS AND DISCUSSION

1.   Blocking Assay
      We recently developed a rapid assay for the
detection and quantitation of antigen binding molecules,
such as ThF (8). This assay depends on the ability of
the factor to inhibit the binding of free antibody to

antigen immobilized on a RIA plate. A second,
radioactive antibody is used to quantitate the amount of
binding. The concentrations of antigen on the plate and
antibody to this antigen must be titrated to determine
the levels that give the greatest sensitivity to blocking
by a small amount of free antigen. A plot of antibody
binding as a function of the concentration of free
antigen can then be used to relate the binding observed
in the presence of factor to an antigen concentration
giving equal blocking. ThF concentration can thus be
expressed in terms of antigen equivalents. In the PPD
system, we could routinely obtain 50-60% inhibition of
binding at 1000 ng/ml of free antigen and 20-30%
inhibition with 100 ng/ml of free antigen in the reaction
of anti PPD antibody to immobilized antigen on a RIA
plate. The titration was repeated each time ThF was
quantitated. We have used the blocking assay to
determine the recovery of blocking activity during
purification of ThF and as a rapid screening assay for
the detection of cells producing ThF as outlined below.

2.   PPD Reactive, IL-2 Dependent Cell Lines
      Although our ultimate objective was to derive T-cell
hybrids that excreted ThF, initially we set out to
establish long-term lines of IL-2 dependent PPD-specific
cell lines. We reasoned that ThF producing cells would
be enriched in the cell line population and that this
should enhance the probability of generating
ThF-producing hybrids. Cell lines were set up by
culturing PPD reactive PBL's with PPD for 4 days and
subsequently transferring these cells into IL-2
containing medium without PPD. Specific blocking
activity could be detected in the culture supernatants
one week after transfer into IL-2 medium. In one
experiment that was monitered frequently, this activity
increased in the first month to 1200 ng/ml antigen
equivalents and then declined to a stable value of about
200 ng/ml. Table 1 shows that after 3 weeks in culture
the cells proliferated specifically in response to PPD.

Table 1.   Proliferative response of an IL-2 dependent
           PPD-stimulated cell line.

HuIL2	Ag (mg/ml)	CPM PPD	CPM CGG	CPM KLH
–	0	10,120	10,120	10,120
–	0.01	63,231	7,843	9,316
–	0.05	82,645	5,794	2,618
–	0.10	94,197	11,653	2,228
+	0	72,760		

Cultures contained 1 x 10^5 PPD blast cells (after 3
weeks in culture w/25% human IL-2) and 5 x 10^5
autologous irradiated HPBL.   After 2 days incubation
cultures were pulsed with 1 µCi/well ^{3}H-TdR and
harvested 24 h later.

   Because the supernatant from the cell line contained
IL-2 it could not be tested directly for antigen-specific
biological activity in the CTL assay.   This material was
purified by affinity chromatography on PPD-Sepharose.
The eluted ThF contained no detectable IL-2 (data not
shown).   It retained blocking activity and specifically
enhanced the CTL response of B6 thymocytes stimulated
with D2 adherent cells when these cells had been pulsed
with PPD (Table 2).   Presumably the role of PPD in this
assay is to bind the ThF to the stimulator thus retaining
it in the assay system.   We have yet to determine the
ultimate cellular target of the ThF.

Table 2.   Biological Activity of ThF-PPD purified from
           the supernatant of a PPD specific IL-2 dependent
           line.

Stimulators ThF Source	Percent Specific Lysis[b] PPD-pulsed	without PPD
Control	7.0	4.5
IL-2 Line[a]	28.0	10.0

a)   ThF-PPD was purified from a PPD-specific, IL 2
     dependent T cell line maintained at 4 x 10^5
     cells/ml.   Fifty ml of supernatant was applied to a
     PPD-sepharose column, and the bound factor was

eluted with 50 ml of 2 M NaCl and dialyzed against
PBS. The factor was tested at a final concentration
of 17 ng/ml PPD equivalents.

b)   Percent specific lysis (E/T = 50/1) of unmodified D2
     targets by CTL generated in cultures of B6
     thymocytes stimulated with PPD pulsed or non-pulsed
     D2 adherent cells. All cultures contained added
     factor or control.

3. T-cell Hybrids
     Three to four weeks after their initiation, IL-2
dependent cells from the lines were fused with HTL-1, a
HAT sensitive variant of a human T-cell leukemia line.
The surface phenotype of HTL-1 is shown in Table 3.
After 2 weeks the supernatant from the fusion wells were
tested for blocking activity and the cells from the
positive wells were cloned by limiting dilution. In our
first 2 fusion experiments the frequency of positive
wells was 1 in 48. Subsequently, this value was
increased to 6 wells in 48 by decreasing the ratio of
lymphocytes to HTL-1 from 10/1 to 2/1 in the fusion
mixture. Table 4 shows the blocking data for
supernatants from one of the positive clones and
subclones derived from it.

Table 3. Surface phenotype of the HTL-1 fusion partner
          by FACS analysis

Marker	Percent Positive
Leu 2	5
Leu 3	75
Leu 4	26
HLA-DR	3
HTLV-1	2

Table 4.   Blocking activity of T-cell hybrid supernatants
           and ThF preparations

Source	Blocking Activity ng/ml PPD
A4 Crude S/N[a]	270
A4 Crude S/N Conc. 5X (Amicon)	571
HTL Crude S/N Conc. 5X	14
A42 Crude S/N	199
Purified ThF from A42 Conc. 40X	8,500
A426 Crude S/N	671
A4263 Crude S/N	428

a)   In all cases, the supernatant was harvested from
     cells were grown to a concentration of 10^6/ml.

b)   A42 supernatant was passed over PPD-Sepharose, bound
     factor was eluted with 0.2 N NH_4OH and
     lyophilized. Test material was reconstituted in PBS
     at 40x concentration based on the original volume of
     supernatant. Recovered blocking activity based on
     the original volume = 212 ng/ml.

Blocking activity in the crude supernatant from A4
could be concentrated using Amicon membranes with a
molecular weight cut off of 10,000 daltons. A
substantial amount of activity was lost in this
procedure. We found that many of our T-cell hybrids lost
function over a period of weeks in culture. Thus it was
necessary to reclone at frequent intervals to maintain
functional hybrids. Clone A42 retained activity and was
studied in detail. As shown in Table 4 the blocking
activity in the supernatant of this clone could be
recovered quantitatively by absorption and elution from
PPD-Sepharose columns. Affinity purified factors from
this hybrid and from a derivative A4263 recloned by
limiting dilution and single cell transfer were active in
the biological assay. Table 5 shows that ThF purified
from the supernatant of A4263 markedly enhanced the CTL
response of B6 thymocytes stimulated with D2 adherent
cells. In the absence of added ThF neither PPD pulsed
nor unmodified adherent cells stimulated this response.
The antigen specificity of the PPD-ThF is indicated by

the selective enhancement of the response to PPD-pulsed
stimulators. Note that stimulation by material purified
from the supernatant of the hybrid A4B2 or the fusion
partner HTL-1 was not antigen specific in that it did not
depend on the presence of PPD on the surface of the
stimulating cell. None of these samples contained
detectable levels of IL-2 as assessed by their inability
to maintain the growth of an IL-2 dependent CTL line.

Table 5. Biological activity of ThF-PPD purified from
the supernatant of T-cell hybrids

| Stimulators | Percent Specific Lysis | |
	PPD pulsed	Without PPD
ThF Source		
0	4.0	1.0
A 4263[a]	22.0	9.2
A 4263[b]	53.0	19.0
A4B2[a]	8.2	8.2
HT1-1 parent	15.2	15.0

a) ThF-PPD was purified from the superantants of cells
grown to a cell density of 10^6/ml. Five hundred
ml of supernatant were passed over a PPD-Sepharose
column, and the bound factor was eluted with 50 ml
of 2 M NaCl and dialysed against PBS. ThF was
tested at 20 ng/ml PPD equivalents.

b) As b, except the bound factor was eluted with 0.2 N
NH_4OH, lyophilized and tested at 80 ng/ml PPD
equivalents.

4.   Presence of MHC markers on ThF-PPD
      Data in Table 6 shows that ThF-PPD from both a PPD
cell line and T-T cell hybridoma A42 bears I-region
determinants. ThF-PPD blocking activity can be removed
by anti HLA-DR antibodies. This characteristic is
consistent with data on ThF from other sources reported
in the literature (1,3,10).

Table 6. Removal of antibody inhibition activity by anti
          HLA-DR antibodies

ThF	Anti HLA-DR	Blocking Activity Recovered ng/ml PPD
IL-2 Line	-	213
	10 µg	15
	60 µg	5
A 42	-	182
	10 µg	36
	60 µg	0
PBS	60 µg	0

ThF from IL 2 line and A 42 hybrid were purified over
PPD-Sepharose columns.

ACKNOWLEDGEMENTS

      This work was supported by a Terry Fox Special
Initiatives Grant from the National Cancer Institute of
Canada. We wish to thank Dr. Denis Burger for the gift of
the HTL-1 cell line and Dr. Michael Weaver for performing
the FACS analysis of its surface phenotype. We also wish
to thank Mrs. Soo Jeet Teh for her able technical
assistance and Susan Heming for typing the manuscript.

REFERENCES

1. Tada, T., and Okumura, K. Adv. Immunol. 28, 1-87
    (1980).
2. Moses, E., Eshhar, Z. and Apte, R.N. Lymphokines 5,
    223-252 (1982).
3. Webb, D.R., Kapp, J.A. and Pierce, C.W. Ann. Rev.
    Immunol. 1, 423-438 (1983).
4. Kilburn, D.G. et al. Nature 277, 474-475 (1979).
5. Fischer, A., Beverley, P.C.L. and Feldmann, M.
    Nature 294, 166-168 (1981).
6. Lanzavecchia, A., Ferrarini, M. and Celada. Eur. J.
    Immunol. 12, 468-474 (1982).
7. Kurnick, J.T. et al. Scand. J. Immunol. 11, 131-136
    (1980).
8. Kilburn, D.G., Crane, S., Altin, M., J. Immunol.
    Methods 67, 193-200 (1984).
9. Krowka, J.F. et al. J. Immunol. in press.
10. Lehner, T. Immunol. 48, 695-702 (1983).

INFLUENZA SPECIFIC CYTOTOXIC T-CELL CLONES AND IMMUNE INTERFERON

B.A. Askonas & P. Pala

National Institute for Medical Research

The Ridgeway, Mill Hill, London NW7.

ABSTRACT

We have examined several aspects of IFN-γ secretion by murine influenza A virus specific cytotoxic T-cell (Tc) clones. IFN-γ secretion is H-2 restricted and depends on contact of Tc with antigen (influenza A infected cells). There is an inverse relationship between IFN production and rapid cellular proliferation of Tc but T-cell mitogens induce IFN at all stages of cell growth. Treatment of Tc with recombinant IFN-γ had no effect on cytolytic activity of cloned Tc or a Tc line. Nor could we find any effect on generation of influenza specific Tc when recombinant IFN-γ is added during the in vitro induction of Tc. Thus we have no evidence that IFN-γ affects Tc proliferation or maturation. The influenza system does not lend itself to test IFN-γ effects on target cells, since it inhibits influenza virus expression on the cell surface of IFN susceptible cells.

INTRODUCTION

Immune interferon (IFN-γ) in addition to its antiviral action is an important regulator of the immune system. Recent studies have shown that interferons enhance NK activity (see review[1]); IFN-γ increases or induces the expression of MHC class I and/or II antigens in certain cell types[2], activates macrophages and enhances production of

IL-1 (Bancroft, Vessey & Askonas, unpublished) and oxygen
radicals with resulting microbicidal activity (e.g.[3,4]). In
addition IFN-γ may serve as one of the B-cell maturation
factors[5,6]. The main source of IFN-γ are activated T-cells,
be they T-helper or cytotoxic T-cells (Tc)[7,8]. Both human
and murine T-memory cells[9,10] as well as T-cell lines or
clones have been shown to have the ability to produce
immune IFN[11-13] while virus infection of T-cells appears to
lead to the release of IFN-α[14]. The multiple action of
IFN-γ prompted us to examine several aspects of IFN-γ
production by influenza specific mouse Tc clones and also
to examine whether IFN itself affects the generation or
cytotoxic activity of Tc.

Tc CLONES AND INTERFERON SECRETION

The advantage of studying cloned T-cells is that we are
dealing with a single T-cell population rather than a mixed
one. It has become clear that Tc clones have the ability
to secrete IFN-γ but only in the presence of T-cell mitogens
or antigen. We have reported previously that IFN secretion
by our Tc clone L4 (grown in IL-2 containing medium in the
absence of antigen) depends on clonal recognition of syngeneic target cells infected with type A influenza virus,
while type B influenza infected or allogeneic A virus
infected target cells do not induce IFN-γ [11]. Secretion of
IFN-γ by Tc thus is antigen dependent and restricted to
class I MHC molecules. However, not all our influenza
specific Tc clones appeared to release IFN-γ although they
showed high levels of antigen specific cytotoxic activity.
Therefore recognition of target cells and their lysis is not
always a sufficient stimulus to induce IFN secretion[15].

This variability in IFN production in a series of
influenza specific Tc clones was assigned to changes in the
growth rate of the Tc clones[16]. Cloned Tc proliferate very
rapidly for a few days post antigenic stimulation. During
this rapid growth phase, further antigen contact does not
lead to IFN release; however, by day 4, the cloned cells
stop dividing and can be maintained viable in IL-2 containing media for up to 2 weeks. Contact with influenza
infected cells during this phase of very slow or non existent
proliferation leads to the secretion of IFN-γ . This may
reflect maturation of the cells. Electron microscopy shows
a great difference in the cytoplasmic organisation between

the rapidly growing Tc and the slow growth phase. Only the
latter Tc have a highly organised endoplasmic reticulum and
Golgi zone in the cytoplasma[15]. Concanavalin A treatment
of the cloned cells overcomes this variability in IFN
release by cloned Tc with growth rate, although some clones
do lose their ability to produce IFN-γ altogether in long
term tissue culture. Con A results in cellular aggregation
and gradual cell death and can also lead to non antigen
specific target cell lysis by binding target and effector
cells together, and thus reflects particularly strong
membrane interactions. There is a similar indication that
rapidly proliferating T-helper cell lines or clones do not
release IFN-γ [17]. This dissociation between T-cell proliferation and IFN-γ release presumably is important since
IFN is thought to have cytostatic potential also for lymphoid
cells and immune responses require expansion of antigen-
specific B- and T-cells. One might expect that in vivo,
during infections, T-cells mature in the tissues where the
pressure for continued growth is less than in vitro with a
continuous supply of excess growth factor and influenza
infected stimulator cells.

At no time has IL-2 on its own induced IFN secretion
by our Tc clones. Since membrane-membrane interactions
appear so essential for IFN secretion by T-cells, we have
examined whether antibody interactions with T-cell surface
proteins other than the antigen receptor, but important in
target cell recognition[18], would affect IFN-γ production.
We studied two influenza specific Tc clones. Monoclonal rat
antibodies to LFA-1 and Lyt-2 bound strongly to both Tc
clones T9/5 and BA4, but either monoclonal antibody strongly
inhibited target cell lysis only of clone BA4; cytotoxicity
of clone T9/5 was only slightly depressed (by 10-15%) by
these antibodies[16]. Capping of the Lyt-2 or LFA-1 molecules
by specific antibodies plus anti-rat immunoglobulin, did not
induce IFN production. However antigen induced IFN secretion was strongly inhibited by anti Lyt-2, while anti-LFA-1
had little effect[16]. Thus the Lyt-2 molecule has a role in
regulation of IFN secretion while LFA-1 is not involved.
The interesting resistance of clone T9/5 to anti-LFA-1
inhibition may reflect a particularly high affinity of its
antigen receptor and shows that LFA-1 is not always essential for target cell recognition.

IS IFN IMPORTANT IN THE PROTECTIVE ROLE OF TC IN
VIRUS INFECTION

The observations that Lyt2+ immune T-cells[19] and type A influenza specific Tc-cell clones can protect mice against lethal infection with influenza A virus or limit virus replication in the lungs of infected hosts[20,21] have raised the question as to whether immune IFN secretion by Tc plays an important role in preventing virus spread in vivo when infected cells are lysed, or in activating macrophages. Lukacher et al.[21] show that protection correlates with the virus specificity of the Tc clone; thus IFN-γ, if important, can act only at short distance to the recognized target cell. It has not been possible to give a final answer as to whether IFN-γ secretion by Tc plays a major role in anti-viral protection, although we had available Tc clones which possessed or lacked the ability to produce IFN-γ at certain phases of growth. However, only a small proportion of Tc clones tested have proved to be protective on adoptive transfer - and many others tested did not influence the course of influenza infection in view of their faulty migration properties regardless of their ability to produce IFN. T-cell clones have been found to lack a surface marker (MEL-14) important in lymphocyte homing. (I. Weissman, personal communication). Overall, it would be surprising if IFN-γ secretion by Tc would not contribute to the prevention of virus spread.

DOES IFN-γ AFFECT THE GENERATION AND CYTOLYTIC
ACTIVITY OF TC?

The effect of pure, preferably recombinant interferons on T-cells requires further investigation and the literature is controversial. To mention a few examples, several studies have reported that purified α/β interferons while inhibiting proliferation of T-cells in mixed lymphocyte reactions, enhanced the generation of human alloreactive Tc in vitro[24] or the specific cytotoxicity of sensitised lymphocytes[25]. High levels of purified IFN α/β preparations were added, but the effects on cytolytic function were small. In mouse, IFN-γ also inhibited TCGF dependent pro-liferation of mitogen induced T-cell blasts[26].

Since IFN-γ is active at very low concentrations on B-cell maturation[5,6] or in macrophage activation (eg.[4]), we

wished to see whether low levels of recombinant IFN-γ would
influence the <u>in vitro</u> induction of Tc or their effector
cytolytic function. Recombinant IFN-γ present in the
culture supernatant of gene transformed CHO (Chinese
Hamster Ovary) cells was a kind donation of Dr. P. Gray,
Genentech, USA, and its level of anti-viral activity re-
assayed in our laboratory since it lost activity on
transport[16]. We incubated Tc clone BA4 (at 2 x 10^5 cells/ml)
for 36 hours in medium containing 0.2 - 2.5 U IFN-γ /ml, or
control CHO cell medium, and then assayed the Tc cytotoxicity
on type B influenza, uninfected and type A influenza
infected P815 or YAC-1 target cells. Table 1 shows that
cytotoxicity remained the same whether or not BA4 cells had
been incubated with 2.5 U IFN-γ . There was no increase in
non-specific killing of B virus infected cells or lysis of
NK target cells. A Balb/c cytotoxic T-cell line kept in
culture for one month was treated overnight with high levels
(30 - 3000 U/ml) of purified mouse α/β (a kind gift of Dr.
A. Morris, Warwick University) but we did not observe any
change in cytolytic activity toward A-influenza infected or
uninfected targets (Table 2).

In contrast to experiments showing B cell maturation in
the presence of IFN-γ [5,6], we could not demonstrate any
effect on the level or kinetics of Tc generation. Spleen
cells from A influenza primed Balb/c mice were stimulated
with homologous virus-infected spleen cells[22]. After two
days, the cultures were treated with 0.2 - 18 U/ml of
recombinant IFN-γ for another 2 days. On day 4, T-cell
cytotoxicity levels were the same in the presence or
absence of IFN-γ. High levels (1000 U/ml) of IFN α/β or
partly purified IFN-γ similarly did not enhance the generation of Tc (not illustrated). We cannot exclude the possibility that a sufficient level of immune IFN is generated in
the polyclonal spleen cell cultures, so that further
addition of IFN-γ has no effect. Farrar et al[27] have
suggested that IFN-γ might act as T-cell maturation factor;
it is clear that pure cell populations and pure lymphokines
need to be examined before any conclusions can be drawn.

Thus we have no evidence that IFN-γ, at concentrations
which activate macrophages or increase antibody secretion,
affects either the induction or cytotoxicity of Tc.
However, one might expect that IFN-γ interaction with
infected cells leading to increased levels of expression of
MHC Class I or II molecules might make the cells more

susceptible to T-cell mediated lysis. This may apply
particularly when such cells express low levels of MHC
molecules on their surface. The influenza system does not
lend itself to test this point since in our experiments IFN
treatment of susceptible targets such as L-cells inhibited
influenza virus infections, while P815 cells for example
were totally resistant to IFN action.

ACKNOWLEDGEMENT

We should like to thank Dr. P. Gray (Genentech, San
Francisco) for sending us supernatants from CHO cells
transformed with a murine IFN-γ expression vector as well
as from control CHO cells.

TABLE 1

Recombinant IFN-γ treatment of Tc clone BA4 does not affect
its cytotoxicity.

Target cells	IFN-γ U/ml	% target cell lysis		
		K/T	2.5	1.3
AX31-P815	–	53	43	31
"	2.5	50	41	30
B/HK P815	–	1	1	0
"	2.5	2	3	0
– YAC-1	–	2	2	1
"	2.5	3	2	2
A/X31 YAC-1	–	2	5	0
"	2.5	2	1	0

The cytotoxicity assay and _in vitro_ culture of the influenza
specific Balb/c Tc clone BA4 have been detailed previously[16].

Target cells were ^{51}Cr-labelled P815 mastocytoma cells
infected with influenza A/X31 or B/HK virus[22] and the murine
NK susceptible YAC-1 cells ($\pm$ A/X31 infection). The recombinant IFN-γ [23] was in supernatants from CHO cells transformed with a cloned murine IFN-γ gene. Anti-viral activity
was titrated as described[16]. The Tc cells were treated with
IFN-γ for 36 hours at 37° before the cytotoxicity assay.
BA4 is a K^d-restricted clone[16]. YAC-1 is of H-2 K^{b}D^d origin
and is highly susceptible to NK cells.

TABLE 2

Overnight treatment of a Balb/c Tc line with IFN-α/β.

IFN-α/β	% Lysis of A/X31 infected targets		
	KT = 5	2.5	1.3
none	69	57	45
30 U/ml	68	64	50
300 U/ml	67	56	N.D.
3000 U/ml	68	59	53

The Balb/c Tc line P 11.0 was derived by stimulating spleen cells from influenza A/X31 virus primed mice three times in vitro with A/X31 infected macrophages[22] over a period of 4 weeks. Target cells were P815 mastocytoma cells infected with A/X31 virus[22]. No lysis of uninfected P815 cells was observed. The antiviral activity of purified IFN-α/β (a kind gift of Dr. A. Morris, Warwick University) was assayed in our laboratory as described previously[16].

REFERENCES

1. Moore, M. In Symp. 35 "Interferons", Society Gen. Microbiology, Cambridge University Press. pp 181-209 (1983).
2. Wong, G.H.W., Clark-Lewis, I., Harris, W.A. & Schrader, J.W. Eur. J. Immunol.14, 52-56 (1984).
3. Schultz, R.M. & Kleinschmidt, W.J. Nature (Lond.) 305, 239-240 (1983).
4. Nathan, C., Murray, H.W., Wiebe, M.E. & Rubin, B.F. J.exp.Med. 158, 670-689 (1984).
5. Sidman, C.L., Marshall, J.D., Schultz, L.D., Gray, P.W. & Johnson, H.M. Nature (Lond.) 309, 801-804 (1984).
6. Leibson, H.J., Gefter, M., Zlotnick, A., Marrack, P. & Kappler, J.W. Nature (Lond.) 309, 799-801 (1984).
7. Krammer, P.M. et al. Immunol. Rev. 76, 5-28 (1983).
8. Wilkinson, M. & Morris, A.G. In Symposium 35 "Interferons", Society Gen.Microbiology, Cambridge University Press. pp. 149-179 (1983).
9. Ennis, F.A. & Meager A. J.exp.Med.154, 1279-1289 (1981).
10. Nakayama, T. Infect. Immun. 40, 486-492 (1983).
11. Morris, A.G., Lin, Y-L. & Askonas, B.A. Nature (Lond.) 295, 150-152 (1982).

12. Klein, J.R., Raulet, D.H., Pasternack, M.S. & Bevan,
     M.J. J.exp.Med.155, 1198-1203 (1982).
13. Matsuyama, M., Sugamura, K., Kawade, Y. & Hinuma, Y.
     J. Immunol. 129, 450-451 (1982).
14. Cooley, M.A., Blackman, M.J. & Morris, A.G. Eur.J.
     Immunol. 14, 376-379. (1984).
15. Taylor, P.M. & Askonas, B.A. In "T Cell Clones" eds.
     H. von Boehmer & W. Haas. Elsevier Science Publishers,
     In press (1985).
16. Taylor, P.M., Wraith, D.C. & Askonas, B.A. Immunol.
     In press (1985).
17. Hecht, T.T., Longo, D.L. & Matis, L.A. J. Immunol. 131,
     1049-1055 (1983).
18. Springer, T.A., Davignon, D., Ho, M-K., Kurzinger, K.,
     Martz, E. & Sanchez-Madrid, F. Immunol. Rev. 68,
     171-195 (1982).
19. Yap, K.L., Ada, G.L. & Mackenzie, I.F.C. Nature (Lond.)
     273, 238-239 (1978).
20. Lin, Y.L. & Askonas, B.A. J.exp.Med. 154, 225-234 (1981).
21. Lukacher, A.E., Braciale, V.L. & Braciale, T.J. J. exp.
     Med. 160, 814-826 (1984).
22. Zweerink, H.J., Askonas, B.A., Millican, D., Courtneidge,
     S.A. & Skehel, J.J. Eur.J.Immunol. 7, 630-635 (1977).
23. Gray, P.W. & Goeddel, D.V. Proc.Natl.Acad.Sci.U.S.A. 80
     5842-5846 (1983).
24. Zarling, J. et al. J. Immunol. 121, 2002-2004 (1978).
25. Lindahl, P., Leary, P. & Gresser, I. Proc. Natl. Acad.
     Sci. U.S.A. 69, 721-725 (1972).
26. Leanderson, T., Hillörn, V., Holmberg, D., Larrson, E-L.
     & Lundgren, E. J. Immunol. 129, 490-494 (1982).
27. Farrar, W.L., Johnson, H.M. & Farrar, J.J. J. Immunol.
     126, 1120-1125 (1981).

THE IL-1 PATHWAY IN T CELL ACTIVATION

Phil Lake, Eve D. Robinson, Mark Brunswick,
Lex Cowsert and Tran C. Chanh

Lombardi Center, Georgetown University
Washington, D.C. 20007

INTRODUCTION

Almost without exception, normal T cells or their progeny require accessory cells (AC) or their products for activation and proliferation induced by mitogens, antigens and soluble anti-idiotypic antibodies. Despite many years of effort, the role of MHC products, interleukin-1 (IL-1) and other possible signalling systems of AC which promote T cell responses remain unclear. In this report we discuss a new IL-1-dependent human T cell activation system which contrasts with and illuminates properties of T cell activation pathways regulated by AC. The results show that IL-1 can promote IL-2 receptor expression on T cells and that signals other than IL-1 are required for T cell responses to lectin mitogens.

CHARACTERISTICS OF IL-1

IL-1 is a macrophage/monocyte-derived protein of 15,000 KD, also known as endogenous pyrogen (EP), epidermal cell-derived-thymocyte activating factor (ETAF), leukocyte endogenous mediator (LEM), lymphocyte activating factor (LAF), serum amyloid A-inducer, mononuclear cell factor and neutrophil releasing factor. It is pyrogenic and has been recently purified to homogeneity (1,2). IL-1 is a single chain polypeptide, which resists endopeptidases although human IL-1 is sensitive to α-chymotrypsin and following antibody-affinity purification shows biological activity at $1x10^{-11}M$ (3). It has at least three variant forms which may differ antigenically in the rabbit. IL-1 resists reduction and alkylation but is denatured by SDS and urea (4). CNBR-treatment inactivates IL-1, producing no active fragments, suggesting methionine residues at the active site.

FUNCTIONS OF IL-1

Most available evidence argues that IL-1 plays a central role in the host's defence against infectious agents. IL-1 is produced by monocytes or macrophages stimulated by constituents of microbial cell walls, such as lipopolysaccharides, peptidoglycans or glucans. The hormone then induces the antibacterial responses of the acute phase proteins which are quickly produced by hepatocytes, such as serum amyloid A (SAA), increases in serum fibrinogen, C reactive protein and others. It produces neutrophilia and induces human neutrophil lysosomal release of lysozyme and lactoferrin in vitro (5). EP/IL-1 may also stimulate bone marrow granulocytic colony formation as part of this inflammatory circuit. IL-1 also acts to enhance B and T cell responses to antigens and this IL-1 effect may be a common focus for the actions of adjuvants of immunity (6); IL-1 or ETAF are chemotactic for PMN and peripheral blood mononuclear cells (7) and induce fever which may be an important mechanism to enhance T cell proliferation responses (8).

IL-1 is also able to stimulate fibroblast growth in vitro (9) and their production of collagenase and prostaglandins. Thus IL-1 may participate in the fibrosis of chronic inflammation, wound healing and scar formation. An IL-1-like factor is also capable of stimulating bone chondrocytes to degrade proteoglycan and collagen, which may be important in inflammatory diseases with bone destruction (10). IL-1 is now recognized as an important component in many B and T cell responses eg., it may be necessary for the progression of B cells from the activated state to DNA synthesis (11,12). In view of the apparent heterogeneity of EP/IL-1 (13,14), the numerous above activities may not all reside in a single molecular species.

IL-1 can also be induced from macrophages or their lines by a range of substances, some of which may relate to injurious processes, such as silica or cell scraping, and by other agents, such as ds-RNA or amphotericin B or by activated T cells (15,16) on interaction with macrophages. Moreover, IL-1 may have a role in the stimulation of T cell development intrathymically (17).

IL-1 action has generally been studied directly by introduction of purified IL-1 preparations into experimental animals or cultures and measuring responses. In addition IL-1 has been anlyzed using antibodies to EP/IL-1 (18,19). These studies showed that B cell proliferation and antibody synthesis was blocked but not the responses of T cells to mitogens PWM, ConA or PHA. Inhibition of IL-1 effects by antibody have also been seen in vivo.

ASSAYS FOR IL-1

Biological activity of IL-1 has been detected in assays of fibroblast proliferation (2), the release of MIF activity from human T cells (20), the enhancement of proliferative responses of accessory cell-depleted PBL to ConA or PHA in man (15,21,22) and the more common murine thymocyte proliferation assay, usually in the presence of PHA (23).

These assays suffer from several problems. The fibroblast and human proliferation assays produce only small response indices (of the order of two-fold) to IL-1. In the human T cell response, this implies that only a fraction of cells capable of responding to lectin and accessory cells, can respond in the presence of lectin and IL-1. This renders analysis of IL-1 receptors and cell metabolism very difficult. Further, as seen in our laboratory, many donors do not show any IL-1-dependent responses to ConA or PHA. The situation is comparable in the thymocyte assay in which most cells die during culture, making analytical and metabolic studies very difficult.

In the course of these studies we observed that responses to the T-cell mitogen, PMA (24), were reconstituted by IL-1 prepared from silica-treated, adherent human PBMC. Further, dose-response analysis showed that responses of E^+ cells could be <u>fully</u> reconstituted by IL-1 while the responses of the same cells to PHA and ConA were only slightly reconstituted (Table 1). These data also show that the failure of IL-1 to reconstitute the PHA and ConA responses was not due to inhibitors present in the IL-1 supernatant since the addition of accessory cells to IL-1 restored the responses.

TABLE 1
Reconstitution of mitogen responses by E^+ cells or IL-1

Mitogen	E^+	$E^+ + E^-irr$	$E^+ + IL-1$	$E^+ + E^-irr + IL-1$
nil	19(2)	318(138)	22(2)	539(61)
PHA	3,104(1052)	181,453(1097)	12,987(2476)	169,404(2018)
PMA	410(99)	41,772(4514)	35,094(2772)	52,546(2711)
ConA	93(32)	57,443(5895)	2,270(614)	73,816(5270)

Response measured to PHA, 0.1%; ConA, 20 µg/ml; PMA, 1 µg/ml. IL-1 was at 10 U per ml. Each cell type was cultured at $2x10^4$ per well.

TABLE 2
Failure to absorb IL-1 by IL-1-responsive PMA-activated T cells

Absorbed at ^{0}C	Test dilution	Proliferative response(CPM) to IL-1 following absorptions with			
		E^+	PBL	PMA-E^+	nil
37^0	1:2	3,832	3,659	3,893	3,822
	1:8	2,741	2,988	4,172	3,014
	1:32	1,739	2,507	2,958	2,204
4^0	1:2	3,011	3,093	3,598	-
	1:8	3,988	2,853	3,633	-
	1:32	2,518	2,099	2,276	-

IL-1 was absorbed with $2x10^7$ cells in 1ml for 2h. At 1:2 IL-1 had approximately one-half maximal units per ml. Control: E^+ + PMA = 149(18), E^+ + IL-1 = 36(18)

The response of T cells to PMA has also been obtained with partly purified IL-1 (kindly provided by Dr. J. Oppenheim) which has no IL-2 activity, indicating that the response is controlled by this monokine and not by other products of adherent cells. Subsequent studies in our laboratory have shown that IL-1 must act within the first 36h of culture for proliferation to result (not shown), indicating a critical time for IL-1 action which lapses after cell activation.

RECEPTORS FOR IL-1

IL-1 is thought to act on target cells via extracellular membrane receptor sites, by analogy with other polypeptide, water soluble and long-acting hormone mediators. However this point has been difficult to establish. Two studies report the absorption of IL-1, first by a murine malignant T cell line which is reactive to IL-1 (25), and more recently by human peripheral blood T cells (20). We have attempted similar absorptions of limiting concentrations of IL-1 using resting T cells or PMA-activated (24h) human T cells at 4^0 and 37^0 for 2h. The results (Table 2) show that no absorption of IL-1 by activated T cells was detectable in this study, using cell concentrations similar to others, and despite the fact that the PMA-activated T cells are reactive to IL-1 during this 24h period. Weak absorption by non-activated E^+ cells was possibly present and is now being studied further. Our results suggest that the IL-1 receptor may exist in very low density on T cells or that the binding affinity for IL-1 is very low and may be reduced further upon cell activation.

MECHANISM OF IL-1 ACTION IN T CELL RESPONSES TO LECTINS AND ANTIGENS

To date little information is available on the immediate specific metabolic consequences of IL-1 signalling to T cells, since homogeneously reactive normal cells, with similar metabolic characteristics have not been available for study. Nevertheless, considerable evidence is available on subsequent cellular events, including the expression of new receptors, secretion of lymphokines and changes in cell cycle phase.

In recent years it has become clear that accessory cells (AC) are essential for T-cell responses to lectin mitogens (26), however the role of Ia, IL-1 and other possible signals from the AC remain unclear. In studies on human T cells a number of authors have shown that IL-1 can replace AC in these responses (15,21,22). However it is unknown, in all of these studies, whether the replacement is complete, partial or minimal, since dose comparisons of AC and IL-1 were never described. In our experience, using

T cells purified by E-rosetting, plastic adherence and Sephadex-G10 passage, it was found that T cells are only slightly reactive to ConA or PHA in the presence of IL-1, usually producing less than 10 percent of their response when mixed with optimal numbers of E^- irradiated cells. Our findings are in agreement with the conclusions of Lipsky et al. (19) using a different approach, with antibody to IL-1.

Thus IL-1 is either only one part of a more complex signal that AC deliver to lectin-stimulated T cells or an entirely different signal which weakly bypasses the normal pathway. It is clear that lectin alone causes G_0 to G_1 transition of resting T cells (21) and expression of new cellular receptors such as the IL-2 receptor. These activated cells respond to IL-2 (15,21) with proliferation.

In murine studies the role for IL-1 in T cell proliferation has been more clearly developed using similar approaches, perhaps since the lectins appear to act differently on murine T cells. Several groups showed that IL-1 functions in these lectin systems to promote T cell proliferation by facilitating the production IL-2 from T cells (27-30).

Glucocorticoids prevent IL-2 production, although they may not inhibit the responses of activated T cells to IL-2. This may cause the known suppression of IL-1 thymocyte responses by dexamethasone. A similar pathway appears to operate for T cell responses to PMA and IL-1, since the addition of antibody to the IL-2 receptor decreases the proliferative response (Table 3). Thus IL-2 appears to be a mediator for proliferation in PMA responses as well.

TABLE 3

Anti-Tac antibody diminishes IL-1-dependent T cell proliferation to PMA

Mitogen	Responding system	Proliferative response CPM		
		nil	Anti-Tac	Control ascites
PMA	PBL	47,442	29,512	49,266
PMA	E +IL-1(1:20)	56,716	39,311	56,145
PMA	E +IL-1(1:100)	50,888	34,967	49,330
nil	CTC+IL-2	2,356	19	2,241

Anti-Tac antibody was used at 3 µg/ml.

   IL-1 also regulates antigen-specific responses by T
cells.   In   several   studies,   antigen-pulsed AC were
inactivated   in   their   ability   to   present   antigen   to T
cells.   The response was then recovered by the addition of
IL-1 to these cultures of human (31) and murine cells (32).

   Most   if   not all of the above requirements   for   IL-1
could   be   explained   by   the induction of IL-2 production.
However, it is possible that IL-1 has additional functions,
eg.   it   has   been   shown   that   IL-2   receptor   density is
increased upon exposure of specific   T cells to antigen and
AC,   leaving   the   densities   of   other   surface   markers
unchanged (33,34).   IL-1 may have a role in this phenotypic
change, which would then   likely   act   to   promote   T   cell
responses via the IL-2 pathway.   This   phenomenon has been
recently shown to be true for a murine   T   cell   clone upon
reaction with anti-idiotype   (35).   IL-1 promotion of IL-2
receptor   expression   has   also   been observed   in   T   cell
responses to PMA (Table 4).   Thus   T cell proliferation in
man   also appears to follow the path of an autocrine   loop,
including the production of, and response   to,   IL-2.   IL-2
itself may be an inducer of IL-2   receptors,   although   the
significance of this finding is unclear (31).

TABLE 4

IL-1 augments expression of IL-2 receptors and T-11
antigens but not HLA-DR or T-1 on PMA-activated T cells.

Fluorescent cells

Donor	Monoclonal antibody	(% positive / mean channel intensity)			
		E^+ only	E^+ +IL-1	E^+ +PMA	E^+ +PMA+IL-1
A	Tac	23/113	8/ 53	38/178*	56/312***
	OKT11	96/112	85/129	97/285*	80/370***
	HB	15/ 83	18/ 88	23/110*	20/110*
	OKT1	75/117	48/102	82/427*	82/306*
B	Tac	16/ 90	11/ 75	32/135*	61/297***
	OKT11	95/176	87/125	89/458*	94/763***
	HB	19/93	20/101	32/145*	30/124*
	OKT1	69/89	97/95	90/466*	87/428*

Cell phenotype after 3d of culture. HB antibody to
HLA-DR. * indicates enhanced antigen expression.

TABLE 5
Inhibition of ConA but not PMA-induced PBL responses with an anti-DR monoclonal antibody

	Proliferative response (CPM) Dilution of antibody ascites		
Mitogen	1:100	1:1000	nil
PMA	21,837	22,572	23,937
ConA(10)	38,905	76,870	76,978
ConA(2.5)	7,336	13,323	41,890
ConA(1)	4,945	7,985	27,705

PBL were stimulated with either PMA (100 ng/ml) or ConA (at 10 to 1 µg/ml) in the presence of antibody 56.105 to HLA-DR antigens.

ROLE OF Ia ANTIGENS

The role of class II MHC antigens in lectin-induced responses and their relation to IL-1 action is not clear. In murine models, anti-Ia monoclonal antibody blocks lectin-induced proliferation (37) in which AC function is replacable by IL-1. This has been confirmed in rat cell responses in which anti-Ia antibodies blocked IL-2 production and cell proliferation, which was reconstituted by IL-1 (38). It is unclear however, if the reconstitution involves responses of the same T cells and the same pathways. Contrary results however were obtained in human studies (15), where no inhibition by monoclonal anti-DR antibody and a rabbit xenoantiserum to DR antibodies was seen in response to ConA. Since the action of monoclonal antibodies are known to be site-specific, several anti-DR antibodies were tested in our laboratory. The results show that responses to ConA but not to PHA were substantially blocked by some, but not all, anti-DR antibodies. Thus the activation of macrophages for T cell signalling with some lectin mitogens may involve DR molecules. An example is shown in Table 5, in which an anti-HLA-DR monoclonal antibody blocks responses of PBL to ConA but not to PMA. These results suggest a relationship between ConA stimulation pathways and HLA-DR molecules, but one which is ConA-dose-dependent (Table 5). Thus at high doses, ConA may compete more effectively with antibody or bypass this interaction, using an alternate path for cell stimulation. PMA responses appear to be independent of these Ia-antibody inhibitory effects as also seen for PHA, even at limiting concentrations (not shown). However this subject is complex as revealed by the AC function of several putatively DR-negative cell lines for T-cell response to ConA and PHA (39). Such cells may employ different signals from those active in normal human E⁻ cells.

SUMMARY

IL-1 is produced by several differentiated cell types and acts on a variety of target tissues important in immunological and inflammatory responses. Investigation of IL-1 action has been limited by bioassays using malignant or heterogeneous cells or assays having low indices of response. Responding cells consist of mixed populations in which only a minority of cells respond. Bioassays with human cells show that IL-1 only minimally replaces accessory cell function to lectin mitogens. We now report that proliferative responses of purified T cells to the phorbol ester mitogen PMA are <u>fully</u> reconstituted by IL-1. IL-1 control of of T cell responses to PMA involves IL-2, since anti-Tac antibody inhibits cell proliferation and since <u>IL-1 acts to augment IL-2 receptor expression</u>. The OKT11 antigen is similarly enhanced in its expression by IL-1, although OKT-1 and HLA-DR are not. Thus T-11 is now seen to be a quantitative activation marker of human T cells. Ia antigens appear to participate in responses of human T cells to low doses of ConA, but appear to be irrelevant in PHA and PMA responses. Thus the role of accessory cells in PMA-induced T cell responses appears to be limited to IL-1 production, while different functions of accessory cells are required for responses to ConA, PHA and possibly other mitogens.

ACKNOWLEDGEMENTS

We thank Dr. T. Waldmann for the anti-Tac antibody and the Office of Naval Research for support. The opinions expressed herein are those of the authors and are not to be construed as those of the Department of the Navy or the Department of Defence.

REFERENCES

1. Mizel,S.B. and Mizel,D., J. Immunol. 126, 834-837 (1981).
2. Schmidt, J.A., J. exp. Med. 160, 772 -787, (1984).
3. Mizel,S.B., Dukovich,M. and Rothstein, J., J. Immunol. 131, 1834-1837 (1980).
4. Mizel, S.B., Molec. Immunol. 17, 571-577 (1980).
5. Klempner, M.S., Dinarello, C.A. and Gallin, J.I. J. Clin. Inv. 61, 1330 (1978).
6. Staruch, M.J. and Wood, D.D., J. Immunol. 130, 2191-2194, (1983).
7. Luger, T.A., Charon, J.A., Colot, M., et al, J. Immunol. 131, 816-820 (1983).
8. Duff, G.W., and Durum,S.K., Nature 304, 449-451, (1983).
9. Schmidt, J.A., Mizel, S.B., Cohen, D. et al., J. Immunol. 128, 2177-2182 (1982).
10. Gowen, M., Wood, D.D., Ihrie, E.J. et al., Nature 306, 378-380 (1983).
11. Howard, M., Mizel, S.B., Lachman, L., et al., J. exp. Med. 157, 1529-1543 (1983).
12. Falkoff, R.J.M., Muraguchi, A., Wong, J.X., et al., Immunol. 131, 801-805, (1983)
13. Mizel, S.B., Oppenheim, J.J. and Rosenstreich, D.L., J. Immunol. 120, 1504-1508 (1978).
14. Murphy, P.A., Cebula, T.A., Levin, J., et al., Infect. Immunol. 34,177, (1981).
15. Palacios, R.,J. Immunol. 128, 337-342, (1982)
16. Rosenstreich, D.L. and Oppenheim, J.J., Immunobiology of the Macrophage, Academic Press, 162-201, (1976)
17. Rock, K.L. and Benacerraf, B., Proc. Natl. Acad. Sci. USA 81, 1221-1224, (1984).
18. Oppenheim, J.J., Luger, T., Sztein, M.B., et al., Self Defence Mechanisms: Role of Macrophages, Elsevier, 127-136, (1982).
19. Lipsky, P.E., Thompson, P.A., Rosenwasser, L.J., et al., J. Immunol. 130, 2708-2714, (1983).
20. Bendtzen, K. and Dinarello, C.A., Scand. J. Immunol. 20, 43-51, (1984).
21. Maizel, A.L., Mehta, S.R., Ford, R.J. et al., J. exp. Med., 153, 470-475, (1981).
22. Koretsky, G.A., Elias, J.A., Kag, S.L., et al., Clin. Immunol. and Immunopathol. 29, 443-450, (1983).
23. Gery, I., Gershon, R.K., and Waksman, B.H., J. exp. Med. 136, 128-142, (1972).

24. Touraine, J.L., Hadden, J.W., Touraine, F. et al., J. exp. Med. 145, 460-465, (1977).
25. Gillis, S. and Mizel, S.B., Immunol. 78, 1133-1137, (1981).
26. Rosenstreich, D.L., Farrar, J.J. and Dougherty, S., J. Immunol. 116, 131-139, (1976).
27. Larsson, E.L., Iscove, N.N. and Coutinho, A., Nature 283, 664-667 (1980).
28. Smith, K.A., Lachman, L.B., Oppenheim, J.J., et al., J. exp. Med. 151, 1551-1556.
29. Shaw, J. Kaplan, B., Paetkaw, V., et al., J. Immunol. 124, 2231-2239, (1980).
30. Farrar, J.J., Mizel, S.B., Farrar, J.F., et al., J. Immunol. 125, 793-798, (1980).
31. Scala, G. and Oppenheim, J.J., J. Immunol. 131, 1160-1166, (1983).
32. Defreitas, EC., Chesnut, R.W., Grey, H.M., et al., J. Immunol. 131, 23-29, (1983).
33. Hemler, M.E., Brenner, M.B., Mclean, J.M., et al., Proc. Natl. Acad. Sci. USA 81, 2172-2175, (1983).
34. Andrew, M.E., Braciale, V.L. and Braciale, T.J., J. Immunol. 132, 839-844, (1984).
35. Kaye, J., Gillis, S., Mizel, S.B., et al., J. Immunol. 133, 1339-1345, (1984).
36. Reem, G.H. and Yeh, N.H., Science 225, 429-430, (1984).
37. Kimura, A. and Ersson, B., Eur. J. Immunol. 11, 475-483, (1981).
38. Gilman, S.C., Rosenberg, J.S. and Feldman, J.D., J. Immunol. 130, 1236-1240 (1983).
39. Wakasugi, H., Harel, A., Dokhelar, M.C., et al., Proc. Natl. Acad. Sci. USA 80, 6028-6031, (1983).

SESSION VIII
T Cell Clones and Anti-Tumour Immunity

Chairpersons: P.W. Askenase and M. Feldmann

The specificity and functional importance of the cellular arc of the immune system in anti-tumour immunity has been hampered both by the failure to identify tumour specific antigens and the use of polyclonal T cell populations. However, the ability to isolate monoclonal populations of T lymphocytes offers the opportunity to reassess the specificity, phenotype and functional role of T cells derived from patients with maligant disease. Dr Vose reported that the frequency of tumour reactive lymphocytes was significantly higher in tumour infiltrating as compared to peripheral blood lymphocytes for a number of different malignancies. The analysis of T cell clones isolated from cocultures of lymphocytes with tumour cells revealed that the majority proliferated in response to autologous tumour and not to allogeneic tumour cells of the same site and histology. Specificity for autologous tumour was also observed for cytotoxic T cell clones. As a cautionary note Dr Vose commented on the importance of separating tumour reactivity from that directed against differentiation antigens for example. Dr Spits described $T4^+$ and $T8^+$ cytotoxic T cells that had been cloned from peripheral blood lymphocytes activated with autologous tumour either from patients with melanoma or B lymphoma. The CTL clones appeared to recognize surface molecules on the autologous tumour cells but not the control cells of many types. Interestingly, lysis of B lymphomas was not MHC restricted. The implications of this observations remain to be more fully explored, but it is possible that these T cells recognise non polymorphic parts of HLA. Lysis of autologous tumour cells was not dependent on T3, T4 or T8 antigens, although some but not all CTL clones could be inhibited by anti-LFA-1 antibodies. Thus different accessory structure appear to be involved in tumour recognition as compared to reactivity to MHC antigens.

Dr Vyakarnam investigated T cell immunity to tumours using a system whereby foreign antigens are coupled to tumour cells to make them more immunogenic. Murine helper T cell clones reactive to the carrier protein in this case PPD were able both to induce antibody and enhance anti tumour immunity. Using the same approach it was

401

demonstrated that PPD reactive human helper (T4$^+$) T cell clones in addition to inducing anti-tetanus antibodies, lysed EBV transformed B cells of the appropriate MHC Class II specificity to which PPD had been coupled by Con A.

Dr Bolhuis described the functional characterisation of cloned cytotoxic lymphocytes that were phenotypically either T3$^-$ or T3$^+$. The T3$^-$ clones displayed higher levels of cytolytic activity and broader target recognition than the T3$^+$ clones. In addition PHA and anti-T3 antibody had no effect on the T3$^-$ clone whereas for T3$^+$ clone non specific unrestricted lytic activity was enhanced and allospecific lysis inhibited. Thus suggesting that the T3 antigen is involved in cytolysis mediated by T3$^+$ cytotoxic T cells.

The analysis of T cell clones has allowed an antigen specific T cell component to be identified in human anti-tumour immunity. Thus the characterisation and functional analysis of these T cells should provide information on the T cell antigens involved in recognition and the regulation of immune responses to tumours, and may permit the elucidation of how tumours usually evade or overcome the immune system; and lead to ideas for new therapeutic strategies.

T CELL CLONES RECOGNISING AUTOLOGOUS TUMOUR CELLS

B.M. Vose

ICI Pharmaceuticals Division plc, Mereside,

Alderley Park, Macclesfield, Cheshire.

INTRODUCTION

The ability to dissect immune parameters in situ by
immunohistology and in vitro by a variety of assays has
resulted in an increasing awareness of the complexity of
the host-tumour relationship. The correlation in some
tumours between infiltration by leukocytes and prognosis
offered preliminary indications of the effectiveness of the
anti-tumour response (1,2). More recently, it has been
possible by staining of sections to show the presence of
macrophages, T helper and T cytotoxic/suppressor cells and
B lymphocytes in a wide range of tumours using specific
monoclonal antibodies. In addition, several groups have
been able to purify T lymphocytes and macrophages from the
tumour and demonstrate proliferative and cytotoxic activity
against autologous tumour cells (reviewed in 3).
Surprisingly, there has been general agreement that cells
of the natural killer cell phenotype, so often championed
as a mediator of anti-tumour surveillance, are poorly
represented in situ and this observation is supported by
functional studies of isolated tumour-infiltrating
lymphocytes (TIL). We now know that the host response to
neoplasia is mediated by heterogeneous effector populations
directed against antigens the nature of which remains, for
the most part, unknown. The ability to sensitise patient
lymphocytes to autologous tumour in vitro, to clone and
expand them in interleukin-2 for several months offered new
opportunities to explore the specificity of the

reactions observed; studies which had previously been
limited by the lack of material. In this report our
experience with the enumeration and cloning of anti-tumour
effectors is detailed.

THE FREQUENCY OF TUMOUR-REACTIVE LYMPHOCYTES

     Using limiting dilution (LDA) techniques (4) we have
addressed the following questions:- 1) does the tumour
represent a site of T lymphocyte activation such that
exposure to mitogen-free preparations of interleukin-2
(IL-2) is sufficient to induce clonal expansion 2) is the
frequency of IL-2 responsive cells increased by inclusion
of autologous tumour cells in the LDA microwells 3) how
many of the T cells that can be expanded represent
precursors of specific cytotoxic precursors or NK-like
cells. Tumour tissue from patients with malignancy of the
lung, breast, colon or ovary was dispersed by treatment
with a mixture of collagenase hyaluronidase and DNAase.
Lymphocytes and tumour cells were separated on
discontinuous gradients of Lymphocyte Separation Medium and
by passage through nylon columns as described previously
(4). Tumour infiltrating lymphocytes (80% UCHT1[+], 40%
OKT4[+], 40% OKT8[+] and 10% TAC[+]) were plated in increasing
numbers in 96 well, round bottomed microtest plates with
2.5×10^4 irradiated (3000R) blood mononuclear cells as
feeders and an optimal concentration of conditioned medium
containing IL-2. Micro-mixed lymphocyte tumour cultures
(MLTC) contained 1.5×10^4 irradiated, freshly isolated
autologous tumour cells. In all experiments nylon column
passed peripheral blood lymphocytes (80% UCHt1[+]. 60% OKT4[+],
25% OKT8[+]   4% TAC[+]) were also cultured under the same
conditions as TIL. Proliferation in wells was assessed by
uptake of ^{3}H-thymidine at day 7 and cytotoxic precursor
analysis was performed with ^{51}Cr-labelled autologous or
allogeneic tumour or K562 on day 10 of culture. In 15
patients examined the mean proliferative frequency in
response to IL-2 was 1/1,920 ± 1,816(SD) in TIL and 1/6,057
± 3,162 (SD) in PBL. There was a broad range of response
frequencies in TIL (1/180-1/5,500) and PBL
(1/1,060-1/12,600) in the different patients but
differences between the two sites were statistically
significant. Responding cells had the T cell phenotype so
that differences between TIL and PBL were not attributable
to proliferation of tumour cells.

Inclusion of autologous tumour cells significantly increased the proliferative frequency of 9/14 PBL and 5/9 TIL such that 1/1,084 ± 512 TIL responded with a range of 1/180-1/4,050). In the lung cancer group response was less varied with between 1/180 and 1/600 TIL responding in the presence of tumour compared with 1/560-1/4,100 expanded in IL-2 alone. These data indicated that the tumour was, indeed, a site of lymphocyte activation (increased number of TAC^+ cells and response to IL-2) and that the frequency of IL-2 responsive cells was increased by cocultivation with autologous tumour cells (4). The tumour is then a rich source of T cells recognising autologous cells.

Further studies examined the frequency of cytotoxic precursors among the MLTC activated cultures. The major cytotoxic activity found in MLTC was directed against autologous tumour cells and represented approximately 1/2-1/4 of proliferating cells in different patients. Expansion of NK-like cells which were cytotoxic for the K562 cell line was also apparent but at a low frequency (< 1/2000). Thus, while the frequencies of response to IL-2, the frequencies of MLTC reactors and autologous tumour cell cytotoxic precursors were highest in the TIL, the frequency of NK precursors was highest in the PBL samples. Similar studies on the frequency of specific cytotoxic precursors have been performed in murine systems and elevation of their frequency in tumour reported (5).

ACTIVATION CONDITIONS FOR THE INDUCTION OF CYTOTOXIC ACTIVITY AGAINST AUTOLOGOUS TUMOUR

Studies over a number of years have shown that, in a proportion of patients, T lymphocytes with cytotoxic activity against autologous tumour in short-term ^{51}Cr release assays can be found in the peripheral blood, tumour-draining lymph node and tumour (6-7). There is now evidence from a number of groups that cytotoxic activity can be induced in previously non-reactive samples by cultivation with autologous tumour (MLTC) (7,8), interleukin-2 (9,10), lectins (11) or with pooled allogeneic lymphocytes from single or multiple donors (MLC) (12,13). With many of these stimulation protocols, cytotoxicity is apparent against a range of NK susceptible and non-susceptible targets and the exact nature of the effector population has remained in doubt. The

difficulties have been compounded by the finding that NK
cells, as well as T cells can expand in IL-2 and that the
former frequently adopt a mature T cell phenotype. Thus,
the establishment that killers are, for example, OKT3[+] does
not in itself indicate the derivation of the cells. From
purified OKT3 large granular lymphocytes (the effectors of
NK) we and others have been able to derive cloned
populations of cells with the ability to lyse K562 and
which express OKT3,4 and 8 but not OKM1 or OKT10 (14,15).
In the activation protocols listed above there are clearly
several possibilities to explain the killing of autologous
tumour. These include 1) The activation and expansion of
specific tumour reactive T cell clones. 2) The expansion
of cells activated in vivo and responsive to IL-2 added to
the culture or produced upon stimulation with lectin or in
MLC. 3) The activation and expansion of alloreactive cells
which would lyse tumour cells as a result of their
expression of inappropriate histocompatibility antigens
(16). 4) Activation of NK cells by IL-2 of γ interferon.
It was in an attempt to study these possibilities that T
cell clones were derived from MLTC and MLC activated
patients lymphocytes and tested for their reactivity
against autologous tumour cells and K562.

CLONAL ANALYSIS OF EFFECTOR CELLS IN CYTOTOXIC AND PROLIFERATIVE ASSAYS

Cloning of tumour-reactive T lymphocytes induced in
MLC or MLTC was performed using the limiting dilution
conditions described above. Patients lymphocytes (1 x
10^6/ml) were cultured with irradiated (3000R) autologous
tumour in RPMI + 10% heat-inactivated autologous plasma in
$25cm^2$ tissue culture flasks at a responder-stimulator ratio
of 5:1. In MLC activation patients lymphocytes were
cultured under the same conditions with irradiated (3000R)
lymphocytes pooled from 4 healthy donors (responder:
stimulator ratio 1:1). After incubation at 37°C for 6 days
blasts were isolated on discontinuous Percoll gradients as
previously described (17) and dispensed into round-bottomed
culture flasks at different dilutions together with 2.5 x
10^4 pooled, irradiated allogeneic feeder cells and IL-2.
After 14 days wells with obvious growth were taken where
10% or less of wells were positive and were considered as
"clones". They were placed in 1ml cultures in RPMI + 10%
human plasma + IL-2 and 2.5 x 10^5 feeder cells. Cells then

grew to a concentration of $5 \times 10^5 - 1 \times 10^6$/ml and could
be maintained for 3-4 months. Thereafter responsiveness to
IL-2 was lost and cultures died. Because of the limited
growth potential of these cells it was not possible to
reclone and the assignation of clonality was made purely on
statistical grounds. Clones were tested for their capacity
to be restimulated by autologous tumour or control cells in
primed lymphocyte tests (PLT) or for cytotoxicity in
short-term ^{51}Cr release assays against a range of targets.

PROLIFERATIVE ACTIVITY OF CLONES

In proliferation assays of pool-MLC activated clones 15
underwent secondary stimulation with the majority (11)
reacting to a single member of the inducing pool. A single
clone was reproducibly restimulated by autologous
monocytes. Three clones were restimulated by more than one
pool member. Since all cultures were derived from wells
seeded with several cells it was not clear whether this was
a true cross-reactivity or simply a result of growth of
more than one cell in the wells. None of the clones
responded to autologous tumour: a finding in accord with
results with bulk cultures of the stimulated T cells (17).
Thus, under these conditions MLC stimulation resulted in
the activation of alloreactive T cells. By contrast,
MLTC-derived proliferative clones (12 isolated) most
frequently responded to autologous tumour and to allogeneic
tumour of the same site and histology. They did not
respond to autologous monocytes or allogeneic lymphocytes
or tumour from different site or from the same site
different histology. A single clone responded to
allogeneic lymphocytes used as feeders in the cloning
procedure but not to autologous tumour and a further single
clone responded only to autologous tumour. Again these
results are similar to those obtained with bulk culture of
MLTC stimulated lymphoblasts reported previously (18) and
emphasis that the MLTC is an efficient way of activating T
cells recognising autologous tumour.

CYTOTOXIC ACTIVITY OF CLONES

MLTC-stimulated clones regularly lysed cells of the
autologous tumour in the absence of similar activity
against allogeneic tumour of the same site and histology,

autologous monocytes, K562 or allogeneic lymphoblasts i.e.
reactivity was tumour specific as far as tested. A similar
situation was found with pool-MLC activated cells where
7/22 clones lysed autologous tumour specifically suggesting
the presence of individually specific antigens or
restriction of killing by histocompatibility. It is not
clear why the MLC was effective in inducing cytotoxic but
not proliferative clones reactive with tumour. After MLC
activation 6/48 clones lysed K562 and other NK susceptible
targets and many clones lysed lymphoblasts from single pool
members. It was, therefore, possible to identify within
the MLC-pool-stimulated population cytotoxic clones
specific for autologous tumour, specific for allogeneic
determinants or with NK-like activity. No correlation
between function and phenotype were apparent in this
series. The presence of tumour-specific killers within the
MLC-stimulated population which did not lyse K562 or
allogeneic lymphoblasts of the pool supports the view that
the mechanism of induction of activity against autologous
tumour cells under this protocol is by expansion of in vivo
activated cells rather than induction of NK-like activity
or sharing of histocompatibility antigens between tumour
and pool members.

NATURE OF THE ANTIGENS RECOGNISED

Work over a number of years has established optimal
conditions for the induction of MLTC reactivity in cancer
patients (19). This work has now been extended to show PLT
and cytotoxic reactivity in cultured T cells and clones
with a high level of specificity for tumour. No cytotoxic
response against freshly isolated cells from autologous
normal lung tissue (6) or against autologous monocytes or
lymphoblasts has been found. However, in a recent
publication the induction of proliferation by autologous
normal tissues (lung, liver and small bowel) as well as
tumour, was reported (20). These data do not negate the
finding with MLTC but do necessitate further investigation
of this complex reaction at the clonal level to attempt to
separate tumour reactivity from that directed against
normal tissue or differentiation antigens (M. Lotze,
experiments in progress). It is only when these studies
have been completed and further investigation of the
apparently specific cytotoxicity against autologous tumour

have been performed that the true significance of the
recognition of autologous tumour cells by T lymphocytes
can be assessed.

ACKNOWLEDGEMENTS

This work was supported by the Cancer Research
Campaign of Great Britain and performed at the Paterson
Laboratories, Christie Hospital and Holt Radium Institute,
Manchester, England. The author is grateful to the many
colleagues who were involved in the studies and to Mavis
Brightwell for preparation of the manuscript.

REFERENCES

1.   Hambin, M.E. Brit. J. Cancer, 22, 383-401, 1968.
2.   DiPaola, M., Angelini, L., Bertolotti, A. and Colizza,
     S. Brit. Med. J., 4, 268-270, 1974.
3.   Vose, B.M. and Moore, M. Seminars in Haematology, in
     press.
4.   Vose, B.M. Int. J. Cancer, 30, 135-142, 1982.
5.   Brunner, K.T., MacDonald, H.R. and Cerottini, J-C. J.
     Exp. Med., 154, 362-373, 1981.
6.   Vose, B.M. Cell Immunol., 55, 12-19, 1980.
7.   Vanky, F.T., Vose, B.M., Fopp, M. and Klein, E. J.
     Nat. Cancer Inst., 62, 1407-1413, 1979.
8.   Vose, B.M., Vanky, F.T., Fopp, M. and Klein, E. Int.
     J. Cancer, 21, 588-593, 1978.
9.   Vose, B.M. and Moore, M. Imm. Lett., 3, 237-241,
     1981.
10. Hersey, P., Bindon, C., Edwards, A., Murray, E.,
     Phillips, G. and McCarthy, W.H. Int. J. Cancer, 28,
     695-703, 1981.
11. Mazumder, A., Grimm, E.A., Zhang, H.Z. and Rosenberg,
     S.A. Cancer Res., 42, 913-918, 1982.
12. Zarling, J.M., Raich, P.C., McKeough, M. and Bach,
     F.H. Nature, 262, 691-693, 1976.
13. Strausser, J.L., Mazumder, A., Grimm, E.A., Lotze,
     M.T. and Rosenberg, S.A. J. Immunol., 127, 266-271,
     1981.

14. Grimm, E.A., Ramsey, K.M., Mazumder, A., Wilson, D.J., Djeu, J.Y. and Rosenberg, S.A. J. Exp. Med., 157, 884-897, 1983.
15. Allavena, P. and Ortaldo, J.R. J. Immunol., 132, 2363-2369, 1984.
16. Bach, F.H., Bach, M.L. and Zarling, J.M. Lancet, I 20-22, 1978.
17. Vose, B.M. and White, W.J. Cancer Immunol. Immunother., 15, 227-236, 1983.
18. Vose, B.M. and Bonnard, G.D. Nature, 296, 359-361, 1982.
19. Vanky, F. and Sjernsward, J. In: Immunodiagnosis of Cancer (eds. Herberman, R.B., McIntire, K.R.), 999-1032 (Dekker, New York, 1979).
20. Grimm, E.A., Vose, B.M., Chu, E.W., Wilson, D.J., Lotze, M.T., Rayner, A.A. and Rosenberg, S.A. Cancer Immunol. Immunother., 17, 83-89, 1984.

CELL SURFACE DETERMINANTS ASSOCIATED WITH THE INTERACTION OF HUMAN CTL CLONES AND AUTOLOGOUS TUMOR CELLS

H. Spits, H. Yssel and J.E. de Vries

The Netherlands Cancer Institute

Plesmanlaan 121, 1066 CX   Amsterdam

INTRODUCTION

Activation of peripheral blood lymphocytes (PBL) of tumor patients by mitogenic lectins (1), allogeneic lymphocytes (2) or autologous tumor cells (3-5) has been shown to result in the generation of cytotoxic lymphocytes that are able to lyse autologous tumor cells in vitro. These findings indicate that in these lymphocyte bulk cultures clones of cytotoxic lymphocytes with auto-tumor reactivity are generated. The aim of the studies described here was 1) to isolate cytotoxic T lymphocyte (CTL) clones with auto-tumor reactivity from mixed lymphocyte tumor cell cultures (MLTC) in which PBL of melanoma of B-lymphoma patients were cocultivated with irradiated autologous melanoma or autologous B-lymphoma cells (6,7); 2) to analyse the specificity of these CTL clones, and 3) to study the specific recognition- and interaction structures associated with CTL clone - autologous tumor cell inter-action.

ISOLATION AND CHARACTERIZATION OF CYTOTOXIC T-LYMPHOCYTE (CTL) CLONES THAT LYSE MELANOMA CELLS

CTL clones with anti-melanoma reactivity were isolated from a mixed leukocyte tumor cell culture in which peri-pheral blood lymphocytes (PBL) from a melanoma patient were cocultured with autologous melanoma cells as described

previously (6). Two CTL clones were selected for further
investigation. CTL clone O-C7 was T4+, whereas CTL clone
O-D5 was T8+. In addition both CTL clones were T3+, but
lacked the markers for NK cells, OKM-1 and HNK. Both clones
lysed efficiently autologous short term cultured melanoma
cells, but failed to react with autologous fibroblasts and
autologous ConA blasts (6). In addition to their reactivity
with autologous melanoma cells, both CTL clones reacted
with approximately 60% of the allogeneic melanoma cells
tested. In contrast, in a panel of target cells derived
from normal and non-melanoma tissues, including many carcinomas and neuroblastomas, O-C7 and O-D5 lysed only 1 and
2/25 cells, respectively. These data indicate that it is
feasible to isolate CTL clones which react in a non-HLA
restricted way with determinants preferentially expressed
on melanoma cells.

T-CELL ANTIGENS INVOLVED IN THE INTERACTION BETWEEN
CLONED CTL AND AUTOLOGOUS MELANOMA CELLS

Previously we have shown that T3, T4 and T8 are involved in the cytotoxic reactivity of T4+ CTL clones
directed against class II MHC antigens, and T8+ CTL clones
directed against class I MHC antigens (8-10). To test
whether these differentiation antigens also play a role in
the activity of CTL against autologous melanoma cells,
blocking studies with monoclonal antibodies were carried
out. As expected antibodies against T3, T8 and LFA-1
blocked the cytotoxic reactivity of CTL clone JR-2-16
directed against HLA-A2 (10), expressed on the O-mel melanoma cells (Table 1). In contrast, none of the anti-T3,
anti-T4, anti-T8 or anti-LFA-1 antibodies inhibited the
reactivity of O-C7 and O-D5 against the autologous O-mel
cells. These results suggest that the interaction and
recognition mechanisms of the anti-melanoma CTL clones
differ from those of CTL clones directed against HLA
antigens.

CHARACTERIZATION OF THE SURFACE DETERMINANTS ON
MELANOMA CELLS RECOGNIZED BY CTL CLONES

The reactivity of the CTL clones against allogeneic
melanoma cells already indicated that the activity of O-C7
and O-D5 is not restricted by HLA products. However, it

Table 1. Effect of Monoclonal Antibodies Directed Against Determinants Expressed on T Lymphocytes on the Reactivity of the CTL Clones with Anti-Melanoma Reactivity

CTL clone	target cell	% inhibition in the presence of			
		α-T3 (n=5)[1]	α-T4 (n=1)	α-T8 (n=3)	α-LFA-1 (n=2)
O-C7 (T4$^+$)	O-mel	-6±3	4±4	NT	13±4
O-D5 (T8$^+$)	O-mel	-11±4	NT	-10±2	5±2
JR-2-16 (T8$^+$)	O-mel	40±5	NT	46±4	38±5
(α-HLA-A2)	JY	74±4	NT	51±5	75±6

[1]nr. of different monoclonal antibodies tested
E/T ratio 5 : 1

could not be excluded that these clones recognize "alien" HLA antigens, which may be expressed on human melanoma cells. Therefore blocking studies were carried out with monoclonal antibodies (m.a.) directed against class I and class II MHC antigens. The m.a. W6/32 (anti-HLA-A,B,C), SPV-L3 (HLA-DC) (11) and Q 5/13 (HLA-DR) (12) did not inhibit the reactivity of the CTL clones against the autologous melanoma cells, in spite of the fact that these m.a. were found to react with the O-mel cells (Table 2). Furthermore, it is shown that the reactivity of CTL clone JR-2-16 (which is specific for HLA-A2) is strongly inhibited by W6/32. These results indicate that the reac-

Table 2. The Effect of Monoclonal Antibodies Directed at Class I and Class II MHC Antigens on the Reactivity of CTL Clones with Anti-Melanoma Reactivity

CTL clone	% ^{51}Cr-release	% inhibition in the presence of		
		Q 5/13 (HLA-DR)	SPV-L3 (HLA-DC)	W6/32 (HLA-A,B,C)
O-C7 (T4$^+$)	53	0	0	4
O-D5 (T8$^+$)	32	3	2	0
JR-2-16 (T8$^+$) (α-HLA-A2)	60	0	0	<u>83</u>

[1]E/T ratio 5 : 1

Table 3. Phenotype and Specificity of CTL Clone BK-5 Cyto-
          toxic for Autologous Melanoma Cells

CTL clone	phenotype	target cells BK-mel	BK-blasts % specific ^{51}Cr-release	BK-fibr	K562
BK-5	T3[+] T8[+]	56	4	13	8[1],46[2]

[1]4 weeks in culture; [2]9 weeks in culture; E/T ratio 2.5:1

tivity of the CTL clones against the autologous O-mel cells
is not directed against "alien" HLA molecules.

In order to characterize the antigenic determinants
expressed on human melanoma cells, monoclonal antibodies
were produced against another short term cultured melanoma
BK. These monoclonal antibodies were selected on their
capacity to inhibit the cytotoxic reactivity of CTL clone
BK-5 which had a reaction pattern comparable to that of
O-C7 and O-D5. BK-5 was T3[+] T8[+] but lacked the markers for
NK cells, OKM-1 and HNK (Table 3). It lysed the autologous
short term cultured BK melanoma cells but failed to react
with autologous BK fibroblasts or BK ConA blasts. Although
this clone initially had no NK-like activity as measured
against K562, it acquired cytotoxic reactivity after prolonged culturing. Panel studies revealed that BK reacted
preferentially with melanoma cells and to a much lower
extent with target cells from normal and non-melanoma
tissue, including many carcinomas and neuroblastomas
(Table 4).

Preliminary studies indicated that one m.a. raised
against BK melanoma cells, designated AMF-6A, was found to
block in two different experiments the cytotoxic reactivity

Table 4. Reactivity of BK-5 Against Allogeneic Melanoma
          Cells and a Panel of Different (Tumor) Target Cells

	nr cytotoxic/nr tested
allogeneic melanoma cells	5/7 (71%)
normal and non-melanoma tumor cells	2/15 (13%)[1]

[1]The two target cells killed by BK-5 were: K562 and U937

Table 5. Effect of Monoclonal Antibody AMF-6A on the
Anti-Melanoma Reactivity of CTL clone BK-5

CTL clone	target cell	W6/32	Q 5/13	SPV-L3	AMF-6A	SPV-L5
		monoclonal antibodies				
		% inhibition of cytotoxicity				
BK-5	BK-mel	5	-11	10	47	32
	K562	-2	-5	3	-7	44
HG-31 (α-HLA-B7)	BK	59	NT	0	4	NT

of CTL clone BK-5 against the autologous BK melanoma cells,
whereas the non-specific cytotoxic reactivity of BK-5
against K562 was not inhibited. A typical experiment is
shown in Table 5. AMF-6A did not inhibit the cytotoxic
reactivity of CTL clone HG-31 (10) which reacted specifically with HLA-B7 expressed on the BK-melanoma cells. In
addition it is shown that the reactivity of CTL clone BK-5
against autologous BK melanoma cells was not inhibited by
the m.a. W6/32 (anti-HLA-A,B,C), Q 5/13 (anti-HLA-DR) or
by SPV-L3 (anti-HLA-DC). However, in contrast to the anti-
melanoma CTL clones O-C7 and O-D5, BK-5 was found to be inhibited by SPV-L5 which reacts with human LFA-1 (13).
Although more inhibition studies with AMF-6A have to be
carried out, these preliminary data suggest that the monoclonal antibody AMF-6A and the CTL clone BK-5 react with
the same determinant expressed on BK-melanoma cells.

Table 6. Distribution of the Antigen Detected by
Monoclonal Antibody AMF-6A

	melanoma	other normal and non-melanoma tumor cells
cultured cells/cell lines (membrane immunofluorescence)	14/14	0/26
frozen sections (immune peroxidase staining)	7/7	2/38 compound naevus perineurium

DISTRIBUTION OF THE ANTIGEN DETECTED BY M.A. AMF-6A

Analysis of the distribution of the antigen detected by AMF-6A showed that it reacted with 14/14 cultured melanoma cells, whereas no reactivity was observed with 25 other normal and non-melanoma tumor cells including many carcinomas and neuroblastomas (Table 6). Additional screening on frozen tissue sections demonstrated that AMF-6A reacted with 7/7 melanomas whereas only 2/38 other tissues were found to react with AMF-6A. Normal skin melanocytes which are regarded to be the normal counterparts of melanoma cells were found to be negative, but a clear positive reaction was found with naevus cells. Also perineurium stained weakly with AMF-6A. This distribution pattern suggests that the antigen detected by AMF-6A can be considered as a normal pigment cell differentiation antigen.

Biochemical analysis in SDS-PAGE of the antigen detected by AMF-6A revealed that this antibody under reduced conditions precipitated a bimolecular complex of one band with a MW of >450.000 D and a second band with an estimated MW of 250.000 D. In addition to the distribution pattern of the antigen described above, these data suggest that AMF-6A reacts with a molecule similar to the chondroitin sulphate proteoglycan described by other laboratories (14-16).

Taken together these results illustrate that CTL clones can recognize and interact with surface determinants preferentially expressed on human melanoma cells. This reactivity seems not to be restricted by HLA, suggesting that the anti-melanoma CTL clones can react with these proteoglycans as such.

ISOLATION AND CHARACTERIZATION OF CTL CLONES WITH ANTI-LYMPHOMA REACTIVITY

CTL clones that lyse preferentially tumor cells of the same histological type could not only be obtained from melanoma patients, but we could also generate a similar CTL clone (MWS-14) from an MLTC in which T cells were repeatedly

activated by fresh non-cultured autologous B lymphoma cells
(7). Analysis to the specificity of two subclones of MWS-14
showed that both subclones, MWS-14-30 and MWS-14-34, were
T3+ T4+ and DR+. They lysed the fresh autologous MWS B-
lymphoma cells efficiently, but had no effect on autologous
ConA blasts or EBV-transformed normal B cells of this donor
(7). MWS-14-30 had NK-like activity as measured against
K562, whereas the NK-like activity of MWS-14-34 was
negligible. This difference in reactivity of both subclones
was possibly related to tissue culture conditions, since
after prolonged culture also MWS-14-34 developed NK-like
reactivity against K562 (not shown).

Panel studies revealed that both CTL clones lysed 7/7
allogeneic B lymphoma cells. In contrast, only 4/31 and
2/31 target cells derived from various normal and non-
lymphoma (both lymphoid and non-lymphoid) tumor tissues
were lysed. The cytotoxic reactivity against the lymphoma
cells could not be attributed to a non-specific intrinsic
susceptibility of lysis by CTL since the lymphoma cells
were found to be very resistant to lysis by MLC blasts, PHA
blasts and cells from a NK-cell clone (7).

Table 7. The Effect of Monoclonal Anti-MHC Antibodies on
the Cytolytic Activity of CTL clones against MWS Lymphoma[1]

CTL clone	% ^{51}Cr- release	% inhibition in the presence of		
		SPV-L3	Q 5/13	W6/32
MWS-14	41	0	0	0
JR-2-19 (DC-1)	25	90	0	2
JR-2-10 (DRw6)	32	0	50	0
JR-2-16 (HLA-A2)	53	0	0	83

[1]HLA phenotype MWS: HLA-A1,2;B8,w52;Cw3,w7;DRw3,6

Table 8. The Effect of Monoclonal Anti-T Cell Antibodies
on the Activity of the T4+ CTL Clones MWS-14 and JR-2-19
                 Against MWS Lymphoma Cells

CTL clone	% ^{51}Cr-release	% inhibition in the presence of		
		SPV-T3b	OKT-4A	SPV-L5
MWS-14	42	0	5	35
JR-2-19	25	72	50	85

THE EFFECT OF M.A. AGAINST CLASS I OR CLASS II MHC ANTIGENS ON THE CYTOTOXIC REACTIVITY OF THE ANTI-LYMPHOMA CTL CLONES

Similar to the anti-melanoma clones it was found that
MHC antigens are not involved in the cytotoxic reactivity
of the anti-lymphoma CTL clones (Table 7). Monoclonal antibodies against class I (W6/32) and class II (Q 5/13, anti-
HLA-DR, and SPV-L3, anti-HLA-DC) inhibited the activity of
CTL clones specific for HLA antigens present on MWS
lymphoma cells but not the activity of the anti-lymphoma
CTL clones MWS-14-30 and MWS-14-34. These results indicated
that the reactivity of MWS-14-30 and MWS-14-34 was not
directed against class I or class II MHC antigens or
"alien" HLA antigens and that their reactivity was not restricted by HLA products.

THE ROLE OF T CELL DIFFERENTIATION ANTIGENS IN THE ACTIVITY OF CTL CLONE MWS-14 AGAINST AUTOLOGOUS LYMPHOMA CELLS

Blocking studies with various m.a. directed against
T3 and a anti-T4 m.a. indicated that T3 and T4 antigens
were not associated with the reactivity of these CTL clones
directed against lymphoma cells (Table 8). In contrast,
anti-T3 and anti-T4 antibodies effectively blocked the
cytotoxic reactivity of the control CTL clone JR-2-19,
which is directed against HLA-DC1 expressed on the MWS
lymphoma cells. Furthermore, the reactivity of the MWS-14
subclones and JR-2-19 could be blocked by anti-LFA-1.
       The notion that T3 was not involved in the cytotoxic
reactivity of the anti-lymphoma CTL clones was supported by
the finding that modulation of the T3 antigen had no effect
on the anti-lymphoma reactivity of MWS-14. After 24 hrs
incubation at 37°C in the presence of anti-T3, the T3
antigen was almost completely modulated (Table 9). However,

Table 9. The Effect of Modulation of T3 on the Activity
of MWS-14 and JR-2-19 against MWS Cells

CTL clone		% cytotoxicity	
	control	T3-modulated	T3-modulated 1 µg/ml ConA
MWS-14	40	30	30
JR-2-19	25	5	23

The cells were incubated with 1:100 diluted SPV-T3b (anti-
T3) for 24 hrs at 37°C and then washed 5 times. 98% of the
T3 antigen was removed from both clones as determined by
FACS analysis.

the cytotoxic reaction of MWS-14 against the autologous
MWS-14 lymphoma cells was not affected. In contrast, modulation of T3 from CTL clone JR-2-19 which is specific for
DC-1 (DRw2, DRw6) expressed on the lymphoma cells resulted
in a strong reduction of its cytotoxic reactivity. The
cytotoxic reactivity of JR-2-19 could be restored by the
addition of ConA indicating that the lack of reactivity was
not due to a general loss of cytolytic reactivity of the
CTL clone.

CONCLUDING REMARKS

It is shown that $T4^+$ and $T8^+$ CTL clones which kill
preferentially autologous and allogeneic tumor cells from
the same histological type can be isolated from peripheral
blood lymphocytes of tumor patients after activation with
autologous tumor cells in vitro. Although some of these
CTL clones were cytotoxic for K562 or acquired NK-like
activity upon prolonged culturing, their reactivity pattern
was too restricted to consider these CTL clones as a
special subset of NK cells. In addition the CTL clones with
anti-tumor reactivity did not react with the m.a. OKM-1 and
HNK which react with NK cells. The CTL clones with anti-
tumor reactivity recognized surface molecules preferentially expressed on melanomas or B-cell lymphomas. It could
be excluded that this cytotoxic reactivity was directed
against "alien" HLA antigens since the monoclonal antibodies directed against class I or class II MHC antigens
were unable to inhibit the cytotoxic reactivity of these

CTL clones with anti-tumor cell reactivity. Preliminary data indicated that the cytotoxic reactivity of a CTL clone against autologous melanoma cells could be inhibited by a monoclonal antibody which possibly reacts with a chondroitin sulfate proteoglycan. This antigen was found to be expressed on all melanomas tested and on naevi cells. Since normal melanocytes were found to be negative, this antigen can be considered as a normal pigment cell differentiation antigen. T3, T4 and T8 antigens that are involved in the cytotoxic reactivity of CTL clones directed against MHC antigens were not associated with the cytotoxic reactivity of the CTL clones with auto-tumor reactivity. However, the reaction of some, but not all of the anti-tumor CTL clones could be inhibited by monoclonal antibodies directed against human LFA-1, indicating that LFA-1 antigens in some cases are required for the expression of cytotoxicity. Taken together these data indicate that we deal here with a novel type of CTL clones, since the recognition and interaction mechanisms required for the reactivity against the antigens preferentially expressed on human tumor cells are different from those involved in the reactivity against MHC antigens.

REFERENCES

1. Grimm, E.A., Ramsey, K.M., Mazumber, A., Wilson D.J., Djeu, J.Y. & Rosenberg, S.A. J. Exp. Med. 155, 1823-1831 (1982).
2. Zarling, J.M., Robins, H.I., Raich, P.C., Bach, F.H. & Bach, M.L. Nature 274, 268-271 (1978).
3. Zarling, J.M., Raich, P.C., McKeough, M. & Bach, F.H. Nature 262, 691-693 (1976).
4. Vanky, F., Gorsky, T., Gorsky, Y., Masucci, M.G. % Klein, E. J. Exp. Med. 155, 83-92 (1982).
5. Mukerdji, B. & McAllister, T.J. J. Exp. Med. 158, 240-245 (1983).
6. De Vries, J.E. & Spits, H. J. Immunol. 132, 510-514 (1984).
7. Yssel, H., Spits, H. & De Vries, J.E. J. Exp. Med. 160, 239-254 (1984)
8. Spits, H., Yssel, H., Thompson, A. & De Vries, J.E. J. Immunol. 131, 673-682 (1983).
9. Spits, H., Borst, J., Terhorst, C. & De Vries, J.E. J. Immunol. 129, 1563-1569 (1982).

10. Spits, H., Breuning, M.H., Ivanyi, P., Russo, C. & De Vries, J.E. Immunogenetics 16, 503-512 (1982).
11. Spits, H., Borst, J., Giphart, M., Coligan, J., Terhorst, C.P. & De Vries, J.E. Eur. J. Immunol. 14, 299-304 (1984).
12. Quaranta, V., Walker, L.E., Pellegrino, M.A. & Ferrone, S. J. Immunol. 125, 1421-1426 (1980).
13. Spits, H., Keizer, G., Borst, J., Terhorst, C., Hekman, A. & De Vries, J.E. Hybridoma 2, 423-437 (1983).
14. Harper, J.R., Bumol, T.F. & Reisfeld, R.A. J. Immunol. 132, 2096-2104 (1984).
15. Hellström, I., Garrigues, H.J., Cabasco, L., Mosely, G.H., Brown, J.P. & Hellström, K.E. J. Immunol. 130, 1467-1472 (1983).
16. Wilson, B.S., Imai, K., Natali, P.G. & Ferrone, S. Int. J. Cancer 28, 293-300 (1981).

T3$^-$ AND T3$^+$ CLONED CYTOTOXIC LYMPHOCYTES: FUNCTIONAL AND

PHENOTYPIC CHARACTERISTICS

R.L.H. Bolhuis and R.J. van de Griend

Rotterdam Radiotherapeutic Institute, Rotterdam and Radiobiological Institute TNO, Rijswijk, The Netherlands.

INTRODUCTION

Cytotoxic effector cells can be divided into two major groups: 1) Natural Killer (NK) cells, lymphocytes from, e.g., peripheral blood, endowed spontaneous with non-specific and MHC' nonrestricted cytolytic activity against NK susceptible target cells such as K562 without deliberate prior antigenic stimulation. Most of these cells also show antibody-dependent cellular cytolysis (ADCC). They generally have the phenotype T3$^-$, B73.1$^+$, T4$^-$, T8$^{-/+}$, T11$^+$, OKM1$^-$ and the morphological appearance of large granular lymphocytes (LGL). Minor subpopulations with partially different characteristics may also exist;
2) cytotoxic T lymphocytes (CTL) having MHC restricted cytolytic activity after prior antigenic stimulation, e.g., after mixed lymphocyte culture (MLC). Their cytolytic activity is directed against target cells presenting the relevant stimulator antigens. Nonspecific cytolytic activity of MLC responder cells against, e.g., K562 but no ADDC, has been reported earlier (1) and has been defined as activated killer (AK) cell activity. They have the phenotype T3$^+$, B73.1$^-$ and usually T8$^+$, T11$^+$, OKM1$^-$. About 10% of cytolytic T-cell clones are reported to be T3$^+$, T8$^-$, T4$^+$ (2).

We have developed a culture system for cloning and rapid expansion of both T3$^-$ and T3$^+$ clones (3) which enabled us to compare the phenotopic and functional characteristics of these two major categories of cytotoxic effector cells. The culture system involves the use of a mixture of feeder cells, i.e., irradiated lymphocytes and cells from an EBV transformed B-cell line (B-LCL) (4). By using this procedure, which also allows rapid expansion of T3$^+$ non-cytotoxic effector cells, we have cloned and expanded T3$^-$ and T3$^+$ effector cells from several normal individuals up to 10^9 cells in about 30- 40 days. Our results show that the clone derived from B73.1$^+$ and B73.1$^-$ fluorescence activated cell sorter cells and from MLC responder cells differ markedly in their cytolytic activities, cell surface phenotypes and their response to activation signals. Moreover, in contrast to T3$^+$ clones, T3$^-$ clones do not respond to certain activation signals. The functional and phenotypic heterogeneity within the group of T3$^-$ and T3$^+$ cloned effector cell types will be discussed.

MATERIALS AND METHODS
Generation of cytotoxic clones
T3 clones were obtained from either total peripheral blood lymphocytes (PBL) or cells enriched for T3$^-$ B73.1$^+$ cells by fluorescence activated cell sorting (FACS) or depletion of high affinity rosette forming cells at 29°C (E29° cells). Clones were obtained by limiting dilution in the presence of two types of irradiated feeder cells, e.g., allogeneic PBL and B-LCL cells as described in detail elsewhere (3, 5).

T3$^+$ clone n-4 was generated from the T3$^+$ fraction in parallel with the T3$^-$ clones. Clone D11 was derived after priming in MLC (6, 7) against the B-LCL BSM and then expanded with feeder cells. Clone G9 was derived from another donor, also after priming against BSM in MLC. Clone R1 was derived from a third donor by priming against APD. All clones were subsequently expanded in 96-well round bottom microtiter plates in a system that contained irradiated (40 Gy) allogeneic PBL (2 x 10^4/well) and irradiated (20 Gy) BSM + APD feeder cells (10^4/well) (for details, see refs. 3 and 4). The HLA phenotypes of the various B-LCL and tumour target cells were:

BSM: A2 Bw62 Cw3 Dw4,R4; APD: A1, Bw60,40.1, C- Dw6,Rw6; WVB: A2 Bw38 C- Dw6,Rw6; WEN: A2,w19 B12,40 Cw3,w5 DR4; LICR-LON: A2,3 Bw35,7 Cw3,w4 DR4,R6; O-Mel: A2,11 B8,w62 Cw3 DR3,4.

Phenotyping with monoclonal antibodies (MAbs)
Cell membrane phenotyping of cloned T cells was carried out by indirect immunofluorescence. Monoclonal antibodies (MAbs) OKT3,4,8,11 and OKM1 were obtained from Ortho Pharmaceutical Corp. (Raritan, NJ, U.S.A.). B73.1, which recognizes virtually all NK cells (8) was a gift from Dr. G. Tinchieri (Wistar Institute, Philadelphia, Pa., U.S.A.). As a second label, we used FITC-labeled goat-

anti-mouse IgG (Nordic, Tilburg, The Netherlands). After washing, the cells were analyzed on a FACS II, Becton Dickinson, Sunnyvale, CA., U.S.A.).

Inhibition or induction of cytolytic activity with MAbs
Cytolytic activity was determined by using ^{51}Cr-labelled target cells (10^3 per well) in a 3 hr assay. Inhibition by MAbs was determined by adding the MAbs to the effector cells and incubating this mixture for at least 30 min at 37°C before adding the target cells. The following dilutions were used: anti-class I (w6/32, Mas 032c), 1:100; anti-class II (HLA, DR 7.5.10.1 from Dr. F. Koning, Dept. of Immuno-Haematology, Academic Hospital, Leiden, The Netherlands), 1:100; anti-T3 (OKT3), 1:100; anti-T8 (OKT8 or FK-18; from Dr. F. Koning, see above), 1:100 or 1:1000, respectively; and anti T4 (OKT4), 1:100.
Induction of cytolytic activity was done by preincubation of effector cells for 30 min at room temperature (continuous shaking) with OKT3 (100 µg/ml/10^6 cells), SPV-T3c (a gift from Dr. H. Spits, Dept. of Immunology of the Netherlands Cancer Institute, Amsterdam, The Netherlands) (10 µl culture supernatant/10^6 cells) or PHA (10 µg/ml/ 5.10^5 cells). The PHA but not anti-T3 was then washed away and effector cells were seeded for cytotoxicity assay.

RESULTS

T3⁻ clones
T3⁻ cytotoxic effector cells were cloned from lymphocytes enriched for T3⁻ B73.1 cells by direct culture under limiting dilution conditions with feeder cells as previously described (9). All T3⁻ clones exerted strong cytolytic activity against a variety of tumour target cells and, without exception, also ADCC activity (40/40 clones tested).
The tumour cells lysed by a single clone included NK sensitive target cells (K562 and T-cell lines Molt4 and HSB); B-LCL cells (APD and BSM); class I negative B cells (Daudi); anchorage dependent target cells (T24 bladder carcinoma cells) and short-term cultured freshly biopsied melanoma cells (O-Mel) as well as LICR-LON human plasmacytoma cells (Table 1).
The majority of the clones showed the phenotype T3⁻, T4⁻, T8⁻, T11⁺, B73.1⁺ and formed rosettes with sheep red blood cells (E$_{sh}$ rosettes), confirming the binding of the OKT11 MAb, and formed rosettes with IgG coated ox erythrocytes confirming the binding of B73.1 MAb and ADCC. One clone (p+16) of 12 tested from one individual did not express T11 antigens and did not form rosettes with E$_{sh}$ and thus

Table 1.

CYTOLYTIC ACTIVITY OF T3⁻ ACTIVATED KILLER CELL CLONES

exp.	clone no.	K562	Molt-4'[1]	P815-IgG[2]	APD	BSM[3]	Daudi	T24	O-Mel
1	− 3	63	62	55	15	16	71		
	− 5	72	69	72	57	43	71	52	
	− 6	75	57	71	45	43	71	28	
	+ 1	66	63	44	24	36	69		
	+ 3	67	68	47	46	50	90		
2	+ 9	44		14	37		45		
	+10	75	45	32	30	35	70	67	65
	+15	66	44	37	8	34	58	75	84
	+16	64	55	37	11	26	36	83	68
	+17	47	25	20	7	27	49	34	59
3	292	28		16			27		
	293	38		41			14		
	299	42		38			41		
	300	60		35			69		
	302	35		28			47		
4	73	65		77			74	16	11
	75	54		75			72	18	14
	76	69		79			77	17	14
	77	75		77			85	53	46
	79	50		75			55	26	13

Results expressed as % ^{51}Cr-release in a 3 hr assay. Effector/target cell ratio 9:1.
[1] Similar results were obtained with the T cell line HSB.
[2] No cytotoxicity was observed against nontreated P815 cells.
[3] Other B-LCL cells such as WVB as well as the plasma cell leukemia derived cell line LICR-LON were also lysed by most of these clones.

had the phenotype of null cells. All T3⁻ clones expressed IL2 receptors as determined with the anti-Tac MAb (data not shown). Another clone showing the general phenotype of the T3⁻ clones additionally expressed T8 antigens on about 50% of the cells. Another clone (RG73) with identical phenotype was also derived from a patient with Tγ lympho-

Table 2.

FREQUENCY OF T3⁻ CYTOTOXIC CLONES GENERATED FROM PBL OF
NORMAL DONORS OR PATIENTS WITH T3⁻ Tγ LYMPHOCYTOSIS

donor	pre-enriched by	phenotype T3$^+$ (%)	B73.1$^+$ (%)	fresh/ frozen	cloning efficiency (%)	no. of clones tested total	T3$^-$CTX$^+$
1	FACS[2]	nt	84	fresh	5	7	7
2[3]	not	8	37	frozen	5	12	12
3	not	68	nt	frozen	<1	10	5
4	not	67	14	frozen	<1	9	0
5	not	67	nt	frozen	<1	8	1
6	not	78	nt	frozen	10	7	1
7	E29°$^-$	21	45	fresh	1	9	3
8	E29°$^-$	19	48	fresh	<1	3	0
9	E29°$^-$	16	30	fresh	1	6	5
10	E29°$^-$	45	11	fresh	<1	9	7
11	E29°$^-$	31	19	fresh	<1	4	0
12	E29°$^-$	12	39	fresh	2	8	8

'CTX$^+$ means: cytolytic activity against K562, P815-IgG as
well as Daudi cells is present.
²B73.1$^+$ cells were obtained by sorting and both B73.1$^+$ and
B73.1$^-$ fractions were cultured with or without leucoagglutinin (1 μg/ml).
³T3$^-$Tγ lymphocytosis patient (11).

cytosis. Most of the clones derived from the B73.1$^-$ fraction expressed the T3 antigen and did not exert lytic activity (see below).
The cloning efficiency (5%) of the T3$^-$ cells, in contrast
to that of T3$^+$ clones (5), was not enhanced by addition of
leucoagglutinin plus feeder cells to the culture medium.
Several T3$^-$ cytotoxic T-cell clone with broad target cell
specificities and various lytic activaties were generated
from 7 out of 12 individuals tested (Table 2). Cells from
two donors (1385 and 1354) were cultured for more than 30
generations with a calculated cell yield of more than 10^9
in about 40 days. The feasability of large scale expansion
of cloned lymphocytes from a panel of randomly choosen
blood donors is under study.

T3$^+$ clones
Clones derived from the B73.1$^-$ cell fraction and cloned
and expanded identically on the T3$^-$, B73.1$^-$ cells showed
the phenotype T3$^+$, B73.1$^-$, T4$^+$ or T8$^+$, OKM1$^-$, T11$^+$. Only

one clone out of 20 (clone n-4) showed appreciable cytolytic activity against various tumour target cells. At E/T
ratio of 20:1 the following lytic activities (% ^{51}Cr-
release) were obtained: 49, 15, 32, 77, 26 and 58 for BSM,
APD, LICR, Daudi, K562 and Molt-4, respectively. Although
this clone did not express the B73.1 antigen and hardly
formed (2%) rosettes with IgG coated ox erythrocytes, it
exerted significant ADCC activity. Some T3$^-$ clones exerted
low levels of lectin dependent cellular cytolysis (LDCC).
T3$^+$ cytotoxic clones were also derived from MLC responder
cells, using as stimulator cells Cw3$^+$ and DRW6$^+$ B-LCLs
(BSM and APD, respectively). The cells were then cloned
and expanded and three of them were studied in detail for
immune specific and nonspecific cytolytic capacity, phenotype and response to MAbs and lectin (D11, G9 and R1). The
clones showed the phenotype T3$^+$, B73.1$^-$, T4$^+$ or T8$^+$, T11$^+$,
OKM1$^-$.
The CTL clones lysed tumour target cells (K562), but
higher effector to target cell ratios were required and
lysis against K562 was not blocked by either anti-T3,
anti-T8 or anti-class I and II MAbs. The tumour target
cell specificities are presented in Table 3. No ADCC was
observed.

Table 3.

CYTOLYTIC ACTIVITY, SPECIFICITY AND SENSITIVITY FOR MAbs
IN CLONE D11 (T3$^+$, T4$^-$, T8$^+$)

target cell	E/T ratio	control	MAbs added		
			anti-class I	anti-T8	anti-T3
BSM	5:1	42	9	32	38
APD	80:1	0			
WEN	80:1	0			
WDV	80:1	0			
LICR	10:1	49	3	42	
Daudi	80:1	0			
O-Mel	20:1	38	4	42	33
Cw3$^+$Ly	20:1	0			
K562	40:1	37	38	41	45
Molt-4	80:1	0			
HSB	80:1	0			

Results as % ^{51}Cr-release in a 3 hr assay.

Clone D11 (Table 3) lysed the stimulator B-LCL BSM, but not lymphocytes expressing identical MHC class I or II antigens. Lysis was not blocked by anti-T3 or anti-T8 MAb, but surprisingly, anti-class-I MAb but not class II MAb blocked lysis of BSM as well as LICR-LON and O-Mel.

$T3^+$,$T8^+$ clone G9 (Table 4) was also primed against BSM cells and showed a similar tumour target cell specificity and level of lytic activities. No ADCC activity was detected. Clone G9 also showed Cw3 antigen specific cytolysis of all $Cw3^+$ B-LCLs and lymphocytes. The lysis of $Cw3^+$ B-LCLs and lymphocytes was inhibited by anti-class I as well as anti-T3 and T8 MAbs.

$T3^+$, $T4^+$ clone R1 (Table 5) showed only a low lytic activity against K562 target cells, but no other tumour target cells were lysed. No ADCC was observed. This clone also showed class II DRW6$^+$ specific lysis of B-LCLs and lymphocytes which could be inhibited by anti-class-II and anti-T3 and anti-T4 MAbs.

Table 4.

CYTLOYTIC ACTIVITY, SPECIFICITY AND SENSITIVITY FOR MAbs IN CLONE G9 ($T3^+$, $T4^-$, $T8^+$).

target cell	E/T ratio	control	MAbs added		
			anti-class I	anti-T8	anti-T3
BSM	3:1	44	1	0	29
APD	80:1	0			
WEN	80:1	60			
WDV	80:1	0			
LICR	10:1	50	6	1	
Daudi	80:1	0			
O-Mel	20:1	59	8	13	
Cw3$^+$ Ly	20:1	40			
K562	40:1	22	19	6	30
Molt-4	80:1	0			
HSB	80:1	5			

Results as % ^{51}Cr-release in a 3 hr assay.

Table 5

CYTOLYTIC ACTIVITY, SPECIFICITY AND SENSITIVITY FOR MAbs
IN CLONE R1 (T3$^+$, T4$^+$, T8$^-$)

target cell	E/T ratio	control	anti-class II	anti-T4	anti-T3
				MAbs added	
BSM	80:1	0			
APD	5:1	50	14	34	35
WEN	80:1	0			
WDV	40:1	30			
LICR	80:1	0			
Daudi	80:1	0			
O-Mel	80:1	5			
DRw6$^+$Ly	20:1	40			
K562	40:1	12			15
Molt-4	80:1	0			
HSB	80:1	0			

Results as % ^{51}Cr-release in a 3 hr assay.

Table 6.

ANTI-T3 M A AND PHA CAN INDUCE NONSPECIFIC CYTOLYTIC
ACTIVITY IN SOME T3$^+$ BUT NOT IN T3$^-$ CLONES AND FRESH NK
CELLS

clone	phenotype	additions	target cells		
			K562	Daudi	BSM
D11	T3$^+$T8$^+$	none	17[c]	0[d]	32[a]
		+ anti-T3	20	23	29
		+ PHA	37	21	32
G9	T3$^+$T8$^+$	none	30[c]	4[d]	55[a]
		+ anti-T3	41	41	34
		+ PHA	58	24	46
R1	T3$^+$T4$^+$	none	8[c]	4[d]	33[a]
		+ anti-T3	6	4	25
		+ PHA	19	13	35
					ADCC
RG75	T3$^-$T8$^-$	none	17[b]	34[a]	42[a]
		+ anti-T3	17	37	35
		+ PHA	19	36	39

E/T ratio a) 3:1; b) 9:1; c) 27:1; d) 81:1.

Responsiveness of $T3^-$ and $T3^+$ clones to activation signals by PHA and anti-T3.

The plating efficiency of $T3^-$, $B73.1^+$ cells was not enhanced by lectins. In contrast, leucoagglutinin significantly increased the plating efficiency of $T3^+$ cells from the average of 5 percent to about 20 percent.

As shown in Table 6, the lytic activity of $T3^-$ clones was not enhanced by PHA or anti-T3 MAbs. In contrast, the lytic activity of $T3^+$ cells can be augmented and induced by both PHA and anti-T3, but not anti-T8 MAbs in a target cell dependent manner. These results suggest that the T3 antigen is involved in the transmission of the activation signal by PHA.

DISCUSSION

We have compared the lytic activities of $T3^-$ and $T3^+$ cloned T cells. The $T3^-$ clones were derived from $B73.1^+$ FACS isolated lymphocytes (5, 8). Most were $T3^-$, $B73.1^+$, $T4^-$, $T8^-$, T11, $OKM1^-$ and thus phenotypically resemble Tγ-lymphocytes (9).

One clone did not express T11 and therefore resembled null cells (9). Two clones derived from the pheripheral blood of a patient with Tγ lymphocytosis were $T3^-$, $B73.1^-$ but showed normal ADCC activity. All $T3^-$, $B73.1^+$ NK cell derived clones exerted strong ADCC (5, 9). Thus, the lack of the T3 antigen, the capacity for ADCC and the high MHC non-restricted lytic activity and wide tumour target cell specificity range clearly distinguishes NK cell derived clones from $T3^+$ CTL with both MHC restricted nonspecific cytolysis. We have demonstrated here that, although $T3^+$ cloned CTL can lyse K562 and other tumour cells, their lytic activity is less and the target cell specificity range is narrower in comparison with $T3^-$ clones as recently described in detail (10). Moreover, $T3^+$ cells can exert non-specific cytolysis without concomitant allospecific cytolysis (e.g., $T3^+$ $T4^-$ $T8^-$ clone, n-4). In addition, PHA and anti-T3 MAb do not influence the plating efficiency or cytolytic activity of cloned $T3^-$ cells, whereas they increase the plating efficiency of $T3^+$ cells and augment and induce the nonspecific, non-MHC restricted lytic activity of cloned $T3^+$ CTL and inhibit the concomitant allospecific lysis of these clones. The anti-T8 MAb may inhibit allo-specific cytolysis but does not induce cytolysis by these clones. Therefore, these data also suggest that the T3 antigen is involved in the induction of IL-2 receptors, in proliferation and in cytolytic activity in $T3^+$ cells.

In conclusion, $T3^-$ cells derived clones activated during cloning and expansion can be distinguished from $T3^+$ CTL activated during MLC followed by cloning and expansion as summarized in Table 7.

Table 7.

DIFFERENCES BETWEEN $T3^-$ AND $T3^+$ ACTIVATED KILLER CLONES

	$T3^-$	$T3^+$
phenotype	$B73.1^+$ $T4^-$ $T8^-$ $T11^+$	$T4^+$ $T8^-$
	$B73.1^+$ $T4^-$ $T8^-$ $T11^-$	$T4^-$ $T8^+$
	$B73.1^+$ $T4^-$ $T8^+$ $T11^+$	$T4^-$ $T8^-$
	$B73.1^-$ $T4^-$ $T8^-$ $T11^+$	
EAγ RFC	yes	no
lytic activity	$ADCC^+$	$ADCC^-$
target cell specificity	broad	narrow
induction of proliferation by PHA and/or anti-T3	no	yes
induction of nonspecific lysis by PHA or anti-T3	no	yes
level of non-specific lytic activity	high	low
specific lytic activity	no	yes

ACKNOWLEDGEMENTS

We thank Dr. M.J. Giphart for providing the various HLA-typed B-LCL cells. We thank Mrs. B.A. van Krimpen, Mr. C.P.M. Ronteltap and Mr. F. Smekens for technical assistance and Mrs. M. van der Sman for typing the manuscript.

REFERENCES

1. R.L.H. Bolhuis and H. Schellekens, Scand. J. Immunol. 13, 401 (1981).
2. A. Moretta, G. Pantaleo et al., J. Exp. Med. 159, 921 (1984).
3. R.J. van de Griend and R.L.H. Bolhuis, Transplantation 38, no. 4, (1984).
4. R.J. van de Griend, B.A. van Krimpen, S.J.L. Bol, A. Thompson and R.L.H. Bolhuis, J. Imm. Methods 66, 285 (1984).
5. R.L.H. Bolhuis, R.J. van de Griend and C.P.M. Ronteltap. Nat. Imm. and Cell Growth Regulation 3, no. 2, 61 (1984).
6. H. Spits, J.E. de Vries and C. Terhorst, Cell. Immunol. 59, 435 (1981).
7. Y. Tanaka, K. Sugamura and Y. Hinuma, J. Immunol. 128, 1241 (1982).
8. B. Perussia, S. Starr, S. Abraham, V. Fanning and G. Tinchieri, J. Immunol. 130, 2133 (1983).
9. R.J. van de Griend, B.A. van Krimpen, C.P.M. Ronteltap and R.L.H. Bolhuis. J. Immunol. 132, 3185 (1984).
10. R.J. van de Griend, M.J. Giphart, B.A. van Krimpen and R.L.H. Bolhuis. J. Immunol. 133, 1222 (1984).
11. R.J. van de Griend and R.L.H. Bolhuis. Blood 65, in press (1985).

Murine and human tuberculin reactive T helper clones: their

role in anti-tumour immunity

Vyakarnam A, Sia D Y and Lachmann P J

Mechanisms in Tumour Immunity Unit, MRC Centre

Hills Road, Cambridge CB2 2QH

1. INTRODUCTION

Helper T (T_H) cells are characterised by the expression of unique cell surface antigens (T4/Leu3a in humans and Lyt 1.2 differentiation antigens in mice) and by their ability to regulate antibody and cell-mediated responses to soluble and cell surface antigenic determinants. We have been interested in mechanisms by which the immune response to antigens on tumour cells can be regulated and in this report describe two distinct methods by which T_H cells can interact with tumour cells.

The first phenomenon describes how murine PPD reactive T_H clones can regulate the immune response to weak cell surface antigens on methylcholanthrene (MCA) induced fibrosarcomas in mice. Previous work from our laboratory has shown that the in-vivo cell-mediated transplantation immunity to certain murine MCA tumours can be enhanced by injecting BCG positive mice with tumour cells coupled to tuberculin (PPD) through the ligand Con A[1-3]. PPD in these studies was shown to function as a carrier determinant potentiating immunity to the native tumour only in those animals which were capable of recognising the carrier. The technique of introducing foreign antigens onto tumour cells so as to make them more immunogenic has been termed Heterogenisation/Xenogenisation, and tumour cells heterogenised with viruses, lectins, or haptens, have been reported by several other workers to induce immune

435

responses to various tumours[4-8]. The hypothesis that we
have used to explain the phenomenon of heterogenisation of
tumour cells with tuberculin is that BCG sensitization
allows expansion of the cell population reactive to PPD to
occur, and that such T cells recruit or augment other T
cells reactive to the tumour in a manner analogous to the
carrier effect in antibody formation[9-10].   In order to
test this hypothesis several murine PPD reactive clones
were prepared and tested for their ability to help both in
induction of antibodies to the soluble antigen NIP and to
enhance the transplantation immunity to the MCA induced-
MC6A tumour.   Some of the results of these experiments
described in detail elsewhere[11] are discussed.

The second phenomenon described in this report is one
whereby PPD reactive human clones, which stimulate
autologous B cells to secrete anti TT antibody are shown to
kill certain tumour targets.   It is clear that lymphocytes
can kill tumour targets in a variety of ways.   This
includes Class-1 MHC restricted killing mediated by antigen
specific cytotoxic T cells and MHC unrestricted killing
mediated by NK cells: - although NK cells are predominantly
large granular lymphocytes (LGL), cloned T cells can under
certain circumstances also kill NK susceptible targets[12-13].   Other forms of killing include ADCC mediated by a
heterogeneous group of cells including lymphocytes,
referred to as 'K' cells, which through their Fc receptors
bind tumour targets coated with specific antibody, and
lectin-mediated killing whereby lectins such as PHA and
ConA can induce T cells to kill tumour targets in a MHC
unrestricted manner[14].

In this report we describe a distinct form of
lymphocyte killing.   Three PPD reactive human clones which
are OKT4 positive, secrete MIF following specific antigenic
stimulation and help in the induction of anti-tetanus
antibodies in autologous B cells[15-16] are shown to kill
Epstein-Barr virus-transformed B cell lines (B-EBV) to
which PPD is attached through the ligand ConA.   Targets
coupled with ConA alone were not killed, and the efficiency
of lysis of targets to which PPD-ConA is attached to
targets pulsed with PPD for 24 hours prior to performing
the killing assay has been compared.   The data also
suggests that this form of killing by T_H clones is
restricted by Class II molecules of the MHC.

2. MATERIALS AND METHODS

Murine clones   The preparation and characterisation of all 8 murine clones has been previously described in detail[11].Also described in the same publication is the murine proliferation assay, helper assay for anti-NIP antibodies and assay for in-vivo transplantation immunity.
Human clones   The isolation and characterisation of line K-1 and clone A1500 F3 have been reported elsewhere[15,17]. Clone 100 F3 was isolated in an identical manner to clone A1500 F3.   Proliferation assays, MIF tests and surface phenotyping were performed as described in detail in these publications[15-17].
Killing assay   Effectors were added to 5×10^3 chromium (51-Cr) labelled targets in individual wells of U bottom microtitre plates to give final effector to target ratios (E:T) of 10:1, 20:1 or 40:1.   All tests were carried out in triplicate for 16 hrs at $37^\circ C$, 5%Co_2 and percent specific lysis were calculated as described previously[16]. Background lysis was taken as counts per minute chromium released by targets cultured on their own and maximum lysis as targets incubated with 4.5% Brij.
Coupling of[^{125}I-PPD-ConA] to targets.   The cross-linking of PPD to ConA was performed exactly as described earlier[2]. The conjugate used in these studies had a molar ratio of PPD:ConA of 2.8:1.   Percentage uptake of conjugate on various tumour lines ranged from 30-35%.   0.2 ug PPD was offered to 1- x 10^6 targets and produced targets which had $3-4 \times 10^6$ moles PPD/cell and $1.1-1.5 \times 10^6$ moles ConA/cell. [^{125}I] labelling of ConA was performed by the iodogen technique[18].   It was mixed with cold ConA to give a final specific activity of 92 cps/ug and 0.8 ug ConA offered to 1- x 10^6 cells.   33% was bound resulting in 1.3×10^6 moles of ConA/cell.   All targets were first labelled with 51-Cr, washed x3 in PBS and then incubated with [^{125}I-PPD-ConA] or [^{125}I-ConA] for 30 mins at $4^\circ C$.   Coupled targets were washed x1 in PBS and resuspended in culture medium for use.

3. RESULTS

I(i) Murine PPD reactive clones - their antigen specificity and surface phenotype.   The tuberculin specificity of a representative clone from a series of 10 clones isolated from BCG sensitized H.2b mice[11] is shown in Fig.1.   The

cells were found to be highly reactive to PPD. The
proliferative response was strictly dependent on Il-2,
required the addition of antigen presenting cells (APC) in
the form of irradiated spleen cells and was restricted by
Class II molecules of the MHC. Thus the clones
proliferated to PPD only when cultured with irradiated
spleen cells derived from recombinant mice showing homology
in the I region with the B10 (H-2b) strain, so that spleen
cells from B10.A.5R mice but not B10.A.2R and Balb/c
derived cells were efficient in inducing proliferation.
Interestingly, the clones proliferate only to PPD derived
from the same strain of Mycobacterium used for in-vivo
sensitization, or to PPD from other strains which are known
to cross-react with M.tuberculosis in in-vivo DTH
reactions. Thus the cells proliferate to PPD human, cross
react with the PPD-avian but do not respond to PPD-Johnin
derived from Mycobacterium para-tuberculosis. This data

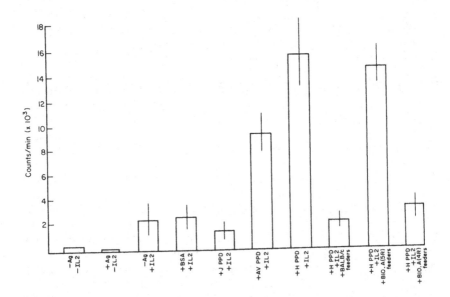

Fig 1 <u>PPD specificity and requirement for APC of murine</u>
<u>clone 11C6</u> 10^4 cloned T cells were cultured with no Il-2,
10% Il-2, 2 x 10^5 autologous or allogeneic irrad spleen
cells and different antigens for 72 hours. Fig represents
mean cpm uptake of ^{3}H-tdr of triplicate cultures.[11] Column
1-7 contain autol APC.

is consistent with previous findings in sheep[19] and with those observed with human clones (as described later), and would suggest that the injection of BCG is itself a powerful method of selecting specifically antigen reactive cells. Table 1 summarises the surface phenotype of the clones - all clones carried markers for T cells, were Thy 1.2 positive and were of the helper phenotype : Lyt 1.2 positive Lyt 2.2 negative.

I(ii). Helper Activity of the clones. Table 2 compares the ability of the clones to induce antibodies to NIP and to enhance the transplantation immunity to the 6A tumour. In vivo helper activity of the clones was studied by adoptively transferring into individual irradiated syngeneic recipients 2×10^6 T cell clones, 2×10^7 B cells from NIP primed animals and 20 ug of the challenge antigen NIP coupled to PPD (NIP-PPD). Recipients were bled 9 days later and their sera tested for anti-NIP antibodies in a Farr assay[11]. The ability to enhance transplantation immunity in vivo was assessed by injecting into each syngeneic BCG negative animal 3×10^6 cloned cells along with 10^7 irradiated 6A cells linked to PPD twice at weekly intervals. A week after the booster injection each animal was tested for its ability to reject a challenge of 10^5 viable 6A cells[11]. The data shows quite clearly that all eight clones tested induce anti-NIP antibodies but only 2 of these enhance the immune response to the 6A tumour. Three interesting features arise from the data in Table 2: First it shows quite clearly that the same T_H cells which augment antibody responses also potentiate in-vivo transplantation immunity to the 6A tumour. Such immunity has previously been shown to be cell-mediated[3] which implies that the same T_H cell can augment both B and T cell

Table 1. Properties of the PPD-reactive T cell clones

Thy 1.2	+ve
Immunoglobulin(Ig)	-ve
Fc receptor	-ve
C3 receptor	-ve
Lyt 1.2	+ve
Lyt 2.2	-ve

responses.   Secondly the data shows that only those T_H cells which give maximum help for antibody responses are capable of augmenting responses to the 6A tumour.   It is possible that T cell activation   requires more potent helper effects compared to B cells.   Thirdly, it is clear that the T_H cells themselves have no effect on tumour

Table 2

Helper Activity of murine clones

Clone	Help for anti-NIP Ab		Help for anti-tumour Immunity	
	Challenge Ag	NIP binding capacity of serum (units/ml)*	Challenge Ag	AR at day 9 of BCG −ve mice**
11C2	NIP-PPD	219	6A	1.26
11C3	"	191	"	1.41
11C4	"	242	"	1.18
11C6	"	496	"	4.16 (10^6)
11C7	"	181	"	1.14
11C8	"	238	"	1.24
11C9	"	417	"	3.22
11C10	"	138	"	1.09
11C6	−	2	−	−
11C6	NIP-CG	8	−	−
11C6 + 6A	−	−	6A	1.17
11C6 + 6A + PPD	−	−	"	<1.5

Note: * Results are mean of assays on three mice.   Ten units of antibody gave 30% binding of 10^{-8}M NIP-CAP[11].
** Results are expressed as Antigenic Ratio (AR) calculated as the growth rate of 6A in unimmunised animals to animals immunised with clones as described.   Groups of three mice were used for each screen of T cell clones.

immunity and serve only to recruit other cells reactive to the tumour: this is shown by the T_H cells not altering the growth of the tumour and the animals showing immunity to a subsequent challenge of viable tumour cells not linked to PPD.

Finally the help mediated by the PPD reactive cells is analogous to the previously described carrier effect in antibody formation[9] on the basis that both for inducing antibody responses and transplantation immunity the antigen needs to be linked to PPD.   In the case of antibody responses the challenge antigen needs to be NIP-PPD (NIP mixed with PPD or coupled to a heterologous carrier eg CG does not induce anti-NIP antibodies[11]).   For transplantation immunity the T_H clones need to be transferred along with 6A linked to PPD.   6A mixed with PPD does not lead to an effective response to the 6A tumour[11].

II (i)   <u>Human PPD reactive clones: their antigen specificity, phenotype and function</u>

The characterisation of clones K-1, and A1500 F3 has already been described in detail elsewhere[15,19].   Figure 2 shows the antigen specificity and requirement for APC of one of the clones. Like the murine clones the human clones clearly failed to cross react with J-PPD and with a range of other test antigens[15].   The proliferative response was however not dependent on exogenous $Il-2$ a finding now common for human antigen specific clones[20,21], required APC in the form of irradiated PBML and was restricted by Class II of the MHC[15]. A search for alternative sources of cells capable of presenting antigen and which could be maintained in culture revealed that B-EBV lines were extremely efficient in inducing T cell proliferation. These cells served solely to present antigen in the context of Class II molecules as shown by the fact that T cell clones cultured with the lines alone failed to proliferate and the specificity of the response to PPD was maintained. Furthermore incubation with an anti-HLA-DR monoclonal (Becton-Dickenson) blocked the proliferative response. All three clones were capable of secreting MIF following PPD stimulation as tested by a highly sensitive assay using the monocytic line U937. The conditions under which MIF secretion occurred was similar to the proliferative response: it was highly PPD specific, and maximal secretion occurred when the clones were cultured with PPD and APC which shared one allele at the D locus with the clones. The clones were of the helper phenotype: T4 positive, T8 negative. Helper activity was measured by co-culturing the clones with autologous B cells in the presence and absence of antigen and CM using the hanging drop technique[22-23]. All three clones were capable of stimulating memory B cells to secrete specific anti-TT antibody when cultured with autologous B cells and TT. The efficiency of such secretion was greatly increased by the addition of CM known to contain B cell growth and differentiation factors. However the addition of CM to cultures of B and T cells in the absence of antigen produced minimal non- specific stimulation thus indicating that maximal triggering of memory B cells required specific antigen and that CM only had an additive effect in the presence of TT. Further details of the helper activity of the clones is being reported in a separate communication[16].

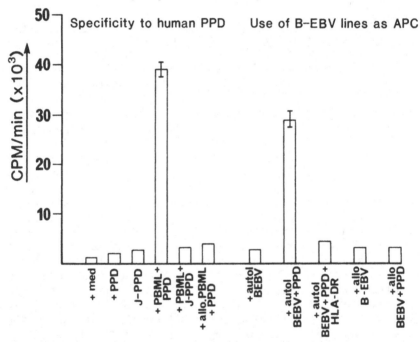

Fig 2 PPD specificity and APC requirement of clone K-1
5×10^3 clones and 2×10^5 APC + 20 ug/ml PPD were cultured in individual microtitre wells. Plates were pulsed with 1 uCi/well ^{3}H-Tdr after 54 hours and harvested 16 hours later. Fig represents mean 3H-tdr uptake of 3 replicate wells.

Table 3   Phenotype and Function of PPD reactive clones

Clone	PPD prolif *(PR)	MIF ** (MI)	% specific lysis of K562 (E.T 10:1)***	T4	T8	T11	DR	Helper Activity# Ag (TT+CM)	Anti TT IgG Ab (ng/ml)
500 A$_1$ F$_3$	30.2	16 (10-28)	12	+	-	+	+	- TT - TT + CM + TT - CM + TT + CM	<1 13 66 155
100 F$_3$	24.1	21 (15-34)	8	+	-	+	+	- +	78 266
K - 1	57.8	19 (15-29)	9.4	+	-	+	+	- +	20 68

* Expressed as Migration Index (MI) with 95% confidence intervals and calculated as percentage of migration of U937 cells incubated with supernatants of clones cultured in the absence of PPD and B-EBV lines.NB MI of supernatants of clones cultured either with PPD or B-EBV lines in each case was >80 and>90 respectively. ** Proliferation ratio (PR) calculated as the ratio of counts per minute (cpm) of ^{3}H-thymidine incorporated by clones cultured with PPD and B-EBV lines to cpm of clones plus medium alone. NB PR of cultures containing clones and PPD or B-EBV lines in each case did not exceed 2.0. *** Figures indicate percentage specific lysis. Medium control was 8.6%.
Phenotype: + indicates >75% strong fluorescence
            -indicates <5% strong fluorescence
\# Clones were incubated with aut B cells +/- TT and CM (conditioned medium)[17,22-23]. Significant difference for the addition of antigen only when autologous T cells were the source of help (p<0.001). B + CM alone gave <5 ng/ml anti TT antibody; +/- for clones 100F3 and K-1 refer to TT +CM and TT - CM respectively.

II(ii) Human PPD reactive T$_H$ clones: their ability to kill tumour targets coupled with PPD.
To see whether the PPD reactive clones could kill tumour targets carrying PPD on their surface, the same B-EBV lines used as APC were coupled with PPD through the ligand ConA. These targets were themselves not susceptible to 'NK' killing either by fresh PBML from individuals who killed K562 efficiently or by activated T cells (PHA stimulated PBML) cultured in Il-2 for 2 weeks (see Table 4). All three PPD reactive T$_H$ clones were tested for their ability

to kill the PPD coupled targets. The clones were
simultaneously tested against targets mixed with PPD and
targets coupled with an equivalent number of molecules/cell
of ConA. The most efficient targets were those to which
PPD had been linked through the ligand ConA. As targets
coupled with ConA alone were not killed efficiently it
would appear that the killing is PPD specific.
Furthermore cells of a different specificity, in this case
autologous PHA stimulated T cells failed to kill the PPD
coupled targets. This also suggests that the ability of
the T_H clones to kill PPD coupled targets is not a function
of the cells being maintained in Il-2 alone.
Interestingly, maximum specific lysis was only 35-40% even
at high effector to target ratios which suggests that
several factors may govern the eficiency of target lysis.
PPD itself needs to be linked to the surface and not added
in free solution to the cultures to induce killing. One
explanation for this may be that the culture period of
killing was inadequeate for sufficient uptake of antigen.
To test this targets were pulsed with PPD for 24 hours
prior to killing. Such targets were capable of inducing
proliferation in the T cell clones in the absence of
additional PPD (data not shown). However, the results
shown in Table 5 indicate clearly that pulsing B-EBV lines
with PPD was not sufficient to induce killing by any of the
three clones.

II(iii) <u>MHC restriction of killing by T_H clones of PPD
coupled targets.</u> The NK susceptible targets K562 and the
EBV-transformed lymphoblastoid line Raji, were coupled with
PPD and the susceptibility to lysis of these targets was
compared with autologous B-EBV lines coupled with PPD.
The results are shown in Table 6. Maximum killing was
clearly induced by autologous B-EBV lines. The inability
to kill K562 or Raji cells linked to PPD suggests that the
killing unlike that mediated by NK cells is under some
genetic control. In order to see whether the restriction
maps to the A, B or D region antigens, killing of
autologous B-EBV cells coupled to PPD was carried out in
the presence of IgG antibodies to the HLA-DR and HLA
(W6/32) framework antigens. Of the two monoclonals
tested the anti-DR monoclonal gave greater inhibition
indicating the importance of D region molecules in killing.
Further data on the involvement of Class II molecules in
killing is being reported in a separate communication.

Table 4
Human PPD reactive T$_H$ clones: their ability to kill tumour targets coupled with PPD

Effectors	K 562** (8%)	Aut B-EBV* (11%)	Aut B-EBV + PPD (10%)	Aut B-EBV -Con A-PPD (18%)	Aut B-EBV -Con A (13%)
K - 1	13	12	10	34 36**	14
500 A$_1$ F$_3$	14	7	8	28 33**	9
100 F$_3$	12	3	4	33 35**	11
PHA - B	46	17	14	12 15**	18
Fresh PBML	40	2	N D	3 4**	12

Figures indicate % specific lysis. E:T = 10:1, 40:1**.
Targets included Aut B-EBV plus 50 ug/ml PPD; Aut B-EBV
linked to 1.3 x 10^6 moles Con A and 4 x 10^6 moles PPD/cell;
Aut B-EBV linked to 1 x 10^6 moles Con A/cell. Figures in
brackets indicate background lysis.

Table 5   Killing of B-EBV targets pulsed with PPD and
linked to PPD

Effectors	Targets	
	B-EBV-PPD 10:1 (15)	B-EBV pulsed with PPD* (12)
K - 1	34	10
100 F$_3$	32	14
500 A$_1$ F$_3$	28	10

*Targets were incubated with 50 ug/ml PPD for 18-24 hours,
washed and labelled with 51-Cr. Figs in brackets indicate
background lysis. All other figs indicate % specific lysis.

Table 6

MHC restriction of killing by PPD T_H clones of tumour

targets linked to PPD

Targets coupled to [PPD- Con A]	Effectors (E:T 10:1)		
	K-1	100 F_3	500 A_1 F_3
K562 (13)	14	8	13
HT-29 (23)	0	2	5
Aut B-EBV (18, 20)	34 (DR 2,6)	33	28
Aut B-EBV + anti DR (15,16)	4	4	8
Aut B-EBV + W6/32 (15,13)	17	18	10

Targets were coupled with 4×10^6 moles PPD/cell and 1.3×10^6 Con A/cell. Targets were incubated with 1/100 dilution of anti DR and W6/32 monoclonal antibodies. Figures in brackets indicate background lysis.

4.DISCUSSION

In these studies we have used a series of well characterised murine and human PPD reactive T_H clones to demonstrate two distinct characteristics of T_H cells: immunoregulation and induction of tumour cell lysis.The helper activity of the murine clones was shown by their ability to augment antibody levels to NIP from NIP-primed B cells stimulated with NIP-PPD. Two of the eight murine PPD reactive T_H clones were also capable of helping other T cells mount an anti-tumour response. The data (see Table 5) thus support the hypothesis put forward in earlier studies that PPD can be used as a carrier determinant to provide immunological help in the induction of transplantation immunity to weak cell surface antigens on certain MCA tumours if it is coupled to tumours and injected into BCG positive mice. The observation that the clones themselves have no effect on tumour growth and that the immunized animals reject a challenge of viable 6A cells not linked to PPD rules out the possibility that the coupling procedure may result in the formation of neoantigens - a frequent occurrence when haptens/carriers are chemically attached to cell surfaces[24]. Instead, the observation that PPD needs to be linked to the tumour cell lends further support to the suggestion that PPD functions by the linked-recognition method of cell-cooperation to induce the antitumour response in an analogous manner to the carrier effect in antibody formation to soluble antigens[9-10]. A further implication of the results in Table 5 is that the same T_H cells can regulate both antibody and cell-mediated responses. While the mechanism by which T_H cells augment B and T cell responses is not fully understood, it is assumed that interaction occurs either by direct cell-cell contact or through the secretion of immunoregulatory soluble mediators. The availablility of PPD reactive T_H clones now makes it feasible to study the interaction between T_H cells and tumour reactive cells, and should facilitate the isolation of the latter population.

The observation that human PPD reactive MIF secreting T4 positive clones which stimulate anti-TT antibody secretion in B cells can also kill autologous B-EBV lines linked to PPD suggests that immunoregulation may not be the sole function of T_H cells. Recently, there has been a report showing that human T4 positive clones specific for measles

virus also kill autologous virus infected targets and that
such killing was Class II HLA restricted[25].
Several interesting features arise from the data on killing
by the human PPD reactive clones: first it would seem that
the killing is specific to PPD, as targets not coupled to
PPD or coupled with ConA alone are not lysed efficiently.
Furthermore, effectors of a different specificity fail to
kill the PPD coupled targets.   It would therefore appear
that the recognition of the target involves the antigen
receptor on the effectors.   Secondly, the killing is
dependent on PPD being covalently attached to the target.
Thus lines pulsed with PPD for 24 hrs prior to the killing
assay and with the capacity to induce T cell proliferation
to PPD were not killed.   Whether this is related to the
ligand ConA remains to be studied by testing targets to
which PPD is linked by alternative lectins for their
susceptibility to lysis by the T_H clones.
Our data suggests that unlike ^{H} MHC unrestricted NK or
lectin induced killing, the killing by T_H clones is gene
tically restricted.   The inhibition of killing by anti - D
region   antibodies   suggests   that   such   killing   may   be
regulated by Class II molecules of the MHC. We are now
studying the MHC restriction of this phenomenon by testing
the effectors against   a range of D region   :matched
targets coupled to PPD.
The overall killing by the T_H clones of PPD coupled Class
II MHC matched targets, although highly significant, was
only moderate even at high effector to target ratios.
Maximum killing achieved was 35-40%.Whether, ineffecient
killing refects the mechanism by which the cells are killed
remains to be studied. Furthermore as killing is Class II
restricted, the degree of lysis may also depend on the
extent to which D region antigens are expressed on the
target and on the susceptibility to cytolysis in general of
the targets used.   So far the phenomenon of killing by T_H
cells has been studied with the human clones.   It would be
of interest to see whether the murine clones with the
ability to regulate B and T cell function also display PPD
specific cytolytic activity and whether this is also mHC
restricted.

References
1.Lachmann, P.J. and Sikora (1978) Nature (Lond) 271, 463.
2.Lachmann, P.J., Vyakarnam, A. and Sikora (1981) Immunol. 42, 329.
3.Vyakarnam, A., Lachmann, P.J. and Sikora (1981) Immunol. 42, 337,
4.Lindenman and Klein (1967) J.exp.Med. 126, 93.
5.Kobayashi, N., Sendo, F., Kaji, K., Shirai, T., Saito, H.,Takeichi, N., Hosokawa M. and Kodama, T. (1970)J.Natl.Cancer.Inst. 44, 11.
6.Martin, W.J., Wunderlich, J.R., Fletcher, F. and Inman, J.K.(1971) Proc.natn.Acad.Sci.USA. 68, 469.
7.Kuzumaki, N., Fenyo, E.M., Klein, E. and Klein, G. (1978)Transplantation 26, 394,
8.Hamaoka, T., Fujiwara, H., Teshima, K., Aoki, H., Yamamoto, H.and Kitagawa, M. (1979) J.exp.Med. 149, 185.
9.Mitchinson N.A. (1971) Europ.J.Immunol. 1, 18.
10.Rajewski, K., Schirrmacher, V., Nase, S. and Jerne, N.K.(1969) J.exp.Med. 129, 1131.
11.Sia, D.Y., Lachmann, P.J. and Leung, K.N. (1984) Immunol.51, 755.
12.Tilden, A.B., Abo, T. and Balsh, C.M. (1983) J.Immunol.130, 1171.
13.Brooks, C.G., Urdadl, D.L. and Henney, C.S. (1983)Immunol.Rev. 72, 43.
14.Perlmann P. and Cerottini, J.C. (1979) in 'The Antigens'edited by M.Sela Vol V, 173.
15.Vyakarnam, N. and Lachmann, P.J. (1984) Immunol. In press.
16.Brenner, M.K., Vyakarnam, A., Strangeways, A.L., Rettie, J.E.and Lachmann, P.J. Manuscript in preparation.
17.Vyakarnam, A., Brenner, M.K., Rettie, J.E. Houlker, C. andLachmann, P.J. (1984) Submitted for publication.
18.Fraker, P.J. and Seck, J.C. Jr. (1978) Biochem.Biophys.Res,Commu. 80, 49.
19.Hopkins, J., McConnell, I. and Lachmann, P.J. (1981)J.exp.Med. 153, 706.
20.Kurnick, J.T. Hayward, A.R. and Altevogt, P. (1981) J.Immunol.126, 1307.
21.Issekutz, T., Chu, E. and Geha, R.S. (1982) J.Immunol129(4), 1446.
22.Brenner, M.K., Newton, C.A., Chadda, H.R., North, M.E.and Farrant, J. (1984) Immunol. 51.
23.Brenner, M.K., Newton, C.A., North, M.E., Weyman. C. and Farrant, J. (1983) Immunol. 50,377.

24.Prager, M.D. and Baetchel, F.S. (1973(Cancer Res. 9, 339.
25.Jacobson, S., Richert, J.R., Biddison, W.E., Satinsky, A., Hartzman, R.J. and McFarland, H.F. (1984) J.Immunol. 133, 754.

Abbreviations
Tuberculin (PPD); Tetanus toxoid (TT); Phytohaemogglutinin (PHA); Concanavalin-A (ConA); Natural Killer (NK); Antibody Dependent Cellular cytotoxicity (ADCC); Major Histocompatibility Complex (MHC); counts per second (CPS); Phosphate buffered saline (PBS); Peripheral blood mononuclear cells (PBML); N-(4-hydoxy-5-iodo-3-nitro-phenacetyl) (NIP); N-(4-hydroxy-5-iodo-3-nitro-phenacetyl)amino caproic acid (NIP.CAP); Autologus (Aut); Allogeneic (Allog); Proliferation (Prolif); Antibody (Ab); Antigen (Ag); Bacillus Calmette Guerin (BCG); Delayed Type Hypersensitivity (DTH); Migration Inhibition Factor (MIF).

Acknowledgements: The authors wish to thank Mr R.G. Oldroyd with help in the preparation of the conjugate [^{125}I-PPD-ConA] and Dr M K Brenner for kindly testing the human clones for helper activity.

INDEX

451